# Mastering MRCS 2

# Mastering MRCS 2

EMQ Practice for the Intercollegiate MRCS 2 conducted by the Surgical Royal Colleges of Great Britain and Ireland


**Sashidhar Yeluri**

Senior House Officer (SHO)
Leeds Basic Surgical Training (BST) Rotation
The Yorkshire School of Surgery (YSS)
St James's University Hospital
The Leeds Teaching Hospitals NHS Trust, Leeds, UK

**Amit Kapoor**

Clinical Research Fellow in Orthopaedics
Wrightington Hospital, Wrightington
Wigan & Leigh NHS Trust, Wrightington, UK

**Sumit Kapadia**

Senior Vascular Fellow
Sir Gangaram Hospital, New Delhi, India

**Brijesh Madhok**

Senior House Officer (SHO) in Orthopaedics
Royal Albert Edward Infirmary, Wrightington,
Wigan and Leigh NHS Trust, Wigan, UK



**Paras Medical Publisher**

*Solutions for Health Care Professionals*

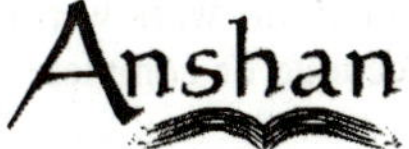

Mastering MRCS 2

*First published in the UK by*

ANSHAN LTD
In 2007

6 Newlands Road, Tunbridge Wells,
Kent. TN4 9AT. UK
Tel/Fax: +44 (0) 1892 557767
e-mail: info@anshan.co.uk
Web Site: www.anshan.co.uk

*Published in arrangement with*
Paras Medical Publisher, 5-1-475 First Floor
Putlibwoli, Hyderabad - 500 095, India.
E-mail: parasmedpub@hotmail.com



ISBN 10: 1 905 74005 0
ISBN 13: 978 1 905740 05 5



British Library Cataloguing in Publication Data
A catalogue record for this book is available from the British Library

# Foreword

I am delighted to be writing the foreword for this new Part 2 MRCS examinations text. The book has been composed very carefully and is targeted at Basic Surgical Trainees preparing for the MRCS examinations. The authors' aim was to provide a book that offers a comprehensive collection of questions that have been put together keeping in mind the changes in the new intercollegiate examination system. The book is exhaustive with the extended matching questions based on a large number of themes covering the entire spectrum of General Surgery. The layout of the text makes it easy for the trainee to practice the questions in a systematic manner. The section on 'examination techniques' allows the trainee to have an insight into finer aspects of preparation that are undoubtedly essential to success in the MRCS exams.

The book has the scope to evolve as more questions are incorporated in future editions.

A great plus for this book, is that it is a multi-authored text that is based on personal experience in preparing for the examination. The book will be a good companion of the trainee approaching the MRCS examination.

Krish Menon, MS FRCS
Consultant in Transplant and Hepatobiliary Surgery
St.James's University Hospital
Beckett Street
Leeds LS9 7TF
United Kingdom

# Foreword

This book *Mastering MRCS 2* represents a substantial and comprehensive collection of example EMQs for the MRCS Part 2 Examination. It has been written by four authors who have all taken the examination in the last two years and, as such, are best placed to provide a representative sample of questions.

A prospective candidate faced with the MRCS Part 2 Examination should have, not only an excellent working knowledge of the subject, but also the ability to perform well in multiple choice questionnaires. This book allows such an individual to assess their own level of knowledge across the subject, exposing any gaps in knowledge and also can be used for multiple choice questionnaire training.

This book *Mastering MRCS 2* will prove invaluable not just to prospective candidates of the MRCS Part 2 Examination, but also for medical students and junior doctors in their foundation years.

Nicholas J London, MA MD, FRCS (Tr & Orth)
Consultant in Trauma & Orthopaedic Surgery
Harrogate District Hospital
Harrogate
United Kingdom
HG2 7SX

# Preface

The syllabus and the MRCS examination of the Surgical Royal Colleges of Great Britain and Ireland has recently undergone a change. The examination is now commonly conducted by all the royal colleges with a common marking and cut off system thereby eliminating variations that existed in the old 'collegiate' system. The new intercollegiate system has been in place for less than 2 years now.

The new part 2 examination replaces the 'systems' module and consists of clinical problem solving extended matching questions/items (EMQ/EMI). While a thorough knowledge is a pre-requisite to pass this prestigious examination, it in no way negates the need for a systematic and 'exam-oriented' approach. Like any other exam, practice is the key to success. Practice books available for this examination are however limited in number. All of us have passed this examination and hence this book is based on our own personal experience of preparing for this examination.

This book is intended to provide a 'flavour' for this examination. It consists of 279 themes and about 1175 questions. I have included the key questions from the most important topic areas. A few questions have no doubt been repeated reflecting the importance given to that particular theme in the examination. I have tried to separate specialties at a few places and have actually 'mixed and matched' at a few places to maintain readership interest. This book should help brush up your knowledge for the examination, help you identify key areas and identify your weaknesses.

I recommend practising through this book like a test keeping your own individual count. Though my estimate is my own guess, I believe candidates scoring 70% at their first attempt of this book should have a good chance of passing this examination. For those who score less-

realize your weaknesses and work on them. That is the whole essence of working through this book.

I have discussed specific examination techniques in a separate section. I welcome suggestions and criticisms. A few mistakes might have crept in and will be most grateful if you write to us with the appropriate corrections. Further, I would like to invite future budding contributors to play a wider role in this book. If you are interested, please write to us with your EMQs for potential consideration of inclusion in future editions. These should reflect your own experience of preparing for this examination. Your name will be acknowledged for the EMQs that are accepted. We look forward to hearing from you.

Thank you once again for your purchase of this book. I really hope you find it useful. On behalf of all the authors, all the best!

— Sashidhar Yeluri

# Contents

1

# Introduction
## (Examination Information)

### COMPOSITION OF THE INTERCOLLEGIATE MRCS EXAMINATION

The intercollegiate MRCS part 1 examination tests you on applied basic sciences. It consists of multiple "true or false" items only. The MRCS part 2 consists of clinical problem solving questions and is based on the extended matching items/questions (EMI/EMQ) pattern. You can take MRCS part 1 at any point after the completion of your house officer training (you do not necessarily have to commence your surgical training before sitting for the exam). However, you should have commenced your surgical training before you are allowed to sit part 2. Though you don't necessarily have to do the parts in order, you will have three and a half years from your first attempt (even if you failed) at part 2 MRCS to complete all parts of your MRCS (even if you chose to take part 2 before 1). For this reason it is advisable to take the parts sequentially or to take parts 1 and 2 together.

Part 2 consists of a total of 180 questions (about 50–60 themes). Each theme will be followed by up to 9–10 choices (they can be as few as 4 in a few themes). A few questions then follow based on that theme. Read the instructions carefully and then select the correct option.

### SYLLABUS FOR THE EXAMINATION

#### *General Surgery*

**The Abdomen**

Abdominal Trauma

- Penetrating abdominal trauma
- Blunt abdominal trauma

- Assessment and management of abdominal trauma
- Specific organ injuries

Common Abdominal Problems
- Abdominal pain
- Abdominal masses
- The acute abdomen

Abdominal Emergencies
- Intestinal obstruction
- Peritonitis and abdominal and pelvic abscess
- Gastrointestinal haemorrhage

Abdominal Hernia
- Inguinal hernia
- Femoral hernia
- Incisional hernia
- Rare hernias

Intestinal Fistulas
- Classification of intestinal fistulas
- Assessment and management

Gastrointestinal Stomas
- Formation and management
- Other stomas
- Gastrostomy
- Ileostomy
- Colostomy

Surgery of the Spleen
- Splenic disease and injury
- Treatment of splenic disease and injury
- Post-splenectomy sepsis

**Upper Gastrointestinal Surgery**
- Diagnosis of oesophageal disorders
- Specific oesophageal disorders (including gastro-oesophageal reflux disease, motility disorders, oesophageal carcinoma, oesophageal diverticulum and oesophageal foreign body)
- Peptic ulcer disease
- Carcinoma of the stomach

Endocrine Disorders of the Pancreas

- Insulinoma
- Gastrinoma
- Neuroendocrine tumours
- Other rare endocrine tumours

**Hepatobiliary and Pancreatic Surgery**

- Jaundice
- Gall stones and gallbladder disease
- Acute pancreatitis
- Chronic pancreatitis
- Carcinoma of the pancreas
- Benign and malignant biliary strictures
- Portal hypertension and ascites

**Colorectal Surgery**

Clinical presentation of colorectal and anal disease

Surgical disorders of the colon and rectum

- Ulcerative colitis and Crohn's disease
- Colorectal cancer
- Diverticular disease
- Faecal incontinence
- Rectal prolapse

Surgical disorders of the anus and perineum

- Pruritus ani
- Fissure-in-ano
- Hemorrhoids
- Fistula-in-ano
- Anorectal abscess
- Carcinoma of the anus
- Pilonidal sinus and abscess

**Breast and Endocrine Surgery**

Common Breast Disorders

- Breast lumps
- Breast pain
- Breast cysts
- Nipple discharge

- Gynaecomastia

Breast Carcinoma
- Risk factors
- Pathology
- Diagnosis
- Treatment
- Breast reconstruction

Surgery of the Thyroid Gland
- Indications for surgery in thyroid disease
- Thyroid cancer (types and management)
- Complications of thyroidectomy

Parathyroid Disorders
- Calcium metabolism
- Clinical presentation of hypercalcaemia
- Investigation of hyperparathyroidism
- Management of hyperparathyroidism

Adrenal Disorders and Secondary Hypertension
- Causes of hypertension
- Conn's syndrome
- Phaeochromocytoma

**Vascular Surgery**

Arterial Surgery
- Peripheral vascular disease and limb ischaemia
- Arterial embolism and acute limb ischaemia
- Arterial aneurysms
- Carotid disease
- Renovascular disease
- Arterial trauma

Venous Disorders of the Lower Limb
- Venous insufficiency and varicose veins
- Venous ulceration
- Deep venous thrombosis and pulmonary embolism

Lymphoedema

**Organ Transplantation**

- Basic principles of transplant immunology
- Clinical organ transplantation
- Organ donation and procurement
- Immunosuppression and prevention of rejection

**Otorhinolaryngology, Head & Neck Surgery**

Ear, Nose & Throat Disorders

- Inflammatory disorders of the ear, nose and throat
- Foreign bodies in the ear, nose and throat

Common neck swellings

- Congenital and rare swellings
- Inflammatory swellings
- Head & neck cancer
- Salivary gland disorders
  - Infections and inflammation of the salivary glands
  - Tumours of the salivary glands
  - Stones of the salivary glands
  - Miscellaneous conditions
- Eye surgery
  - Trauma to the eye
  - Common eye infections
- Endoscopy

**Oral and Maxillofacial Surgery**

Maxillofacial Trauma

- Classification of facial fractures
- Presentation of maxillofacial fractures
- Assessment and investigation
- Treatment of facial fractures

Common conditions of the Face, Mouth & Jaws

Principles of Soft Tissue Repair of Mouth, Face, Head & Neck

**Paediatric Surgery**

Principles of Neonatal & Paediatric Surgery

- History and physical examination of the neonate and child
- Maintenance of body temperature

- Assessment of respiratory and cardiovascular function
- Metabolic status
- Fluids, electrolytes and the metabolic response
- Vascular access

Correctable Congenital Abnormalities

- Congenital abnormalities of GI tract
- Congenital heart disease
- Abdominal wall defects
- Diaphragmatic hernia
- Neural tube defects
- Urological abnormalities

Common Paediatric Surgical Disorders

- Pyloric stenosis
- Intussusception
- Inguinal hernia and hydrocele
- Undescended testes
- Torsion of the testes

Orthopaedic Disorders of Infancy and Childhood

- Gait disorders
- Hip problems
- Knee disorders
- Foot disorders

## *Plastic & Reconstructive Surgery*

Burns

- Classification and pathophysiology
- Initial assessment and management
- Treatment including secondary surgery
- Burns of special areas (i.e., face, eyes, hands, perineum)

Soft Tissue Infections

Principles of Hand Trauma (tendon, nerve, nail bed)

Hand Disorders

- Dupuytren's contraction
- Carpal tunnel syndrome

Benign Skin Lesions

Malignant Skin Lesions (Basal Cell Carcinoma, Squamous Cell Carcinoma, Malignant Melanoma)

Principles of Skin Cover
- Split skin grafts
- Full thickness skin grafts
- Local flaps
- Distant flaps
- Free transfer flaps

Principles of Microvascular Surgery

Wound Healing

Traumatic Wounds
- Principles of management
- Gunshot and blast injuries
- Stab wounds
- Human and animal bites

Management of Skin Loss
- The wound
- Skin grafts
- Skin flaps

## *Neurosurgery*

Neurological Trauma
- Head injuries
- Spinal cord injuries
- Paralytic disorders
- Nerve disorders

Surgical Disorders of the Brain
- Clinical presentation of the intracranial mass
- Tumours of the nervous system
- Epilepsy
- Congenital and developmental problems

Intracranial Haemorrhage (Subarachnoid, Intracerebral and Subdural)

Brain Stem Death

- Diagnosis and testing for brain stem death
- Principles of organ donation

Surgical Aspects of Meningitis

- General features of meningitis
- Surgical considerations

Rehabilitation

- The rehabilitation team
- Pain management
- Rehabilitation

## *Trauma & Orthopaedic Surgery*

Skeletal Fractures

Pathophysiology of fracture healing

- Classification of fractures
- Principles of management of fractures
- Complications of fractures
- Management of joint injuries
- Common fractures and joint injuries
  - Upper limb
  - Lower limb
  - Trunk, pelvis and vertebral column

Soft Tissues Injuries and Disorders

- Nature and mechanism of soft tissue injury
- Management of soft tissue injuries

Common Disorders of the Extremities

- Disorders of the hand
- Disorders of the foot

Degenerative and Rheumatoid Arthritis

- Osteoarthritis
- Rheumatoid arthritis
- Other inflammatory conditions
- Surgical treatment of joint diseases

Infections of Bones and Joints

- Osteomyelitis
- Other bone infections

Locomotor pain
- Low back pain and sciatica
- Pain in the neck and upper limb

Bone Tumours and Amputations
- Primary bone tumours
- Metastatic bone tumours
- Amputations

General
- Imaging techniques
- Neurophysiological investigations

## *Urology*

Urological Trauma
- Renal, ureteric, bladder, urethral, penile and scrotal trauma

Urinary Tract Infections and Calculi

Haematuria
- Classification, aetiology and assessment
- Tumours of the genitourinary tract

Urinary Tract Obstruction
- Urinary retention
- Disorders of the prostate

Pain and Swelling in the Scrotum
- Scrotal skin conditions
- Non malignant testicular swellings
- Inflammatory conditions
- Testicular torsion
- Testicular tumours

Chronic Renal Failure
- Dialysis
- Principles of transplantation

Aspects of Pelvic Surgery
- Gynaecological causes of acute abdominal pain

- Pelvic inflammatory disease
- Disorders of urinary continence

### *Cardiothoracic Surgery*

Haemodynamic Control

- Haemodynamic principles
- Cardiovascular homeostasis
- Pharmacological haemodynamic control

Cardiac Surgery

- Surgical disorders of the heart vessels and heart valves
- Cardiopulmonary bypass

Thoracic Trauma

- Pathophysiology of thoracic trauma
- Presentation, assessment and management
- Specific thoracic injuries

Thoracotomy and Chest Drainage

- Assessment and preparation
- Indications for thoracotomy
- Chest drainage and pericardiocentesis

Surgical Disorders of the Lung

- Lung cancer
- Other indications for lung resection

Complications of Thoracic Operations

- General complications
- Specific complications

Pneumothorax and Empyema Thoracis

## EXAMINATION CENTERS

**England**

London 7(2 Centres), Birmingham/ Coventry, Manchester, Newcastle, Leeds, Bristol

**Wales**—Cardiff

**Ireland**—Dublin

**Scotland**—Edinburgh, Glasgow

**Malta**

**Middle East**—Oman, Abu Dhabi, Syria, Riyadh

**Africa**—Malawi, Cairo

**India**—Chennai (Edinburgh college), Mumbai (Edinburgh college), Kolkata (England college)

**Sri Lanka**—Colombo, **Thailand, Nepal, Malaysia-** Kuala Lumpur, **Singapore**, **Myanmar, Hong Kong**

## SCHEDULE FOR 2006/2007

| *Date of Examination* | *Closing Date for Application* |
|---|---|
| 16 January 2006 | 28 October 2005 |
| 25 April 2006 | 24 February 2006 |
| 11 September 2006 | 30 June 2006 |
| 15 January 2007 | 27 October 2006 |
| 24 April 2007 | 23 February 2007 |

## HOW TO REGISTER

Candidates can obtain application forms and detailed examination regulations by viewing any one of the 4 Royal College's websites. The websites also provide specific information regarding fees and venues.

### *Fees*

The cost of registration for the Intercollegiate MRCS exam is £195 for MRCS Part 1 and £195 for MRCS Part 2.

## EXAMINATION MARKING/RESULTS

There is no standard pass mark. There is a standard setting procedure using the Angoff method whereby for every examination, a group of health professionals judge which questions they believe candidates should be able to answer correctly and a pass mark is then set accordingly for that paper. You are thus competing with everybody who sits the examination with you.

Results are normally available on the respective college website within 3 weeks from the examination and posted to you in another week's time. The Edinburgh college does not give you your marks if you pass. However, the English college does.

## IMPORTANT ADDRESSES

1. **The Royal College of Surgeons of Edinburgh**
   The Adamson Centre
   3 Hill Place
   Edinburgh
   EH8 9DS
   Tel: 44 (0) 131 668 9222
   Fax: 44 (0) 131 668 9218
   Enquiries: mail@rcsed.ac.uk or information@rcsed.ac.uk
   Website: www.rcsed.ac.uk

2. **The Royal College of Surgeons of England**
   35/43 Lincoln's Inn Fields
   London WC2A 3PE
   Tel: 44 (0) 207 869 6281
   Fax: 44 (0) 20 7869 6290
   Enquiries: exams@rcseng.ac.uk
   Website: www.rcseng.ac.uk

3. **The Royal College of Physicians and Surgeons, Glasgow**
   232-242 St. Vincent Street
   Glasgow
   G2 5RJ
   Tel: 44 (0) 141 221 6072
   Fax: 44 (0) 141 221 1804

Enquiries: exam.office@rcpsglasg.ac.uk
Website: www.rcpsg.ac.uk

4. **The Royal College of Surgeons, Ireland**
123 St. Stephen's Green
Dublin 2
Ireland
Tel: 00 353 1402 2232
Fax: 00 353 1402 2454
Enquiries: examinations@rcsi.ie
Website: www.rcsi.ie

## EXAMINATION TECHNIQUE

The part 2 examination consists of 50–60 themes each consisting of 2–5 questions for a total of 180 questions. You have 3 hours to answer these 180 questions, which means 1 minute for each question. It is hence very important to maintain a good speed and pace your examination accurately. Remember, you have to mark your computer readable mark sheet as well in this one minute.

Candidates tend to make 2 big mistakes as far as this examination is concerned:

1. Not reading question correctly
2. Not marking properly.

Always read the question very carefully. There could be a world of difference between the next appropriate step and the most appropriate step. For example in a patient presenting with upper gastrointestinal bleeding, the next appropriate step might be intravenous access and fluid resuscitation; but the most appropriate step might be an upper GI endoscopy.

You must also decide on a game plan to mark your answer sheet. I think the best way to do it is to mark your answer sheet after each theme. Hurrying up to transfer your answers to your mark sheet in the end could introduce costly mistakes. Never underestimate this part of the examination.

The best thing about this examination is the absence of negative marking. Hence do not leave any question unattempted. If you are not sure about any answer, make an educated guess. But be sure to attempt all questions.

The best way to go about the examination is to read each theme very carefully. Read the title of the theme first and then the instructions. Quickly glance over the options that have been given, making a mental note of them. Then read each question carefully. Find out the most appropriate answer based on the instructions. Quickly re-glance over the options to rule out other answers. Then mark your answer by the side on the question paper. Complete the entire theme and then transfer all the answers for that theme to the marking sheet, taking care. You have to shade the respective box. Mark all answers you are sure about, as well as all answers you are completely unsure about (using an educated guess). Leave questions you think you need more time to think about for the end. Mark these questions with a big circle on the question sheet for your attention in the end. Spare some time thinking on these questions in the end.

In the very unlikely event of finding some time in the end, there might be a temptation to read and and re-read your answers over and over again. Resist that temptation. However, if you are strongly convinced about changing an answer, please do. But remember, do not change a guess for another guess. First thoughts and guesses are usually the best.

Remember that these questions are not designed to trick or confuse you. You will always read them correctly as long as you read them carefully. Take each question at its face value.

I hope you find the selection of questions in this book useful. It consists of 279 EMQs and 1175 questions. They should provide a flavour for the examination, help assess your knowledge, identify important subject areas and identify potentially weak areas. I have tried to include explanations for all answers where necessary. That should help improve your understanding of the matter under discussion. But that in no way negates the need for a thorough, systematic reading of a standard textbook.

Try and finish this book at a stretch at least a month before the examination date. That should help give you sufficient time in the end to concentrate on the most important subject areas for the examination.

## 1. THEME : VASCULAR DIAGNOSIS

OPTIONS

A. Venography
B. Colour-flow duplex
C. Computed Tomography (CT) angiography
D. Magnetic Resonance (MR) angiography
E. Ankle Brachial Pressure Index (ABPI)
F. Air plethysmography
G. Arteriography

*Which is the most appropriate investigation for the following patients? Select an option from those listed above. Each option can be used once, more than once or not at all.*

1. A 59-year-old man, a heavy smoker, had an 8-month history of cramps in the left calf on walking. He noticed a small painful ulcer in his great toe, which is not healing for the past one month.

2. A 67-year-old female underwent emergency laparotomy with resection of an obstructive mass of the sigmoid colon 5 days ago. Today her left thigh and leg appear markedly swollen with induration of the calf.

3. An ultrasound of a 63-year-old man showed an aortic aneurysm of 6.5-cm diameter.

4. A 56-year-old male presented with superficial necrosis of the right foot. He is on irregular treatment for diabetes mellitus for the past 14 years. On examination, his popliteal pulse is palpable, whereas dorsalis pedis and posterior tibial pulses are not palpable.

## 1. ANSWERS

1. **G - Arteriography.** Rest pain, ulceration and gangrenous changes following claudication are classical of critical limb ischaemia, which is best evaluated by an arteriography. It may be diagnostic as well as crucial in planning interventions. It can also be useful therapeutically to treat arterial stenosis by endovascular angioplasty. Colour-flow duplex is an operator-dependent technique with a sensitivity of 70–90% and specificity of 90–98% for identification of femoro-popliteal arterial stenosis. It may be the preferred initial investigation as it is non-invasive.

2. **B - Colour-flow duplex.** This patient most probably has deep venous thrombosis (DVT), the risk factors being advanced age, malignancy, major operative procedure and immobilization. Contrast venography, although the 'gold standard' for evaluation of acute and chronic DVT, is used less frequently after the advent of duplex imaging. Ascending or descending venography may be useful to detect valvular incompetence. Colour-flow duplex scan has a 95 to 98% sensitivity and specificity for detection of DVT, although it is less sensitive for isolated calf vein thrombosis.

3. **C - Computed tomography angiography.** Ultrasound is a useful screening as well as follow-up tool for abdominal aortic aneurysms. CT angiography is the optimal imaging method for evaluation prior to abdominal aortic aneurysm repair. Spiral CT and three-dimensional reconstruction provide important details of anatomical extent of aneurysm and its relation to surrounding structures.

4. **D - MR angiography.** This patient also has peripheral arterial occlusive disease with critical ischaemia. He needs further evaluation to decide regarding revascularisation. In a diabetic patient, renal failure is not uncommon. MR angiography eliminates the risk of contrast nephropathy and identifies patent distal vessels with high accuracy. ABPI is a simple and rapid test for assessment of limb ischaemia. An ABPI< 0.9 indicates presence of lower limb arterial disease, whereas a value below 0.5 is suggestive of critical limb ischaemia and imminent gangrene. It is unreliable in presence of incompressible vessels in diabetes and renal failure. Plethysmography is a non-invasive method of detecting blood volume changes in extremity and is infrequently used for evaluation of venous reflux and venous pressure in venous insufficiency.

## 2. THEME: ACUTE LIMB ISCHAEMIA: DIAGNOSIS

OPTIONS

A. In situ thrombosis
B. Embolic occlusion
C. Bypass graft occlusion
D. Popliteal aneurysm
E. Popliteal entrapment
F. Deep venous thrombosis
G. Popliteal artery injury
H. Compartment syndrome

*Which is the most likely diagnosis in the following patients? Select an option from those listed above. Each option can be used once, more than once or not at all.*

1. A 62-year-old man with a past history of left thigh and calf claudication presented with rapidly increasing foot pain at rest since yesterday. Examination revealed absent popliteal and distal pulses in both legs. There was mild sensory impairment over dorsum of his toes, but no motor weakness.

2. A 40-year-old lady presented to the emergency department with rapid onset of persistent right leg pain, paraesthesias and foot coldness for 6 hours. Her past medical history was significant for postpartum dilated cardiomyopathy. On examination, the leg was cold, with absent femoral and distal pulses.

3. A 70-year-old male presented with a 3-day history of severe right leg pain with coldness of right foot. On examination, the right popliteal and pedal pulses were not palpable. The left popliteal pulse was prominent.

4. A 65-year-old woman developed leg pain 6 hours after total knee replacement. Her past history was significant for hypertension. Her ipsilateral foot was warm, but no pulses were found distal to the femoral. The first web space was numb.

5. A 32-year-old man met with a vehicle accident with resultant injury to left leg. His X-ray showed an undisplaced fracture of the tibial condyle, for which a plaster slab was given. Eight hours later, he developed severe pain, which was not relieved after removal of the plaster slab. His calf was swollen, tender and tense on palpation. The dorsalis pedis and posterior tibial pulses were palpable.

## 2. ANSWERS

1. **A - In situ thrombosis.** In situ thrombosis is the final stage in progression of an atherosclerotic arterial lesion. This is considered the most common cause of acute limb ischaemia. Because of the gradual progression of atherosclerosis, collaterals may have developed. Hence, thrombosis presents more insidiously and less dramatically than an acute embolus. Important clues include history of claudication, mild ischaemia and bilateral absence of pulses.

2. **B - Embolic occlusion.** Embolic occlusion presents with sudden onset of profound ischaemia. The source of emboli is usually cardiac-mural thrombus following myocardial infarction, dilated cardiomyopathy or rheumatic mitral valvular disease. Less commonly, proximal arterial aneurysms or atherosclerotic plaques may be responsible for distal emboli. Such microembolism can result in the 'blue-toe' syndrome with palpable pulses. Large emboli typically lodge at an arterial bifurcation, especially the common femoral and popliteal arteries. Important clues include rapid worsening of ischaemia and history of cardiac disease.

3. **D - Popliteal aneurysm.** Popliteal aneurysms may be bilateral in 50% of patients. Their clinical presentations range from an asymptomatic pulsatile mass to severe lower extremity ischaemia. Acute thrombosis occurs in nearly 40% of patients, while distal embolisation is found in 25%. Important clues include elderly age and prominent contralateral popliteal pulse. Occasionally a prominent ipsilateral popliteal pulse may be present in spite of thrombus within the aneurysm.

4. **G - Popliteal artery injury** Popliteal artery injury can result from various orthopaedic knee procedures, like arthroscopic procedures, knee replacement, high tibial osteotomy or inappropriate screw placement during fracture fixation. The hints in this case are: knee surgery and absent pulses postoperatively. The temperature of limb may be warm due to postoperative condition or poikolothermia (an acutely ischaemic limb often takes on the temperature of the surrounding).

5. **H - Compartment syndrome.** Raised intracompartmental pressure may follow blunt soft tissue or bony injury, especially the leg. The condition may worsen with the application of a plaster cast. Hence, a plaster slab is preferred for such injuries. Severe pain, often out of proportion to the signs is classical of compartment syndrome. Important clues in this patient include history of trauma, bony injury, severe pain, tense calf and present pulses.

## 3. THEME: DIAGNOSTIC INVESTIGATIONS

OPTIONS

A. Colour-flow duplex
B. Arteriography
C. Spiral CT with 3-dimensional reconstruction
D. MR angiography
E. Transcutaneous oximetry
F. ABPI

*Which is the investigation of choice in the following conditions? Select an option from those listed above. An option can be used once, more than once or not at all.*

1. Prediction of amputation level

2. Femoro-popliteal bypass graft surveillance

3. Aortic dissection

4. Vascular malformation

## 3. ANSWERS

1. **E - Transcutaneous oximetry**

$TcPO_2$ measurement reflects the perfusion and metabolic state of the target tissues. Normal measurement ranges from 40 to 70 mm Hg. At foot level, $tcPO_2$ < 20 mm Hg is diagnostic of limb-threatening ischaemia. The main application of this test is in determination of the healing potential of wounds and prediction of successful amputation level.

2. **A - Colour-flow duplex**

Duplex surveillance of infrainguinal arterial bypass grafts is a major component of postoperative care following vascular reconstructions. Low Peak Systolic Velocity (PSV < 40 cm/sec) and absence of diastolic forward flow are highly predictive of impending graft failure. ABPI, although simple, rapid and widely performed, is not a reliable method to detect graft stenosis.

3. **C - Spiral CT with 3-dimensional reconstruction**

This is the study of choice for aortic dissection. Both true and false lumens are well opacified, along with the aortic branches. MR angiography may not demonstrate aortic dissection well if one lumen is thrombosed or calcified. However, MRA with or without gadolinium enhancement may be preferred in presence of renal failure when iodinated CT contrast media are contraindicated.

4. **D - MR angiography**

MRI with MR venography is considered the diagnostic test of choice for low-flow vascular malformations. In high-flow arteriovenous malformations, arteriography may be necessary following MRI and MRV, to show the exact angiotexture or feeding vessels, which is essential for treatment planning.

## 4. THEME: DOPPLER CHARACTERISTICS

OPTIONS

A. Antegrade systolic flow with diastolic flow reversal
B. Antegrade systolic and diastolic flow
C. Peak systolic flow of 240 cm/sec
D. Peak systolic flow of 30 cm/sec
E. Antegrade systolic flow with loss of diastolic flow reversal

*Which of the above-mentioned Doppler flow patterns is found in the following conditions? An option can be used once, more than once or not at all.*

1. Normal internal carotid artery

2. Internal carotid stenosis > 70%

3. Normal popliteal artery after exercise

## 4. ANSWERS

1. **B - Antegrade systolic and diastolic flow**

The normal pattern of flow in peripheral arteries is typicallytri- or biphasic (pulsatile, high-resistance flow) with a strong antegrade component during systole, followed by end-diastolic flow reversal of short duration. A return to forward flow (3rd phase) during late diastole may be occasionally present.

In contrast, a low-resistance flow with antegrade flow in both systole and diastole is detected in vessels that supply critical organs (brain, kidneys).

2. **C - PSV = 230 cm/sec**

In arterial stenosis, a high-velocity jet is produced at the stenosis due to turbulence and loss of laminar flow. As the severity of stenosis increases, the most consistent change is an increase in the PSV. Haemodynamically significant stenosis (> 50% lumen diameter narrowing) causes an 80–100% increase in the PSV. A PSV >125 cm/sec is a reliable indicator of significant internal carotid stenosis, whereas PSV >230 cm/sec suggests a stenosis > 70%. The ratio of internal carotid to common carotid artery PSV (normally < 1.8) has also been found to be a useful marker of stenosis. A ratio > 4.0 is highly diagnostic of > 70% stenosis.

3. **B - Antegrade systolic and diastolic flow**

A low-resistance pattern is also found in normal vessels following exercise. The normal response to exercise is intense peripheral vasodilatation and decrease in peripheral resistance, which produces a characteristic continuous forward flow, with a good velocity. Such a pattern may also be seen in severe peripheral arterial disease distal to a stenosis or an occlusion. In this condition, ischaemic vasodilatation contributes to the reduction in the peripheral resistance. The extreme pattern of flow in arteries distal to an occlusion is a low velocity, slow waveform (*parvus et tardus*).

## 5. THEME: DUPLEX SCANS

OPTIONS

A. Inspiratory increase and expiratory decrease in flow
B. Inspiratory decrease and expiratory increase in flow
C. Loss of phasic flow
D. Swirling flow
E. Retrograde flow on Valsalva maneuvre
F. High-velocity flow persistent on Valsalva maneuvre

*Which of the above-mentioned patterns is found in the following conditions? An option can be used once, more than once or not at all.*

1. Normal subclavian vein

2. Pseudoaneurysm

3. AV fistula

4. Sapheno-femoral junction incompetence

## 5. ANSWERS

1. **A - Inspiratory increase and expiratory decrease in flow**
Normal venous flow is phasic with respiration. In the lower extremity, flow decreases with inspiration and increases with expiration. During inspiration, intra-abdominal pressure rises, thus compressing the inferior vena cava and decreasing the lower extremity venous outflow. The opposite occurs in the upper limb veins. The negative intrathoracic pressure during inspiration causes an increased venous flow.

2. **D - Swirling flow**
The typical pattern of swirling flow (yin-yang sign) is classical of a pseudoaneurysm arising from a localized tear in the arterial wall.

3. **F - High-velocity flow persistent on Valsalva maneuver**
An arteriovenous fistula is characterized by high-velocity, artery-like flow signals in the vein, which persist even during the Valsalva maneuver.

4. **E - Retrograde flow on Valsalva maneuver**
In normal veins, flow is diminished or interrupted without retrograde flow during the Valsalva maneuver. Incompetent veins show retrograde flow in response to the Valsalva maneuver. A retrograde flow > 0.5 seconds is termed as significant reflux.

Continuous flow without respiratory variation (loss of phasic flow), absence of augmentation and continuous flow during Valsalva maneuver suggest a proximal obstruction.

## 6. THEME: VASCULAR PHARMACOLOGY – ACTION OF ANTICOAGULANTS

OPTIONS

A. Direct inactivation of thrombin
B. Inhibition of Factor Xa
C. Indirect inactivation of thrombin
D. Reduced synthesis of Factors II, VII, IX, and X
E. GP IIa/IIIb inhibition

*For each of anticoagulant drugs listed below, select the most likely mechanism of action from the list of options above. An option can be used once, more than once or not at all.*

1. Unfractionated heparin

2. Low-molecular-weight heparin (LMWH)

3. Warfarin

4. Hirudin

## 6. ANSWERS

1. **C - Indirect inactivation of thrombin**

The anticoagulant effect of standard (Unfractionated) heparin depends on its binding with antithrombin. The heparin-antithrombin complex inhibits factors IIa (thrombin), IXa, Xa, XIa and XIIa.

2. **B - Inhibition of Factor Xa**

LMWH interact with antithrombin and cause indirect inhibition of factor Xa and IIa. But the activity against factor IIa is very less compared to heparin. Thus the bleeding rates are lower for LMWH.

3. **D - Reduced synthesis of Factors II, VII, IX, X**

Oral anticoagulants like warfarin are vitamin K antagonists, which reduce the synthesis of vitamin K dependent procoagulant factors II, VII, IX and X. As they also reduce the synthesis of anticoagulant protein C, they produce an initial procoagulant state. Hence, heparin should be overlapped with warfarin until the prothrombin time reaches a therapeutic range.

4. **A - Direct inactivation of thrombin**

Hirudin and Argatroban are direct thrombin inhibitors, which are useful in patients with heparin-induced thrombocytopenia.

Recently, direct factor Xa inhibitors (Antistatin) and indirect factor Xa inhibitors (Pentasaccharides, e.g., Fondaparinux) have also been used as safer anticoagulants.

## 7. THEME: VASCULAR PHARMACOLOGY – CIRCULATION ENHANCING DRUGS

OPTIONS

A. Haemodilution
B. Vasodilatation
C. ADP platelet receptor inhibition
D. GP IIa/IIIb platelet receptor inhibition
E. Phosphodiesterase III inhibition
F. Enhancement of muscle metabolism
G. Lipid-lowering action

*Select the mechanism of action of the following drugs, from the options listed above. An option can be used once, more than once or not at all.*

1. Clopidogrel

2. Cilostazol

3. Naftidrofuryl

4. Abciximab

## 7. ANSWERS

1. **C - ADP platelet receptor inhibition**
Antiplatelet drugs like aspirin and clopidogrel are widely used in patients with vascular disease. Low-dose aspirin inhibits platelet cyclooxygenase 1 (COX 1), thus reducing thromboxane A2 dependent platelet function. Clopidogrel selectively inhibits ADP-induced platelet aggregation, with no direct effects on arachidonic acid metabolism.

2. **E - Phosphodiesterase III inhibition**
Cilostazol, a phosphodiesterase III inhibitor, has been used successfully in patients with intermittent claudication.

3. **F - Enhancement of muscle metabolism**
Naftidrofuryl is believed to increase production of adenosine triphosphate (ATP) and reduce lactate accumulation in ischaemic tissues, especially muscles. Thus the muscles become more resistant to ischaemia.

4. **D - GP IIa/IIIb platelet receptor inhibition**
Glycoprotein (GP) IIa/IIIb platelet receptors on platelet surface are the final common pathway of platelet aggregation, regardless of the initiating stimulus. Monoclonal antibodies against the receptor (e.g., abciximab) have been used in patients who are judged to be at a moderate or high risk of percutaneous transluminal angioplasty (PTCA)-associated ischaemic complications.

Vasodilators like nifedipine and verapamil may have some role in vasospastic conditions like Raynaud's phenomenon.
Prostaglandins, with vasodilatory and antiplatelet effects have been used for treatment of critical limb ischaemia, especially in non-reconstructible vascular disease.

## 8. THEME: VASCULAR PHARMACOLOGY – MONITORING

OPTIONS

A. Thrombin time
B. Bleeding time
C. Activated Plasma Thromboplastin Time (aPTT)
D. Prothrombin Time (PT)
E. Anti-Factor Xa activity
F. Clotting time

*How are the following anticoagulant drugs monitored during therapeutic use? Choose an option from the list of options above. An option can be used once, more than once or not at all.*

1. Unfractionated heparin

2. LMWH

3. Warfarin

## 8. ANSWERS

1. **C - aPTT**

The anticoagulant effect of heparin is monitored by aPTT when usual therapeutic doses are used and by the ACT (activated clotting time) when higher doses are used in association with percutaneous coronary interventions and cardiac surgeries. An aPTT of 1.5 to 2.5 times the control value is accepted as a therapeutic range.

2. **E - Anti-Factor Xa activity**

LMWH usually do not require regular monitoring. But in certain conditions like severe obesity or renal failure, the anti-factor Xa activity is measured to guide the dose of LMWH, as these patients are prone to over-dosing when weight-adjusted dosing regimens are used.

3. **D - Prothrombin time**

The PT test responds to a reduction of the vitamin K-dependent procoagulant factors that are reduced by warfarin. Hence it is used for monitoring of patients on these oral anticoagulants. The PT ratio is converted into an International Normalized Ratio (INR), which is more reliable and remains similar even if different methods are used for the test. Optimal therapeutic range is different for various indications. Commonly, for long-term secondary prevention of venous thrombosis, an INR of 2.0–3.0 is found acceptable.

## 9. THEME: EXTREMITY VASCULAR TRAUMA – MANAGEMENT

OPTIONS

A. Discharge on analgesics
B. Admit for observation
C. Angiography
D. Exploration and vascular repair
E. Fasciotomy
F. Anticoagulation

*Select the most suitable plan of management for the following patients, from the options listed above? An option can be used once, more than once or not at all.*

1. A 30-year-old man injured his leg in a vehicular accident. On examination, there was bruising in his left calf. The distal pulses were palpable. No fracture was detected on X-rays.

2. A 62-year-old female underwent right femoral artery embolectomy under local anaesthesia today morning. She complains of increasingly severe pain in the calf postoperatively. Her calf is tense and tender. She has pain on passive plantar flexion and cannot dorsiflex her foot. The dorsalis pedis and posterior pulses are palpable.

3. Three days following a femur fracture, a rapidly increasing pulsatile thigh swelling is noticed in a 26-year-old male. The dorsalis pedis and posterior tibial pulses are palpable.

4. An 18-year-old male was hit by a speeding car, sustaining injury to his right knee. X-rays did not demonstrate any bony injury. He developed severe pain in the right foot a few hours later. On examination, the right foot is cold and the popliteal and pedal pulses are not palpable. There is loss of sensation over the 1st and 2nd toes.

## 9. ANSWERS

1. **B - Admit for observation.** Patients with blunt soft tissue trauma and haematoma are at risk of compartment syndrome. Hence they should be kept under close observation.

2. **E - Fasciotomy.** Compartment syndrome can also develop following surgical correction of acute limb ischaemia, as in this lady. This is termed as the 'ischemia-reperfusion syndrome'. Release of anaerobic metabolites, superoxide and hydroxyl radicals during reperfusion leads to tissue damage by peroxidation of cell membrane lipids, which increases microvascular permeability and thus the intracompartmental pressure. Severe pain, often out of proportion to the signs and worsened by passive muscle stretch is suggestive of compartment syndrome. Normal compartment pressures are lower than 10 mm Hg. When it exceeds 30 mm Hg, tissue perfusion is reduced to critical levels. In a hypotensive patient, a compartment pressure that is less than 20 mm Hg below the diastolic blood pressure should prompt surgical intervention.

The indications of fasciotomy include:

a. Compartment syndrome with nerve dysfunction or muscle weakness
b. Massive soft tissue injury and swelling
c. Delayed vascular repair
d. Prophylactic fasciotomy in elective tibial operations

3. **C - Angiography.** This patient most likely has a pseudoaneurysm from the superficial femoral, profunda femoris artery or its branches in the thigh. In a stable patient with suspected arterial injury, but non-limb threatening ischaemia, diagnostic arteriography can be performed to evaluate the exact site and extent of injury.

The indications of preoperative angiography in extremity vascular trauma include:
(a) Distal ischaemic deficit, (b) Expanding or pulsatile haematoma, (c) Diminished pulses, (d) Penetrating injuries in proximity to neurovascular structures.

4. **D - Exploration and vascular repair.** This patient has an arterial injury with threatened viability (cold foot, loss of sensation). His typical history (high-impact direct injury to the knee) and absence of fracture on radiographs should lead to a suspicion of knee dislocation, which might have spontaneously reduced. This condition often causes contusion of the popliteal artery and distal pulses may be palpable initially. But with time, a thrombus develops and distal pulse deficits are detected if specifically looked for. In presence of limb-threatening ischaemia, further diagnostic tests are unnecessary. Hence, surgical exploration may be performed on clinical grounds. Preoperative angiography may be used for delineation of arterial injuries.

## 10. THEME: VASCULAR TRAUMA – MANAGEMENT

OPTIONS

A. Angiographic evaluation
B. Primary amputation
C. Immediate exploration and repair
D. Quadruple ligation
E. Endovascular management

*Select the most suitable plan of management for the following patients, from the options listed above. An option can be used once, more than once or not at all.*

1. Absent radial and ulnar pulses after reduction of fracture supracondylar humerus.
2. Extensive crush injury of leg.
3. Haemodynamically stable patient with penetrating injury of neck.
4. Left iliac arteriovenous fistula in a patient who has undergone laparotomy and bowel resection twice following gun shot injury of abdomen.

## 10. ANSWERS

1. **A - Angiographic evaluation**

Supracondylar humerus can occasionally injure the brachial artery. Sometimes, the radial pulse at wrist may be palpable even in presence of brachial artery injury, due to the abundant collaterals in the upper limb. Pulse deficits should be evaluated by angiography to detect the site and extent of injury.

2. **B - Primary amputation**

Primary amputation following lower extremity injury is indicated when vascular repair is not technically feasible or the limb has irreversible ischaemia. Consideration of immediate amputation should be based on soft tissue destruction, muscle loss and bony injury.

3. **A - Angiographic evaluation**

Penetrating injuries of the neck can cause carotid or vertebral artery injury, which often leads to neurological deficits. In order to identify arterial injury, four-vessel angiography is recommended in all such patients in a stable condition. CT scan with contrast enhancement is also a useful investigation to detect vascular trauma as well as associated injuries to the remaining neck structures.

4. **E - Endovascular management**

Gunshot injuries are associated with damage to various abdominal viscera apart from vascular structures. Arteriovenous fistula is usually detected as a late complication, often presenting with unilateral limb swelling or congestive cardiac failure. In a patient who has already undergone multiple laparotomies, endovascular covered stent placement is an attractive, minimally invasive and preferred alternative to surgery.

## 11. THEME: IATROGENIC VASCULAR INJURIES

OPTIONS

A. Surgical repair
B. Conservative management
C. Endovascular covered stent
D. Endovascular coil embolisation
E. Ultrasound guided compression

*What is the most appropriate treatment option for the following patients? An option can be used once, more than once or not at all.*

1. A 4-cm diameter femoral pseudoaneurysm, detected in a 62-year-old female who had undergone coronary angioplasty two days ago.

2. Localized haematoma in a 52-year-old man who underwent diagnostic aortofemoral angiography yesterday.

3. A 36-year-old man was admitted in the ICU for management of acute respiratory failure following fulminant hepatitis. 8 days later, a 10 x 6 cm sized pulsatile mass was noted in the right supraclavicular fossa. Treatment history was significant for attempted right subclavian venous access.

4. A 56-year-old lady underwent coronary artery bypass one year ago. An intra-aortic balloon pump (IABP) insertion was performed then, for postoperative cardiogenic shock. She presented with a one-month history of pain in her right foot. On examination, a thrill is palpable in the right groin. Popliteal and distal pulses are feeble.

## 11. ANSWERS

1. **E - Ultrasound guided compression**

Percutaneous diagnostic and therapeutic arterial and venous access procedures can lead to complications like haematoma, pseudoaneurysm and arteriovenous fistula. Small femoral pseudoaneurysms (< 6 cm diameter) are best treated by Ultrasound Guided Compression (UGC).

2. **B - Conservative management**

Small, non-expanding haematomas often develop following angiography in patients on antiplatelets and anticoagulants. They can be successfully managed conservatively with close surveillance. Large haematomas with compression effects or tense haematomas with skin changes should be considered for early surgical drainage and repair.

3. **C - Endovascular covered stent**

Although UGC is applicable to superficial pseudoaneurysms, it may not be possible at sites where compression cannot be achieved. Hence a subclavian aneurysm needs prompt surgical or endovascular management. In a critically ill patient like this man, endovascular covered stent is a better option with low risks and morbidity compared to open surgery. Endovascular coil embolisation may be of value in small pseudoaneurysms or those arising from arterial branches.

4. **A - Surgical repair**

The most likely diagnosis in this lady is a femoral arteriovenous fistula (AVF) following arterial access during IABP insertion. An AVF can present with local symptoms (limb swelling, distal ischaemia) or systemic symptoms (high-output failure). Surgical ligation of fistula with repair of the artery and vein is the preferred treatment procedure in this location. However, endovascular covered stents have been successfully used in aorto-caval, iliac and superficial femoral AVF.

## 12. THEME: CLASSICAL ARTERIOGRAPHIC FINDINGS

OPTIONS

A. Takayasu's arteritis
B. Buerger's disease
C. Fibromuscular dysplasia
D. Atherosclerosis
E. Embolus
F. Raynaud's phenomenon

*For each of the following arteriographic findings, identify the most probable disease from the options listed above. An option can be used once, more than once or not at all.*

1. Large vessel stenosis, occlusion and aneurysms

2. Abrupt cut-off of an arterial bifurcation

3. String of beads appearance

4. Multi segmental distal arterial occlusion with corkscrew collaterals

5. Filling defect in an artery

## 12. ANSWERS

1. **A - Takayasu's arteritis**

Takayasu's arteritis is an inflammatory and obliterative arteritis commonly affecting the aorta and its branches. Arteriography shows vessel occlusion or stenosis, aneurysm formation and collaterals around occlusions.

2. **E - Embolus**

An acute occluding embolus in an artery may be detected as an abrupt cut-off without noticeable collaterals. Often, the distal run-off is not visualized owing to thrombus within the arteries.

3. **C - Fibromuscular dysplasia**

This is an uncommon disease, which affects the renal and carotid arteries. It is characterized by involvement of the arterial intima and media, producing alternate segments of stenosis and aneurysmal dilatation—the 'string of beads' appearance.

4. **B - Buerger's disease**

Buerger's disease (thromboangitis obliterans) typically involves the small and medium-sized arteries of lower limbs and occasionally the upper limbs. Angiography shows segmental occlusion of infrapopliteal arteries with large, tortuous corkscrew collaterals.

5. **E - Embolus**

A non-occluding embolus in an artery is detected as a filling defect on arteriography.

Atherosclerosis, a degenerative disease with accumulation of lipids, cells and tissue debris in the intima, can give rise to stenosis or obstruction of arteries. It is usually widespread and may involve abdominal aorta, carotid, coronary, renal, iliac or superficial femoral arteries.

## 13. THEME: VASCULAR GRAFTS

OPTIONS

A. Arterial autograft
B. Venous autograft
C. Knitted dacron
D. Woven dacron
E. Thin walled PTFE
F. Ringed PTFE
G. Umbilical vein allograft
H. Stent-graft

*For each of the following conditions, select the most preferred graft from the options provided above. Each option can be used once, more than once or not at all.*

1. Femoro-distal bypass

2. Axillo-bifemoral bypass

3. Left coronary artery bypass

4. Arteriovenous graft

## 13. ANSWERS

1. **B - Venous autograft**

For infrainguinal arterial bypasses, autogenous vein is the conduit of choice. Long saphenous vein is most commonly utilized for this purpose. For an above-knee bypass, some surgeons consider thin-walled PTFE as an acceptable alternative. But for below-knee bypasses, PTFE has poor patency rates. Hence vein is preferred in this instance. If no adequate venous conduit is available, PTFE may be used in combination with a distal interposition vein cuff.

2. **F - Ringed PTFE**

An axillo-bifemoral bypass requires a long graft, which is placed subcutaneously and crosses the hip joint. An externally supported (ringed) PTFE is preferred for this extra-anatomic bypass as it is resistant to kinks and external compression. An internally supported PTFE graft is also available for this purpose.

3. **A - Arterial autograft**

The commonest arterial autograft in use is the left internal mammary artery for left coronary artery bypass. It has a patency rate superior to that of saphenous vein grafts.

4. **E - Thin walled PTFE**

An arteriovenous graft is a subcutaneously placed graft as a bridge between a donor artery and a recipient vein. It is used as an access procedure for chronic haemodialysis if arteriovenous fistulae are not successful. PTFE is most commonly used for this purpose.

Knitted or woven Dacron (polyester) grafts are preferred for thoracic or abdominal aortic surgeries. PTFE has also become popular for this use.

Glutaraldehyde stabilized human umbilical cord vein allograft may be used for lower limb revascularization when autologous vein is unavailable or unsuitable.

A stent-graft is an endovascular device that is a combination of prosthetic graft and a vascular stent. It has been increasingly used in endovascular treatment of large-vessel aneurysms, pseudoaneurysms and arteriovenous fistulae.

## 14. THEME: BASIC VASCULAR OPERATIONS

OPTIONS

A. Endarterectomy
B. Embolectomy
C. Bypass
D. Thrombectomy
E. Sympathectomy
F. Conservative

*For each of the following patients, choose the most likely single treatment from the list of options provided above. Each option can be used once, more than once or not at all.*

1. A 67-year-old male underwent arteriography for critical limb ischaemia. The superficial femoral artery was occluded from origin and the popliteal artery reforms behind the knee, with patent two-vessel runoff in leg.

2. Two episodes of transient amaurosis fugax occurred in a 71-year-old lady. Her carotid color-duplex revealed 80% stenosis of left internal carotid artery.

3. A 34-year-old lady with rheumatic mitral stenosis presented with a 6-hour history of severe pain in left lower limb. Her femoral and distal pulses are not palpable. The ipsilateral foot is cold, cyanosed and with reduced sensation. Contralateral pulses are palpable.

## 14. ANSWERS

1. **C - Bypass**

The preferred treatment for this long segment occlusion would be a femoro-popliteal bypass. Vein is the conduit of choice. In absence of suitable vein, PTFE may be used for this purpose.

2. **A - Endarterectomy**

This patient has a symptomatic significant carotid stenosis. Carotid endarterectomy is the 'gold-standard' treatment for this disease, especially for stenosis greater than 70%. Percutaneous angioplasty and stenting is emerging as a minimally invasive alternative to surgery.

3. **B - Embolectomy**

The most likely aetiology for acute limb ischaemia is an embolus of cardiac origin. In view of the threatened viability, surgical femoral embolectomy should be performed as an emergent procedure.

## 15. THEME: HISTORY OF VASCULAR SURGERY

OPTIONS

A. Coote
B. Hauer
C. DeBakey
D. Von Winiwarter
E. Fogarty
F. Dotter
G. Carrel
H. Virchow
I. Buerger

*For the historical achievements given below, select the responsible clinician from the list provided above. Each option can be used once, more than once or not at all.*

1. Description of thromboangitis obliterans

2. Nobel laureate

3. Pathogenesis of thrombosis

4. First removal of cervical rib

5. Introduction of balloon catheter technique for arterial thromboembolectomy

6. Introduction of concept of percutaneous transluminal arterial dilatation

## 15. ANSWERS

1. **I - Buerger**

Although thromboangitis obliterans is synonymous with Buerger's disease, Von Winiwater first described a similar endarteritis in 1879.

2. **G - Carrel**

Alexis Carrel and Guthrie described the principles and techniques of the modern vascular anastomosis. Carrel was awarded the Nobel Prize in 1912 for description of the 'triangulation technique' for end-to-end vascular anastomosis.

3. **H - Virchow**

He described the famous triad, responsible for deep venous thrombosis in 1859. It includes endothelial injury, stasis of venous blood and a hypercoagulable state.

4. **A - Coote**

He described the first successful excision of a cervical rib in 1861.

5. **E - Fogarty**

Thomas Fogarty, in 1963, introduced his balloon catheter for removal of thromboembolic material from sites proximal and distal to the arteriotomy with a minimum of invasiveness and tissue dissection.

6. **F - Dotter**

Charles Dotter, a radiologist conceptualized percutaneous balloon angioplasty in 1964. But it was Gruentzig who advanced and popularized this technique.

## 16. THEME: MANAGEMENT OF ABDOMINAL AORTIC ANEURYSM

OPTIONS

A. Watchful waiting
B. Pharmacotherapy with ultrasound follow-up
C. Aorto-biiliac stent-graft placement
D. Fluid resuscitation followed by CT scan
E. Immediate transfer to operation theatre
F. Inclusion endoaneurysmorrhaphy

*For each of the conditions described below, select the most likely single management from the options listed above. Each option can be used once, more than once or not at all.*

1. A 61-year-old man underwent an ultrasound examination for a one-month history of vague abdominal discomfort. An infrarenal AAA, 6.5 cm in diameter was detected. His CT scan with 3-dimensional reconstruction confirmed the aneurysm with concentric intraluminal thrombus. There was a 90-degree angulation of the aneurysm neck. His past medical history was not significant.

2. A 70-year-old male with a one-day history of lower back pain was brought to the emergency department in a state of shock. On arrival, his pulse was 120/min and the supine blood pressure 80 mm Hg. On per abdominal examination, an ill-defined pulsatile mass was palpable in the epigastric region.

3. A 65-year-old male was under regular ultrasound surveillance for a 4-cm diameter AAA detected one year ago. His recent ultrasound shows the aneurysm diameter to have increased to 5 cm. His past medical history is significant for hypertension and COPD.

4. An ultrasound study in a 54-year-old obese male detected gallstones and an AAA of 3.5 cm diameter. His only complaint was of recurrent dyspepsia. Past medical history was not significant.

## 16. ANSWERS

1. **F - Inclusion endoaneurysmorrhaphy**
Symptomatic, large AAA (> 6 cm diameter) should be electively repaired. Excess angulation at the neck precludes successful endovascular repair. As this patient is otherwise fit, he should be considered for open repair with inclusion endoaneurysmorrhaphy using a prosthetic graft.

2. **E - Immediate transfer to OT**
The likely cause for hypotension and shock is a ruptured AAA. Aggressive fluid resuscitation may promote further bleeding by increasing the blood pressure. Although CT scan would establish the diagnosis of a ruptured AAA, it may cause a significant delay in treatment. Haemodynamically unstable patients with clinically apparent AAA should undergo immediate, emergent surgery. CT scan may be helpful in a haemodynamically stable patient to determine the presence of rupture.

3. **C - Aorto-biiliac stent-graft placement**
A rapid expansion rate (> 0.5 cm in 6 months) is a predictor of a high risk of rupture. Also, COPD and hypertension are additional predictors of rupture. In presence of favourable anatomy, endovascular repair is preferred. Inclusion criteria include: (a) normal aorta between aneurysm and renal artery > 15 mm, (b) angulation of proximal neck >120°, (c) non-tortuous iliac arteries.

4. **B - Pharmacotherapy with ultrasound follow-up**
For patients with low-risk AAAs (small diameter, without other risk factors for rupture), medical management and periodic ultrasound measurements are recommended. Propranolol, a β-blocker, reduces the blood pressure, and also has a direct effect on extracellular matrix and increases tensile strength. Doxycycline functions as an antibiotic for eradication of *Chlamydia* infection and is also a non-specific inhibitor of matrix-metalloproteinases.

## 17. THEME: AAA – AETIOPATHOLOGY

OPTIONS

A. Reduced activity of Matrix Metalloproteinases (MMP) in the aortic wall
B. Increased activity of Matrix Metalloproteinases (MMP) in the aortic wall
C. Increased number of elastin fibers in aortic wall
D. 4.5 cm diameter AAA with thick rim of thrombus within the aneurysm sac
E. 5 cm diameter AAA with minimal eccentric thrombus

*For the questions given below, identify the most likely option from the list provided above. Each option can be used once, more than once or not at all.*

1. Proposed aetiological factor

2. High risk for rupture

3. Low risk for rupture

## 17. ANSWERS

1. **B - Increased activity of Matrix Metalloproteinases (MMP) in the aortic wall**

The aetiology of AAA is termed as degenerative or non-specific. Many aetiological factors have been proposed in the causation of AAA:

a. Reduction of elastin layers
b. Medial thinning and intimal thickening
c. Decrease in collagen and elastin content in the aortic wall
d. Absence of vasa vasorum in infra renal aorta
e. Increased proteolytic activity (MMPs, especially MMP 9)
f. Transmural inflammatory response to infection by *Chlamydia pneumoniae* is also proposed as a causative factor

2. **E - 5 cm diameter AAA with minimal eccentric thrombus**

The risk factors for AAA rupture include:

a. Aneurysm diameter. Larger aneurysms (>6 cm diameter) have a high risk of rupture, nearly 25% at one year.
b. Expansion rate of >5 mm per six months or > 1 cm per year is also an accepted predictor of the high risk for rupture.
c. Hypertension and COPD are independent predictors of rupture.
d. Eccentric saccular aneurysms represent greater rupture risk than more diffuse, cylindrical aneurysms.
e. Intraluminal thrombus also has an effect on rupture risk. Thrombus has been suggested to reduce aneurysmal wall tension. So thin walled aneurysms without thrombus are more likely to rupture than aneurysms with thick intraluminal thrombus.

3. **D - 4.5 cm diameter AAA with thick rim of thrombus within the aneurysm sac**

## 18. THEME: AAA – IMAGING

OPTIONS

A. Colour-flow duplex
B. Spiral CT scan
C. MR angiography
D. Ultrasound
E. Arteriography

*For each of the following conditions, select the most likely imaging technique from the options listed above. Each option can be used once, more than once or not at all.*

1. Screening for AAA

2. Follow-up of a AAA 3.5 cm in diameter, detected on screening

3. Pre-treatment evaluation of a 6.5 cm diameter AAA in a diabetic patient with a S. creatinine of 1.9 mg%.

## 18. ANSWERS

1. **D - Ultrasound**

Because asymptomatic AAAs are often not discovered until they rupture, the potential benefit of screening programs has been accepted. Simple ultrasound is recommended for this purpose. In a large screening of 16,000 patients aged 65 years and above, a 4% prevalence of AAA > 3 cm diameter was noted.

2. **D - Ultrasound**

Although diameter measurement by CT scanning is more accurate, ultrasound is commonly used as it is rapid, less invasive, less expensive and obviates the need for contrast. CT scan may be used as the final determinant for evaluation of borderline-sized AAAs.

3. **C - MR angiography**

MRA may be valuable in the pre-treatment evaluation of patients with AAA who have compromised renal function and iodinated intravenous contrast agents are contraindicated.

## 19. THEME: AORTIC SURGICAL EXPOSURES

OPTIONS

A. Transperitoneal
B. Right retroperitoneal
C. Left retroperitoneal

*For each of the following conditions, select the most preferred approach for surgical repair from the list given above. Each option can be used once, more than once or not at all.*

1. Juxtarenal AAA

2. Ruptured AAA

3. AAA in a 60-year-old male, who has undergone abdomino-peroneal resection for malignancy of rectum 3 years ago

4. AAA with bilateral iliac aneurysms

## 19. ANSWERS

1. **C - Left retroperitoneal**

Exposure of sufficient normal aorta proximal to a juxtarenal AAA may be difficult via a transperitoneal approach. Left retroperitoneal exposure, with anterior displacement of left kidney facilitates suprarenal exposure. However, this can also be achieved through a transperitoneal approach with medial visceral rotation.

2. **A - Transperitoneal**

In emergency situations, when prompt proximal control of aorta is required, a long midline transperitoneal approach can be accomplished rapidly. If normal infrarenal aorta above the aneurysm is visible, it can be clamped immediately. But usually the presence of haematoma precludes a direct visualization of aneurysm neck. In this condition, the aorta can be rapidly exposed and clamped just beyond the diaphragm, via the lesser omentum.

3. **B - Right retroperitoneal**

Presence of an abdominal stoma (left sigmoid colostomy in this instance) is a relative contraindication for a transperitoneal approach. Right retroperitoneal exposure may be suitable when such problems rule out the left approach.

4. **A - Transperitoneal**

This approach gives an excellent view of both iliac arteries in addition to the aorta.

## 20. THEME: COMPLICATIONS OF AORTIC SURGERY

OPTIONS

A. Conservative
B. CT scan guided drainage
C. Prolonged antibiotic administration
D. Graft excision with extra-anatomic bypass
E. Reoperation

*For each of the following patients, select the most likely single treatment from the list provided above. Each option can be used once, more than once or not at all.*

1. A 62-year-old man had undergone aorto-biiliac interposition Dacron graft for repair of AAA two years ago. He presented with vague abdominal discomfort for 3 months. His CT scan shows a 3 x 2 cm sized perigraft fluid collection. The total WBC count is normal and the blood culture is sterile.

2. A 60-year-old man presented with two episodes of moderate haematemesis in the past one week. His upper GI endoscopy performed elsewhere showed mild gastritis. His past medical history is significant for an AAA repair 5 years ago.

3. A 56-year-old female underwent transperitoneal repair of an infrarenal AAA with iliac aneurysms three days ago. Today, two patches of purplish discolouration are noted in her left leg. The pedal pulses are palpable.

4. A 67-year-old male was operated a week ago for a ruptured AAA. His bowel function has returned but he has passed four bloody stools since yesterday. His total leucocyte count is 20,000 cells/mm$^3$. The nurse has noticed a mild increase in respiratory rate since today morning.

## 20. ANSWERS

**1. D - Graft excision with extra-anatomic bypass**

This patient most likely has developed a late prosthetic infection, characteristic of *Staphylococcus epidermidis.* Patients present months to years after graft implantation with local complications (anastomotic pseudoaneurysm, perigraft fluid cavity or discharging sinus). Typically, there are no systemic signs of sepsis (fever, leucocytosis and bacteremia). Axillo-bifemoral bypass grafting through uninfected tissues should be followed by total excision of the infected aortic graft. In situ replacement with debridement may be an alternative in such low-grade graft infections.

**2. D - Graft excision with extra-anatomic bypass**

Any patient with gastrointestinal bleeding and an aortic graft should be considered to have graft infection and graft-enteric fistula unless proved otherwise. The classic triad of aortic graft-enteric fistula includes gastrointestinal fistula, fever and abdominal pain. It may present two days to 15 years after graft replacement. A complete endoscopic examination including 3rd and 4th parts of duodenum may be helpful in diagnosis. Contrast-enhanced CT is also a useful test to demonstrate perigraft air or fluid, pseudoaneurysm or leakage of contrast. Graft excision with extra-anatomic bypass is the recommended approach for this difficult situation.

**3. A - Conservative**

This patient probably has patchy skin necrosis due to atheroemboli, which may be released into the circulation during aneurysm mobilization or clamping. As the major leg vessels are patent, an expectant management is sufficient. LMWH and low-molecular weight dextran have also been recommended in such conditions.

**4. E - Reoperation**

Important clues to bowel ischaemia in this patient include (a) bloody diarrhoea, (b) tachypnoea, possibly as a compensatory effect in response to metabolic acidosis and (c) leucocytosis.

Fiberoptic colonoscopy should be performed urgently to prove the diagnosis. Reoperation is usually necessary. All compromised bowel, commonly the sigmoid colon, must be resected. Primary anastomosis is contraindicated. Hence colostomy with Hartmann's pouch or distal mucus fistula construction is necessary.

## 21. THEME: CHRONIC LOWER LIMB ISCHAEMIA – PATHOLOGY

OPTIONS

A. Atherosclerosis
B. Cystic adventitial disease
C. Buergers' disease
D. Popliteal artery entrapment
E. Arterial thrombosis
F. Raynaud's syndrome
G. Neurogenic claudication

*For each of the following patients, select the most likely cause of limb ischaemia. Each option can be used once, more than once or not at all.*

1. A 68-year-old male with a history of previous myocardial infarction presents with pain in left foot for the past 20 days. He has had calf pain with walking for 2 years, but the recent pain even wakes him from sleep. Popliteal and distal pulses are not palpable.

2. A 40-year-old male smoker presents with a one-month history of painful ulceration over his right great toe. On examination, the foot is swollen and the skin shiny. The popliteal pulse is palpable, while the pedal pulses are absent. He had two previous episodes of painful swelling of his leg veins, which resolved spontaneously.

3. A 62-year-old male presents with a 3-year history of aching pain in both thighs, brought on by walking to a distance and relieved on resting for 5 minutes. His pedal pulses are palpable at rest.

4. A 28-year-old football player complains of cramping pain in left calf while playing. On examination his popliteal and pedal pulses are palpable, but they diminish on active plantar flexion of the foot.

## 21. ANSWERS

1. **A - Atherosclerosis**

Intermittent claudication and critical limb ischaemia are the classic manifestations of lower limb ischaemia. Although atherosclerosis is a generalized disease, it is usually segmental in its distribution. It typically develops at arterial bifurcations and areas of posterior fixation or acute angulation. The distal superficial femoral artery at adductor hiatus is the most common site of atherosclerotic disease, although it can involve iliac, common femoral, superficial femoral origin and popliteal arteries too.

2. **C - Buerger's disease**

Critical limb ischaemia in young patients can be due to presenile atherosclerosis, arterial thrombosis or Buerger's disease. Important clues in this patient include (a) age <45 years (b) smoking (c) history of thrombophlebitis (d) infra-popliteal arterial involvement.

3. **A - Atherosclerosis**

The history of aching thigh pain precipitated by exercise and relieved by rest is suggestive of arterial intermittent claudication. Good collateral channels that form in response to a chronic unisegmental occlusion or stenosis can usually provide adequate blood flow distally, which produces a pulse at rest. However, the pulse will disappear when patient is asked to walk up to his claudication distance.

4. **D - Popliteal artery entrapment**

It is an uncommon disorder in which popliteal artery passes medial to and beneath the medial head of the gastrocnemius muscle, with subsequent compression of the artery. It is manifested by unilateral claudication in young adults. Pulses may be present or absent at rest. Often the pulses disappear on active plantar flexion or passive dorsiflexion of foot.

## 22. THEME: CHRONIC LOWER LIMB ISCHAEMIA – TREATMENT

OPTIONS

A. Non-interventional management
B. Endovascular balloon angioplasty
C. Anatomic bypass
D. Extra-anatomic bypass
E. Lumbar sympathectomy
F. Amputation

*For each of the following patients, select the most likely single treatment. Each option can be used once, more than once or not at all.*

1. A 34-year-old male presents with a 6-month history of cramp like pain in his right calf, on walking for nearly 1000 metres. His popliteal and distal pulses are not palpable. His serum homocysteine level is 50 μmol/ L.
2. A 67-year-old male with a previous history of percutaneous angioplasty of coronary artery presents with right thigh claudication for the past three years. His claudication distance has reduced to less than 50 metres. On examination, a bruit is detected over his right femoral artery. The popliteal and pedal pulses are feebly palpable.
3. A 42-year-old male smoker underwent an arteriographic evaluation elsewhere for severe rest pain in the first and second toes of left foot. There was occlusion of anterior tibial artery at its origin. No distal reformation could be visualized on subtracted images. The presence of few tortuous collaterals in leg was noted.
4. A 75-year-old male has a 4-week history of painful ulceration of right forefoot. He had previously undergone coronary artery bypass twice in the last decade. His latest echocardiography reported an ejection fraction of 24%. His peripheral angiography shows occlusion of right common iliac artery at origin, with reformation of common femoral artery. The superficial and profunda femoral arteries are patent. The contralateral iliac and femoral arteries are patent.

## 22. ANSWERS

**1. A - Non-interventional management**

Lower limb ischaemia in this person is probably due to hyperhomocysteinaemia, resulting from congenital defects in homocysteine metabolism. The most common variant is cystathione β synthase (CBS), which presents with coronary, carotid, and peripheral atherosclerosis or venous thromboembolism at an early age. Arterial reconstruction should be avoided in this patient with functional limb ischaemia, which is not limb threatening. Non-interventional management is thus preferred and includes cessation of smoking, risk factor modification, exercise therapy and pharmacotherapy (antiplatelet agents, cilostazol, and naftidrofuryl). Long-term administration of folic acid, vitamin $B_6$ and $B_{12}$ is also recommended for hyperhomocysteinaemia.

**2. B - Endovascular balloon angioplasty**

This patient has a disabling claudication, which is likely to interfere with his daily activities. He should be offered revascularisation to alleviate his symptoms. A bruit over the femoral artery is probably due to a haemodynamically significant iliac stenosis. Following an angiographic evaluation, short iliac stenosis is best treated by percutaneous balloon angioplasty. Primary stenting is debatable, but is definitely indicated for post angioplasty dissection or residual stenosis >30%.

**3. E - Lumbar sympathectomy**

The most likely cause in this patient is Buerger's disease. If after a proper angiographic evaluation, no distal target vessels can be detected, vascular reconstruction might not be possible. Lumbar sympathectomy may offer relief in the symptoms in such 'non-reconstructible' vascular diseases. Obviously, cessation of smoking and medical management is complementary to this technique.

**4. D - Extra-anatomic bypass**

This patient would be at a high risk for an aortofemoral bypass surgery. Hence an extra-anatomic femoro-femoral bypass is considered the operation of choice for unilateral iliac artery occlusion in older, high-risk patients.

## 23. THEME: FIVE YEAR GRAFT PATENCY RATES

OPTIONS

A. 40–60%
B. 20–40%
C. 60–80%
D. 80–90%
E. 90–100%

*For each of the following conditions, select the most likely 5-year patency rates. Each option can be used once, more than once or not at all.*

1. Femoro-popliteal (above-knee) reversed vein bypass performed for ischaemic ulceration
2. Aorto-bifemoral PTFE bypass performed for disabling claudication
3. Endovascular angioplasty and stenting performed for a 2-cm long, 80% stenosis of common iliac artery in a 62-year-old male with disabling claudication.
4. Femoro-tibial in situ vein bypass performed for limb salvage.

## 23. ANSWERS

A graft is considered to have primary patency if it has uninterrupted patency without any further intervention. This reflects the natural history of the procedure. When interventions are performed for failing grafts before occlusion, the term assisted primary patency rate is used. If graft patency is restored after occlusion, this is termed as secondary patency rate.

1. **C - 60–80%**

The 5-year primary patency rates of femoro-popliteal vein bypasses are 60–80%. The range is wide due to difference in the status of distal runoff. Prosthetic above knee bypasses, often used as an alternative to venous conduit, have a patency rate of 50–70%.

2. **D - 80–90%**

A bifurcated aorto-bifemoral PTFE bypass graft usually has excellent primary patency in absence of distal disease. Primary rates of 80–90% at 5-years and 70–75% at 10-years are reported.

3. **C - 60–80%**

Percutaneous angioplasty for iliac stenosis has a primary patency rate of 60–80% at five years. The rates may differ according to length of lesion, type of ischaemia and runoff rates.

4. **B - 40–60%**

Primary patency rate for femoro-distal vein bypasses is 40–60% at five years. Prosthetic bypass for infra-popliteal reconstruction is associated with poor patency rates of 15–30%. Hence venous conduit is recommended below the knee. In absence of suitable vein, prosthetic grafts should be combined with vein collar or distal arteriovenous fistula to enhance patency rates.

## 24. THEME: VASCULAR GRAFT OCCLUSION

OPTIONS

A. Graft stenosis
B. Idiopathic thrombosis
C. Neointimal hyperplasia
D. Progression of atherosclerotic disease
E. Poor runoff
F. Graft kink

*For each of the following patients, select the most appropriate cause of graft failure from the list provided above. Each option can be used once, more than once or not at all.*

1. A 72-year-old female underwent femoro-popliteal (above-knee) PTFE bypass for rest pain today morning. She complains of severe pain in right foot for the past two hours. Her popliteal and pedal pulses are not palpable at present. The registrar confidently recollects that the pulses were palpable three hours ago. On further inquiry, she had received an epidural top-up followed by transient hypotension (systolic blood pressure of 90 mm Hg), which was corrected within half-hour by rapid intravenous fluids.

2. A 63-year-old male who had undergone left femoropopliteal vein bypass two years ago, presented with an 8-day history of painful ischaemic ulcers over left foot. The posterior tibial pulse is not palpable.

## 24. ANSWERS

1. **B - Idiopathic thrombosis**

The causes of early graft failure (within 30 days of operation) are technical flaws like graft kink, retained valve cusp, poor run-off or poor inflow site selection. Idiopathic thrombosis often develops in prosthetic grafts, precipitated by hypotension or a transient fall in cardiac output. Graft kinks or twists are common in vein grafts, but uncommon in prosthetic grafts.

2. **C - Neointimal hyperplasia**

An intermediate cause of graft failure (30 days to two years) is most commonly due to neointimal hyperplasia (NIH). Although NIH is formed at the proximal as well as distal anastomotic site, the distal one is more vulnerable to occlusion owing to the smaller diameter of the distal artery.

After 2 years, progression of atherosclerotic disease process in the inflow or outflow tract of arterial reconstruction becomes the predominant cause of graft failure.

## 25. THEME: UPPER LIMB ISCHAEMIA

OPTIONS

A. Atherosclerosis
B. Hypothenar hammer syndrome
C. Connective tissue disease
D. Thoracic outlet syndrome
E. Takayasu's arteritis
F. Fibromuscular dysplasia

*For each of the following patients, identify the most likely cause of upper limb ischaemia from the list given above. Each option can be used once, more than once or not at all.*

1. A 59-year-old male was admitted for inguinal hernia repair. The systolic blood pressure in left arm was measured to be 80 mm Hg, while in the right arm it was detected to be 130 mm Hg. There is no previous history of pain in right upper limb. Medical history is positive for coronary artery disease

2. A 32-year-old female was detected to have asymmetry of blood pressure between right and left arms when she presented to a physician for a month history of fever and myalgia. She had two previous episodes of transient dizziness a week ago. Her left subclavian, brachial, radial and ulnar pulses are not palpable. She has no previous history of pain or colour changes in left upper limb.

3. A 27-year-old female presented with intermittent episodes of pallor and paraesthesias of left thumb and index finger for two months. Five days ago, she developed severe pain in the tip of index finger, followed by spontaneous ulceration. The left subclavian pulse is more prominent compared to the right.

4. A 44-year-old automobile mechanic presents with a 3-month history of numbness and paraesthesias in his right ring and little fingers. He noticed a small painful swelling in his palm three days ago. On examination, radial and ulnar artery pulses are palpable at wrist. A 2 cm diameter, tender pulsatile swelling is palpable over the right hypothenar eminence.

## 25. ANSWERS

**1. A - Atherosclerosis**

Important clues include (a) age (b) positive history of coronary artery disease (c) asymptomatic left upper limb ischaemia. The commonest site of atherosclerosis is left subclavian origin. It can present with upper limb claudication or manifest itself by microembolisation—'blue finger syndrome'—with palpable wrist pulses. Occasionally macroembolisation can cause acute limb ischaemia.

**2. E - Takayasu's arteritis**

This condition is seven times more common in females than males. It usually occurs in patients < 40 years of age. Other clues include (a) history of fever and myalgia, which are signs of systemic inflammatory process (b) history of dizziness, probably due to carotid or vertebral artery involvement. Ocular symptoms like blurred vision, amaurosis fugax and diplopia may often be the presenting features.

**3. D - Thoracic outlet syndrome**

Important clues include (a) Episodes of Raynaud's phenomenon, (b) Ischaemic ulceration in radial artery territory, (c) Prominent subclavian pulse, possibly due to post-stenotic dilatation or aneurysm. Microemboli are especially common in the thumb and index finger, probably due to the straightforward pathway through the radial artery in contrast to the ulnar artery. Often arm claudication may be absent. The shower of microemboli may last for months before major embolic complications occur. Proximal embolisation in mid brachial artery may present as acute limb ischaemia.

**4. B - Hypothenar hammer syndrome**

This rare cause of hand ischaemia is typically found in mechanics who use the palm of the dominant hand to push or strike objects. The ulnar artery in the hypothenar eminence is prone to repetitive trauma that can lead to aneurysm formation and microembolisation in the ulnar artery distribution areas.

## 26. THEME: UPPER LIMB ISCHAEMIA – TREATMENT

OPTIONS

A. Carotid-subclavian bypass
B. Brachial embolectomy
C. Endarterectomy
D. Transaxillary rib excision
E. Supraclavicular rib excision
F. Cervicothoracic sympathectomy
G. Amputation

*For each of the following patients, select the most likely single treatment. Each option can be used once, more than once or not at all.*

1. A 62-year-old male presented with a two-day history of severe pain and paraesthesias left hand. He was admitted a month ago for myocardial infarction. On examination, the left hand is cold and cyanosed. Brachial and distal pulses are not palpable.

2. A 54-year-old male with a two-year history of aching pain in left arm on working, presented with a painful ulcer over the left index finger since 10 days. His hand is warm, but fingers cold. Brachial and distal pulses are not palpable.

3. A 36-year-old lady presented with intermittent episodes of pallor and paraesthesias of left thumb and index finger for two months. Five days ago, she developed severe pain in the tip of index finger, followed by spontaneous ulceration. The left subclavian pulse is more prominent compared to the right. Her X-ray shows presence of bilateral cervical ribs.

4. A 32-year-old female noticed episodic bluish discolouration of her finger tips in response to cold for the past two years. She is on irregular medical treatment for the same. She is referred for painful digital ulcerations in her right hand. Her radial and ulnar pulses are palpable.

## 26. ANSWERS

1. **B - Brachial embolectomy**

The most likely cause of acute limb ischaemia is an embolus from a cardiac source. Brachial embolectomy can be successfully performed under local anaesthesia. Other causes of acute-on-chronic ischaemia like embolism from proximal subclavian aneurysm or from a proximal atherosclerotic plaque should also be remembered.

2. **A - Carotid-subclavian bypass**

Important clues to left subclavian artery stenosis or occlusion include (a) Long history of claudication, (b) Critical limb ischaemia, (c) Absent pulses. Traditional surgical management is by carotid-subclavian bypass or subclavian-carotid transposition. Endarterectomy of subclavian artery origin is difficult and can be achieved only via a midline sternotomy. Obstruction proximal to vertebral artery origin may give rise to the 'subclavian steal syndrome', i.e., reversal of flow through the vertebral artery, which steals blood from the cerebral circulation. This may present as dizziness on excess use of the arm.

3. **E - Supraclavicular rib excision**

Arterial thoracic outlet syndrome is best treated via a supraclavicular approach. The cervical rib can be excised along with the scalenus anticus muscle. The subclavian artery can be evaluated for aneurysm or mural thrombus and reconstruction carried out through this approach.

4. **F - Cervicothoracic sympathectomy**

Vasospastic Raynaud's syndrome classically presents with cold-induced colour changes in digits. Oral medications like nifedipine may be effective in obtaining symptomatic relief. Cervicothoracic sympathectomy may occasionally be performed for reduction of rest pain and healing of ulcers.

## 27. THEME: INVESTIGATIONS FOR CEREBROVASCULAR DISEASE

OPTIONS

A. Arteriography
B. Colour-flow duplex
C. CT scan
D. CT angiography
E. Transcranial Doppler
F. No further investigations

*For each of the following patients, select the initial investigation from the list provided above. Each option can be used once, more than once or not at all.*

1. A 59-year-old male presents with two episodes of sudden onset weakness of right upper limb, which resolved spontaneously within a few minutes. At present, he has no focal neurological deficit. No cervical bruit is audible.

2. A 63-year-old female is planned for a coronary artery bypass for triple vessel disease. Her colour-flow duplex showed a 70% stenosis of left internal carotid artery. There is no previous history of transient ischaemic event.

3. A 67-year-old female presented with disabling claudication of left thigh, for which an angiography is planned. Her previous history is positive for a left sided hemiparesis 6 years ago from which she has fully recovered. Colour-flow duplex shows a 70% stenosis of the right internal carotid artery.

4. A 70-year-old male is brought to the emergency with sudden onset left hemiplegia of two-hour duration. His vital signs are maintained.

## 27. ANSWERS

1. **B - Colour-flow duplex**

Carotid duplex examination is the most widely performed initial investigation for patients with transient ischaemic attack, amaurosis fugax and cervical bruit. Various criteria have been developed for diagnosis of internal carotid artery stenosis. A peak systolic velocity (PSV) > 125 cm/sec is considered to be suggestive of a haemodynamically significant stenosis (>50% lumen diameter narrowing).

2. **D - CT angiography**

This patient with an asymptomatic carotid stenosis of 70% needs further accurate evaluation to decide regarding the need for carotid endarterectomy along with coronary artery bypass grafting (CABG). CT angiography is a non-invasive, accurate investigation with results comparable to invasive angiography. The risk of peri-operative stroke in patients undergoing CABG increases to nearly 10-times in presence of carotid stenosis >75%. The combination of age >60 years plus carotid stenosis >75% is associated with a peri-operative stroke risk of 15% as compared with 0.6% in similar age-group patients without carotid stenosis.

3. **A - Arteriography**

In this patient who is planned for an angiographic evaluation of his lower-limb arteries, carotid angiography can be performed in the same session. Although this is invasive and associated with a procedural neurological complication of 0.5–1.0%, it can be useful therapeutically. Carotid angioplasty and stenting with cerebral protection, is fast emerging as an alternative to surgical management of carotid stenosis.

4. **C - CT scan**

All patients with acute cerebrovascular stroke should undergo CT scanning to differentiate between haemorrhagic and ischaemic stroke. Specialist stroke centers may consider thrombolytic therapy for early ischaemic stroke, in absence of intracranial bleed and hypertension.

## 28. THEME: MANAGEMENT OF CAROTID ARTERY LESIONS

OPTIONS

A. Thromboembolectomy
B. Endarterectomy
C. Angioplasty with stenting
D. Bypass
E. Best medical management
F. Ligation
G. Thrombolysis

*For each of the following patients, select the best possible treatment from the list given above. Each option can be used once, more than once or not at all.*

1. A 62-year-old male presented with a two-hour history of left hemiplegia. His vital signs are maintained. His CT scan shows loss of cortical ribbon in right temporal cortex.

2. A 65-year-old female had three episodes of left transient amaurosis fugax in the past week. Her colour-flow duplex shows a left internal carotid artery stenosis of 20% and a right internal carotid stenosis of 30%.

3. A 74-year-old male had undergone right carotid endarterectomy 6 years ago. He presents with an episode of transient left upper limb paresis. His colour-flow duplex is suggestive of 80% stenosis of the right internal carotid artery.

## 28. ANSWERS

1. **G - Thrombolysis**

Patients with acute ischaemic cerebrovascular stroke can be considered as potential candidates for thrombolytic therapy. Prompt restoration of flow within 3–4 hours can restore brain viability and neurologic function. Important exclusion criteria for thrombolysis include:

a. Possible haemorrhage on CT scan
b. Systolic BP > 185 mm Hg
c. Head trauma in previous 3 months
d. Gastrointestinal or genitourinary bleed in past 3 weeks
e. Isolated, mild neurological deficits
f. Rapidly improving deficit

2. **E - Best medical management**

Evidence has failed to demonstrate benefit of carotid endarterectomy for patients with < 50 % stenosis. Long-term medical management is thus preferred in this patient. Antiplatelet agents like aspirin, ticlopidine and clopidogrel are widely used. Anticoagulants like warfarin are used in presence of embolisation from cardiac source.

3. **C - Angioplasty with stenting**

Restenosis > 50% may occur in 1–3% of patients following carotid endarterectomy. Re-operation in these patients is associated with a higher risk of neurological events and cranial nerve palsy. Endovascular carotid angioplasty and stenting (CAS) is an effective, minimally invasive treatment, which is not associated with cranial nerve damage.

Protected CAS is used frequently in:

a. High-risk patients
b. High lesions
c. Re-stenosis
d. Post-radiation lesions

With increasing evidence, this technique is also being used in symptomatic or asymptomatic stenosis in low-risk patients.

## 29. THEME: SWELLINGS IN VASCULAR SURGERY

OPTIONS

A. Aneurysm
B. Pseudoaneurysm
C. Haematoma
D. Abscess
E. Carotid body tumour
F. Enlarged lymph node mass
G. Lymphocele

*For each of the following patients, select the most likely cause of swelling from the list provided above. Each option can be used once, more than once or not at all.*

1. A 63-year-old male noticed a swelling in his right groin 15 days ago. He had undergone aorto-bifemoral bypass for ischaemic limb ulceration two years ago. There is no history of fever. On examination, there is a 4 x 3 cm sized cystic, pulsatile swelling in right groin crease at the site of previous surgical scar.

2. An 80-year-old female presents with a 10-year history of gradually increasing swelling on the right side of neck, without any other symptoms. There is no history of trauma or previous intervention. A cystic, pulsatile swelling is palpable along the anterior border of sternocleidomastoid muscle.

3. A 75-year-old male complained of discomfort caused by a swelling near the angle of his jaw. It had been present for many years without any discomfort. On examination, a 6 x 5 cm sized, firm, non-tender, pulsatile mass is palpable below the angle of mandible. It is laterally mobile but fixed vertically. Oral examination appears normal.

## 29. ANSWERS

1. **B - Pseudoaneurysm**

Any pulsatile swelling at the site of vascular anastomosis should lead to the suspicion of an anastomotic pseudoaneurysm. This can often be a consequence of a low-grade infection with *S. epidermidis*. It should never be incised suspecting an abscess, without a duplex examination.

2. **A - Aneurysm**

Important clues include (a) Elderly age, (b) Long duration, (c) Asymptomatic, (d) No prior intervention, (d) Cystic and pulsatile.
Further investigations will confirm the aneurysm.

3. **E - Carotid body tumour**

Important clues include (a) Elderly age, (b) Long duration, (c) Asymptomatic, (d) Firm consistency, (e) Lateral mobility with vertical fixity as the mass is attached to the carotid bifurcation.

Malignant deposits in lymph nodes may often demonstrate transmitted pulsation and firm to hard consistency. But they may be laterally as well as vertically mobile if not fixed. In advanced cases, they will be immobile in all directions.

## 30. THEME: RENAL AND MESENTERIC VASCULAR DISEASE

OPTIONS

A. Conservative
B. Angioplasty with stenting
C. Bypass
D. Embolectomy
E. Endarterectomy

*For each of the following patients, select the most likely treatment from the list of options given above.*

1. A 61-year-old male underwent coronary angioplasty for angina pectoris. He has a 6-year history of poorly controlled hypertension despite being on a combination of three antihypertensive medications. His renal angiography shows a 70% ostial stenosis of right renal artery, while left is relatively spared of disease. The infrarenal aorta shows mild atherosclerotic plaques.

2. A 34-year-old female was admitted three days ago in the cardiac ICU for management of cardiac failure and atrial fibrillation due to rheumatic mitral stenosis. She complains of sudden onset of peri-umbilical pain with abdominal distension since today morning. On per abdomen examination, minimal tenderness in umbilical region is detected. There is no guarding or rigidity.

3. A 65-year-old female underwent emergency laparotomy for a two-day history of increasing abdominal pain and marked abdominal tenderness. At laparotomy, the jejunum and ileum appear dusky and dull, with feeble peristalsis. The superior mesenteric pulse in mesentery base is absent.

## 30. ANSWERS

1. **B - Angioplasty with stenting**

Atherosclerotic renal artery stenosis can present as uncontrolled hypertension or progressive renal failure. Often, it may be asymptomatic. Percutaneous angioplasty is a minimally invasive procedure with good patency rates and has reduced the need for surgical renal revascularization.

2. **D - Embolectomy**

Important clues to mesenteric artery embolic occlusion include: (a) History of rheumatic heart disease, (b) Atrial fibrillation, (c) Sudden onset of abdominal pain, (d) Symptoms out of proportion to signs. She needs an urgent laparotomy to avoid bowel infarction. An embolus usually lodges beyond the first few branches of superior mesenteric artery (SMA). Hence on laparotomy, the jejunum is frequently spared. Revascularization should precede bowel resection. SMA embolectomy can be performed through the base of the small bowel mesentery.

3. **C - Bypass**

Important clues to mesenteric artery thrombotic occlusion include (a) Elderly age, (b) Rapid aggravation of bowel ischaemia, (c) Absent SMA pulse.

Nearly 50% of patients may have a past history of chronic post-prandial abdominal pain. In SMA thrombosis, the bowel is usually ischaemic throughout its length, with sparing of only stomach, duodenum and distal colon. Simple embolectomy may not be sufficient enough to achieve good flow. Hence a SMA bypass with inflow from iliac artery or infra-renal aorta, using a venous conduit may be required.

## 31. THEME: ACUTE LIMB SWELLING

OPTIONS

A. Haematoma
B. Cellulitis
C. Deep venous thrombosis
D. Lymphoedema
E. Ruptured Baker's cyst
F. Gastrocnemius muscle rupture

*For each of the following patients, select the most likely cause of lower limb swelling from the list of options provided above. Each option can be used once, more than once or not at all.*

1. A 60-year-old male presents with sudden swelling and pain in right leg and foot since three days. He also developed high-grade fever yesterday. There is no history of trauma. He denies any previous history of similar swelling. On examination, there is pitting oedema of leg and foot with warm, erythematous skin. His random blood sugar is 390 mg%.

2. A 62-year-old female is on regular medical treatment for osteoarthritis of knees. She noticed a small swelling behind her left knee a month ago, which gradually increased in size. Since yesterday, she has developed severe pain and swelling of her left calf. On examination, there is tenderness in her calf. The pedal pulses are palpable.

3. A 30-year-old female underwent an emergency Caesarian section for her first delivery five days ago. She complains of swelling and heaviness in her left thigh and leg since yesterday. Her left calf circumference is 4 cm greater than her right.

## 31. ANSWERS

1. **B - Cellulitis**

Important clues include (a) Suspected diabetes mellitus, (b) Oedema, (c) Signs of hyperaemia. Inflammation of skin may follow minor trauma or occur spontaneously. This condition is especially common in patients with diabetes or cirrhosis. The common causative organisms are streptococci and *Staphylococcus aureus*.

2. **E - Ruptured Baker's cyst**

It is a degenerative herniation of synovium through the knee joint capsule and is the commonest non-vascular swelling in the popliteal fossa. It is usually found in association with osteoarthritis, rheumatoid arthritis or gout. Acute rupture may occur with trivial trauma and present with severe pain and swelling in calf.

3. **C - DVT**

Important clues include (a) Postpartum condition, (b) Spontaneous onset of swelling, (c) Calf circumference > 3 cm compared with the asymptomatic side.

The factors responsible for development of DVT (Virchow's triad) is vessel wall injury, abnormalities of blood flow especially stasis and hypercoagulable state. DVT in pregnancy or postpartum period has been attributed to an acquired prothrombotic state in combination with impaired venous outflow due to uterine compression of veins. In this patient, an operative procedure is also a contributory factor.

## 32. THEME: RISK FACTORS FOR DVT

OPTIONS

A. Venous injury
B. Blood stasis
C. Primary hypercoagulable state
D. Secondary hypercoagulable state

*For each of the following conditions, select the most important pathophysiological mechanism responsible for venous thrombosis from the list of options provided above. Each option can be used once, more than once or not at all.*

1. A 62-year-old female undergoing left hip replacement with left iliofemoral deep vein thrombosis (DVT).

2. A 58-year-old male with carcinoma lung developed right femoro-popliteal DVT.

3. Right calf DVT in a 70-year-old male with cerebrovascular stroke and right hemiparesis.

4. Right subclavian vein thrombosis following central line insertion for haemodialysis.

## 32. ANSWERS

1. **A - Venous injury**

Elderly patients undergoing hip arthroplasty are particularly prone to iliac venous thrombosis due to direct venous injury. Other contributory factors include perioperative immobilization and transient hypercoagulable state due to release of tissue factor during surgery.

2. **D - Secondary hypercoagulable state**

Patients with malignancy are at a higher risk of venous thrombosis due to a secondary hypercoagulable state. Increase in plasma fibrinogen levels and thrombocytosis are the most common abnormalities.

3. **B - Blood stasis**

Immobilization or muscle paresis predisposes to stasis of blood in the soleal veins, which is associated with an increased risk of DVT.

4. **A - Venous injury**

The use of central venous cannulation has been associated with an increasing frequency of DVT. In the upper limbs, nearly 65% of thrombi are related to central venous catheters. The catheter associated vascular injury is considered an important factor in the causation of thrombosis.

There is a high incidence of DVT following surgery. The reasons are multifactorial: (a) Perioperative immobilization, (b) Venous injury especially in hip or pelvic surgeries, (c) Hypercoagulable state, probably due to release of tissue factor causing thrombin activation and increased plasminogen activator inhibitor levels.

Primary hypercoagulable states include factor V Leiden, hyperhomocysteinemia and deficiencies of antithrombin, protein C and protein S. These may be responsible for the so-called idiopathic DVT in which no apparent cause can be found.

## 33. THEME: THROMBOPROPHYLAXIS

OPTIONS

A. Warfarin
B. LMWH
C. Intermittent pneumatic leg compression (IPC)
D. Aspirin
E. None
F. LMWH with intermittent leg compression

*For each of the following patients, select the most likely method for prevention of venous thromboembolism from the list of options provided above. Each option can be used once, more than once or not at all.*

1. A 60-year-old male with suspected periampullary malignancy, to undergo a Whipple's procedure tomorrow.
2. A 26-year-old male planned for inguinal hernia repair.
3. A 34-year-old female with cervical cord tumor planned for tumour excision tomorrow.
4. A 56-year-old male undergoing TURP.
5. Laparoscopic cholecystectomy in a 39-year-old female with chronic cholecystitis.

## 33. ANSWERS

1. **F - LMWH with IPC**

This patient is at a high-risk for venous thromboembolism, with multiple risk factors including age, malignancy and major surgery. Pharmacological methods (LMWH or low dose heparin) are recommended in combination with the use of mechanical devices (IPC or graduated compression stockings) in the perioperative period.

2. **E - None**

In low-risk general surgery patients who are undergoing a minor procedure, are < 40 years of age and have no additional risk factors, no specific thromboprophylaxis methods are recommended other than early mobilization.

3. **C - IPC**

In patients who are at a high risk of bleeding or high complication rates following bleeding should receive mechanical thromboprophylaxis methods like graduated compression stockings (GCS) or intermittent pneumatic compression (IPC). Patients undergoing spinal cord or intracranial surgeries are at a high risk of venous thromboembolism, although bleeding in these locations can have disastrous consequences. Hence mechanical methods are considered safer and equally effective.

4. **E - None**

For patients undergoing transurethral or other low-risk urological procedures, only early and persistent mobilization has been recommended.

5. **E - None**

Reduced venous return due to pneumoperitoneum predisposes to venous stasis. But laparoscopic cholecystectomy is being performed rapidly and also associated with a short hospital stay. Hence early mobilization can be possible. Routine thromboprophylaxis is not necessary. But in patients with additional risk factors, LMWH or IPC or GCS is recommended.

## 34. THEME: THROMBOEMBOLISM DIAGNOSIS

OPTIONS

A. Fat embolism
B. Venous thromboembolism
C. Tumour emboli
D. Paradoxical embolism
E. Amniotic fluid embolism

*For each of the following patients, identify the most likely diagnosis from the list of options given above. Each option can be used once, more than once or not at all.*

1. A 28-year-old male met with a vehicular accident yesterday with resultant fracture of right femur shaft and undisplaced pelvic fracture. The next evening you have been called to see this patient who is restless and tachypnoeic for the past two hours. He is conscious but disoriented. His respiratory rate is 34 per minute and his $SaO_2$ is 96% on nasal oxygen. There are no audible crepts on respiratory examination. His X-ray chest appears grossly normal.

2. A 63-year-old obese lady underwent left hip replacement 7 days ago. Prophylactic LMWH was started the 2nd postoperative day because of concern of perioperative bleeding. Since today evening, she complains of uneasiness and discomfort while breathing. Her vitals are maintained and her $SaO_2$ is 98% on room air. Her left thigh appears swollen compared to the right.

## 34. ANSWERS

### 1. A - Fat embolism

Important clues include (a) Long bone and pelvic trauma, (b) Symptoms occurring the next day after trauma, (c) Respiratory and cerebral symptoms.

This may follow major trauma or prosthetic joint implantation, typically 1–5 days later. Respiratory distress (dyspnoea, tachypnoea, and hypoxaemia), cerebral features (restlessness, confusion, and coma) and petechial rash comprise the classic triad. Chest radiography may be normal initially although bilateral fluffy shadows may appear.

### 2. B - VTE

Important clues include (a) Age, (b) Obesity, (c) Hip surgery, (d) Inadequate thromboprophylaxis, (e) Thigh swelling, (f) Mild respiratory symptoms. It should be remembered that VTE could occur despite thromboprophylaxis.

## 35. THEME: THROMBOEMBOLISM – TREATMENT

OPTIONS

A. Thrombolysis
B. Thrombectomy
C. Anticoagulation
D. Intermittent pneumatic compression
E. Caval interruption procedures

*For each of the following patients, select the most likely single treatment from the options listed above. Each option can be used once, more than once or not at all.*

1. A 56-year-old male underwent emergent laparotomy with suturing of duodenal perforation a week ago. The nurse noticed swelling of his left calf since yesterday. A colour-flow duplex confirmed thrombosis extending from popliteal to superficial femoral vein. The common femoral vein is patent and compressible.

2. A 62-year-old male presented to the emergency a week ago with massive haematemesis. Endoscopic control of bleeding from an active peptic ulcer was successful. He was then nursed in a high-dependency unit. He developed sudden swelling and pain of the left lower limb since yesterday. His pain has worsened today. The calf appears tense and there is mild bluish discolouration of the foot. His colour-flow duplex shows iliofemoral venous thrombosis without extension into the inferior vena cava.

3. A 28-year-old male presents with a 4-day history of swelling of right lower limb. He also has mild discomfort and difficulty while walking. His pedal pulses are palpable. His colour-flow duplex shows thrombus in femoral and external iliac veins. There is no history of trauma or immobilization.

4. A 60-year-old female operated 15 days ago for malignancy of caecum was detected to have right iliofemoral DVT a week ago. She was treated with continuous intravenous heparin with oral warfarin for 5 days and discharged subsequently on 5 mg of warfarin, with a recent INR of 2.2. She is brought to the emergency department today complaining of severe breathlessness. A V/Q scan shows high probability of pulmonary embolism.

## 35. ANSWERS

1. **C - Anticoagulation**

The DVT in this high-risk patient can be successfully managed by anticoagulation. Intravenous heparin with APTT monitoring or subcutaneous unmonitored LMWH have been compared and found to be equally efficacious. The advantages of LMWH include twice-daily doses, home based administration, higher bioavailability, predictable response and lower risk of bleed when compared to unfractionated heparin.

2. **B - Thrombectomy**

This gentleman has developed phlegmasia cerulea dolens following extensive iliofemoral DVT. It is important to intervene and prevent compartment syndrome or venous gangrene. The recent history of upper gastrointestinal bleeding is a contraindication for thrombolytic therapy. Hence, thrombectomy will be necessary to clear the extensive clots.

3. **C - Anticoagulation**

Idiopathic DVT, especially in younger healthy adults may have a thrombophilic aetiology. This patient can be managed successfully by anticoagulation. He should also be evaluated to find a cause for his hypercoagulable state.

The duration of anticoagulation in a patient with a first episode of idiopathic DVT should be 6–12 months.

4. **E - Caval interruption procedures**

This patient has developed PE despite being on adequate anticoagulation. Most would advocate placement of an inferior vena cava (IVC) filter for this indication. Other indications for IVC filter placement include:

a. DVT/PE with contraindication to anticoagulation.
b. Bleeding complications with force discontinuation of therapy.
c. After pulmonary embolectomy.
d. Extensive free-floating iliofemoral thrombus.
e. Prophylactic use is emerging as a relative indication in patients with polytrauma or major hip surgery who remain at high risk of thromboembolism but do not actually have the disease.

## 36. THEME: CHRONIC UNILATERAL LEG SWELLING

OPTIONS

A. Primary lymphoedema
B. Secondary lymphoedema
C. DVT
D. Primary varicose veins
E. Post-thrombotic syndrome
F. Klippel-Trenaunay syndrome
G. Parkes-Weber syndrome

*For each of the following patients, select the most likely aetiology for chronic limb swelling from the options provided above. Each option can be used once, more than once or not at all.*

1. A 38-year-old female presents with an 8-month history of aching discomfort in her right leg, especially towards the end of the day. She also noticed swelling of the right foot at night, which disappears in the morning. Her previous medical history is positive for swelling of right lower limb during her last pregnancy 6 years ago for which no specific treatment was taken. Her right ankle shows pitting odema with few pigmented spots.

2. A 20-year-old female presents with a 5-year history of painless swelling of left leg and foot. She had no problems earlier, but now has noticed a warty texture of her foot skin, which causes pain on wearing shoes. There is uniform, non-pitting oedema of the leg and foot, with thick, hyperkeratotic skin of toes.

3. An 18-year-old female presents with disfigurement of her left lower limb since childhood. There is a limp while walking, but no pain in the affected limb. On examination, the left lower limb is longer and greater in circumference than the right. Multiple tortuous veins are seen along the lateral thigh and leg, with a purplish-pigmented patch over the thigh. There is no bruit or thrill over the dilated veins. Pedal pulses are palpable.

## 36. ANSWERS

1. **E - Post-thrombotic syndrome**
Important clues include (a) Past history of lower limb swelling, (b) Symptoms of chronic venous incompetence, (c) Hyperpigmentation at ankle. The other typical features of post-thrombotic syndrome include ulceration over medial malleolus, with thick, hyperpigmented skin (lipodermatosclerosis). It should be remembered that similar symptoms and signs might also be present with superficial venous incompetence. Hence, the term post-thrombotic syndrome may be replaced by chronic venous insufficiency.

2. **A - Primary lymphoedema**
It is classified as congenital (age < 1 year), praecox (age < 35 years) and tarda (age > 35 years). Secondary lymphoedema may follow malignant disease, previous surgery, irradiation or infection (commonly filariasis).

The important clues in this case include (a) Long duration of swelling, (b) Spontaneous onset, (c) Skin changes (d) Non-pitting oedema.

The oedema may be pitting initially, but with time it becomes non-pitting due to fat and increasing subcutaneous fibrosis. The skin gradually thickens and becomes less elastic. It may not be possible to pinch up a fold of skin of foot. Hyperkeratosis and warty projections or verrucae give rise to the pigskin appearance. Lymphoedema of foot causes a 'buffalo-hump'. Although skin ulcers are uncommon, this condition is highly sensitive to fungal infections.

3. **F - Klippel-Trenaunay syndrome**
This is a congenital venous malformation of the lower limb, where the embryonic lateral venous complex of leg persists and connects with the profunda vein in the thigh or the internal iliac vein in pelvis.

The deep venous system of leg is often hypoplastic so that the malformation acts as the primary venous outflow from the leg.

Important clues include (a) History since childhood, (b) Limb lengthening, (c) Atypical lateral varicosities, (d) Port wine stain, (e) Absence of thrill or bruit.

Bruit and thrill may be present in congenital arteriovenous malformation (Parkes-Weber syndrome). In this instance, the varices may be pulsatile and the distal arterial pulses diminished.

## 37. THEME: VARICOSE VEINS – AETIOLOGY

OPTIONS

A. Idiopathic
B. Post-thrombotic
C. Arteriovenous fistula
D. Arteriovenous malformation
E. Venous malformation

*For each of the following patients, identify the most likely aetiology of varicose veins from the options given above. Each option can be used once, more than once or not at all.*

1. A 28-year-old male presents with a 6-month history of prominent, tortuous veins over left leg with a non-healing ulcer at the ankle. On examination there is a scar over the left groin with a palpable thrill. He had a penetrating gunshot injury 7 years ago for which debridement had been done elsewhere.

2. A 32-year-old female presents with aching discomfort in her legs, which started and increased during her first pregnancy, 4 years ago. On examination, there are bilateral multiple, tortuous veins in the anterior and medial aspect of leg as well as thigh. There is no pigmentation or ulceration at ankle. Pedal pulses are palpable.

3. A 38-year-old female presents with swelling of left leg for 6 months. There are few dilated, tortuous veins in the leg with thick, hyper-pigmented skin at the ankle. Past medical history is significant for treated postpartum iliofemoral DVT 6 years ago.

## 37. ANSWERS

1. **C - Arteriovenous fistula**

The probable cause is an arteriovenous fistula of the femoral vessels secondary to gunshot injury. The importance of recognizing this rare condition is that primary treatment should be aimed at the arteriovenous fistula and not the varicose veins. Following surgical repair of the arteriovenous fistula, compression stockings can be prescribed to reduce the venotensive changes.

2. **A - Idiopathic**

This is the commonest cause of varicose veins. Probable contributory factors include (a) Female sex, (b) Familial history, (c) Obesity, (d) Prolonged standing. These primary varicose veins are due to valvular failure, either primary degenerative change in the valve leaflets or secondary to developmental weakness of vein wall.

3. **B - Post-thrombotic syndrome**

There is a high prevalence of post-thrombotic syndrome in patients with iliofemoral DVT. Severe manifestations of chronic venous insufficiency may be due to valvular reflux or persistent venous obstruction or a combination of both. Apart from few varicose veins, the other features of CVI include lipodermatosclerosis, ulceration, oedema, varicose eczema and atrophie blanche.

## 38. THEME: VARICOSE VEINS – INVESTIGATIONS

OPTIONS

A. Hand held Doppler
B. Duplex
C. Ascending venography
D. Descending venography

*For each of the following patients, select the most likely single diagnostic test from the list of options provided above. Each option can be used once, more than once or not at all*

1. A 30-year-old female with varicose veins over medial aspect of leg and thigh. Her mother and sister have also been operated earlier for similar complaints.

2. A 39-year-old male who underwent saphenofemoral ligation with stripping and multiple avulsions 6 years ago presents with recurrent varicosities in leg.

3. A 26-year-old female with varicose veins over posterior aspect of calf and popliteal fossa.

## 38. ANSWERS

1. **A - Hand held Doppler**

Although few institutes use preoperative duplex in all patients with primary varicose veins, most consider a hand held Doppler to be a sufficient diagnostic technique for primary uncomplicated long saphenous vein incompetence. Saphenofemoral incompetence can be diagnosed with > 95% accuracy in such cases.

2. **B - Duplex**

Duplex scanning is useful in assessment of recurrent varicose veins. The causes of recurrence include (a) Type I recurrence – intact saphenofemoral junction, (b) Type II recurrence – obliterated saphenofemoral junction, in which the source of reflux can be thigh perforators or neovascularisation.

The majority of recurrent varicose veins are due to a failure to carry out flush saphenofemoral ligation and/or removal of long saphenous vein as a source of perforator incompetence at the first operation.

Varicography (contrast injected directly into a varix) may often be necessary to delineate the anatomy of recurrent varicose veins.

3. **B - Duplex**

In contrast to the saphenofemoral junction, the saphenopopliteal junction has a highly variable level of termination. In nearly 50% of cases, the termination of short saphenous vein is within 5 cm of the knee joint crease. But it may terminate higher in a femoropopliteal vein or the vein of Giacomini. Hence, preoperative localization and marking of saphenopopliteal junction should be performed by a duplex examination.

## 39. THEME: TREATMENT OF VENOUS DISEASE

OPTIONS

A. Bypass
B. Ligation with stripping
C. Subfascial Endoscopic Perforator Surgery (SEPS)
D. Sclerotherapy
E. Compression therapy
F. Linton's operation

*For each of the following patients select the most likely single treatment from the list of options provided above. Each option can be used once, more than once or not at all*

1. A 39-year-old male underwent left saphenofemoral ligation with stripping with multiple avulsions. He noticed two unsightly dilated veins in the left leg. On duplex examination, there is no evidence of intact saphenofemoral junction or long saphenous vein in thigh. The saphenopopliteal junction is competent.

2. A 52-year-old male presents with a 3-week history of spontaneous ulceration over medial aspect of left ankle. On examination, there is oedema with hyperpigmentation surrounding the ulceration. Pedal pulses are palpable. Duplex scan shows popliteal venous reflux with incompetent Cockett perforators.

3. A 33-year-old female presents with prominent and tortuous veins over right leg since two years. Her color-flow duplex shows saphenofemoral junction incompetence without perforator or deep venous incompetence.

## 39. ANSWERS

1. **D - Sclerotherapy**
This patient most likely has persistent and not recurrent varicose veins. Such varices can be successfully treated with injection sclerotherapy.

2. **C - SEPS**
Deep venous incompetence with perforator incompetence is responsible for CVI, a significant cause of morbidity. Compression therapy has been the mainstay of treatment of CVI. Perforator incompetence had been classically treated by the Linton subfascial perforator ligation, which has been abandoned because of its associated wound complications. Currently, SEPS is the treatment of choice for this purpose.

3. **B - Ligation with stripping**
Primary saphenofemoral incompetence with long saphenous varicose veins is best managed by saphenofemoral ligation and stripping of long saphenous vein till knee level. Varices in leg can be avulsed out through small stab incisions. The recent advances in varicose vein management include endovenous radiofrequency or endovenous LASER obliteration of long saphenous vein.

## 40. THEME: LEG ULCERS

OPTIONS

A. Neuropathic
B. Ischaemic
C. Venous
D. Marjolin's ulcer
E. Meleney's ulcer
F. Pyoderma gangrenosum

*For each of the following patients, select the most likely aetiology of leg ulceration. Each option can be used once, more than once or not at all.*

1. A 68-year-old male, on treatment for diabetes mellitus, presents with a spontaneous painless ulcer over the plantar aspect of foot. On examination, it is a 2 x 1 cm sized punched out ulcer. The foot is warm and pedal pulses are palpable. His sensation over the sole is reduced.

2. A 60-year-old male presented with recurrent ulceration above the medial malleolus, in association with hyperpigmentation and oedema. He has recently noticed that the ulcer bleeds readily on change of dressings. On examination, there is a 3 x 2 cm sized ulcer over the gaiter area with everted edges and indurated base.

3. A 39-year-old male presents with a two-year history of prominent tortuous veins in his left leg, for which no specific treatment was taken. Since the past month, he has developed an ulcer above the medial malleolus with surrounding pigmentation.

## 40. ANSWERS

1. **A - Neuropathic**

Diabetic foot disease can be the result of neuropathy, macroangiopathy, microangiopathy, infection or a combination of these processes.

Important clues include (a) Painless, (b) Pressure point ulcer, (c) Palpable pulses, (d) Reduced sensation. Arterial ulcers are usually painful and occur over the toes.

2. **D - Marjolin's ulcer**

Venous ulcers following chronic venous insufficiency occur typically around the medial malleolus (gaiter area). Long-standing ulcers can undergo malignant transformation to squamous cell carcinoma (Marjolin's ulcer). Important clues include (a) Long history, (b) Recent onset of bleeding, (c) Everted edges.

3. **C - Venous ulcer**

Venous ulcers account for nearly 80% of leg ulceration. They are usually painless and shallow. They can be a result of chronic venous insufficiency, due to reflux or obstruction of superficial and/or deep venous systems. The theories proposed to be responsible for venous ulceration are (a) Fibrin cuff theory, (b) White cell trapping theory.

## 41. THEME: ACUTE NEONATAL CONDITIONS

OPTIONS

A. Exomphalos major
B. Exomphalos minor
C. Ectopia vesicae
D. Necrotising enterocolitis
E. Mid gut volvulus
F. Gastroschisis
G. Hirschsprung's disease
H. Oesophageal atresia

*For each of the patients described below, select the most likely diagnosis from the list of options above. Each option may be used once, more than once, or not at all.*

1. A male infant born at term is found to have a massive sac protruding through a large abdominal defect. The sac contains liver, spleen and intestines.

2. A preterm baby in the special care baby unit presents with bloody diarrhoea, and a distended abdomen. Plain abdominal X-ray shows generalized bowel dilatation with multiple fluid levels.

3. A 6-hour-old female infant is found to regurgitate all of its feeds. She is pouring saliva continuously from the mouth.

4. An absolutely normal male infant presents at 6 weeks with bilious vomiting and abdominal distention.

5. A term male infant is found to have an incomplete development of the infra-umbilical part of the anterior abdominal wall with exposed bladder and epispadiac penis.

## 41. ANSWERS

1. **A - Exomphalos major.** Presence of a large defect with sac is exomphalos major. Exomphalos minor is arbitrarily defined as a defect less than 4 cm in diameter. Gastroschisis is protrusion of the intestines through the abdominal wall, usually to the right of the umbilicus and classically without a covering membrane.

Clues include the presence of a large sac and the presence of liver and spleen.

2. **D - Necrotising enterocolitis.** This often fatal disorder occurs in newborn babies, who are almost invariably the premature or seriously ill in special care baby units. Pathophysiology probably involves ischaemia of the large bowel wall, which then becomes invaded by gas-producing bacteria.

Initially, there is adynamic bowel obstruction. This later progresses to large bowel necrosis, perforation and generalized peritonitis.

Plain abdominal X-ray initially shows generalized bowel dilatation with multiple fluid levels. Later, when bowel necrosis sets in, gas shadows may be seen in the bowel wall.

Clues include preterm baby in a special care baby unit, bloody diarrhoea.

3. **H - Oesophageal atresia.** Always suspect atresia in early feeding problems.

Clues may include regurgitation of all feeds, frothy mouth (continuously pouring saliva from mouth), attacks of cyanosis and coughing on feeding and polyhydramnios during pregnancy.

4. **E - Midgut volvulus.** Acute onset of these features in a previously well infant should arouse clinical suspicion to the possibility of a midgut volvulus.

5. **C - Ectopia vesicae.** Clues may include the incomplete development of infraumbilical abdominal wall, the exposed bladder, absent umbilicus, presence of epispadias in a broad and short penis. Bilateral inguinal herniae may be present; the prostate and seminal vesicles are rudimentary. In the female infant, the clitoris is bifid and labia minora are separated anteriorly. The pubic bones may be widely separated with resulting posterior rotation of the hip joints.

## 42. THEME : ACUTE NEONATAL CONDITIONS

OPTIONS

A. Exomphalos major
B. Gastroschisis
C. Tracheo-oesophageal fistula
D. Imperforate anus
E. Exomphalos minor
F. Duodenal atresia
G. Hirschsprung's disease
H. Volvulus neonatorum

*For each of the patients described below, select the most likely diagnosis from the list of options above. Each option may be used once, more than once, or not at all.*

1. A term neonate is born with bare bowels protruding through an abdominal wall defect.

2. A month old baby is brought with chest infection. Mother complains of respiratory distress encountered during feeding her baby.

3. A term male baby infant presents with bilious vomiting and abdominal distention. There has been no passage of meconium.

4. A term neonate is born with a 3 cm defect in the abdominal wall with herniation of a sac covered umbilical cord.

5. A term neonate presents with bilious vomiting immediately after birth. Nursing staff inform you that the baby has passed meconium. On examination the abdomen is scaphoid.

## 42. ANSWERS

1. **B - Gastroschisis**

Bare bowels (absence of a covering membrane) are suggestive.

2. **C - Tracheo-oesophageal fistula**

Congenital atresia of the oesophagus is usually associated with the above fistula. In 85% of cases, it is the lower segment that communicates with the trachea. Attacks of coughing and cyanosis occur on feeding. Aspiration pneumonia is a common complication.

3. **G - Hirschsprung's disease**

Delayed passage of meconium along with features of abdominal obstruction should alert one to the possibility of this disease. Some patients present in later life with chronic constipation.

4. **E - Exomphalos minor**

5. **F - Duodenal atresia**

The obstruction of duodenal atresia is usually below the entry of the CBD, resulting in bilious vomiting. Important feature here is the passage of meconium, which helps differentiate this condition from Hirschsprung's disease.

Clues may include an X-ray picture of 'double bubble' appearance and the presence of scaphoid abdomen. 20% of infants with duodenal atresia have Down's syndrome. Duodenal atresia is associated with a number of common anomalies including OA, anorectal malformations and cardiac, urinary tract and vertebral abnormalities.

## 43. THEME: NEONATAL CONDITIONS

OPTIONS

A. Diaphragmatic hernia
B. Meconium ileus
C. Hirschsprung's disease
D. Intussusception
E. Congenital cystic disease of the lung
F. Exomphalos major
G. Exomphalos minor
H. Umbilical hernia
I. Pneumothorax
J. Necrotising enterocolitis

*For each of the patients described below, select the most likely diagnosis from the list of options above. Each option may be used once, more than once, or not at all.*

1. A newborn baby develops respiratory distress soon after birth. Examination reveals cyanosis and a scaphoid abdomen. Air entry is decreased on the left side.

2. A premature infant presents with bloody diarrhoea and features of intestinal obstruction. He also manifests features of septic shock.

3. A newborn baby diagnosed with cystic fibrosis presents with abdominal distention and bilious vomiting. Examination may reveal thickened loops of hypertrophied bowel. X-ray shows distended coils of bowel with a few fluid levels.

4. A newborn baby presents with abdominal distention, bilious vomiting and a failure to pass meconium. Rectal examination allows an explosive release of air and meconium.

5. Parents are concerned that their baby boy develops a swelling in the region of the belly button while crying.

## 43. ANSWERS

1. **A - Diaphragmatic hernia**

80% of diaphragmatic hernias occur on the left side. Diagnosis is now frequently made before birth on antenatal ultrasound screening. Cyanosis, mediastinal shift and an empty (scaphoid) abdomen are important clues. Diagnosis is easily confirmed on chest X-ray.

2. **J - Necrotising enterocolitis**

3. **B - Meconium ileus**

Meconium ileus is an obstruction of the distal ileum by thick, viscid meconium. It occurs in 5–10% of newborn infants with cystic fibrosis. Clues may include the association of cystic fibrosis and a mottled ground glass appearance on X-ray.

4. **C - Hirschsprung's disease**

This is a congenital abnormality of part of the bowel which affects all of the intramural autonomic nerves. Ganglion cells (neurons) are absent from the inter-myenteric and submucosal plexuses. Diagnosis is made from the observation on contrast enema of a 'conical appearance' and is confirmed with mucosal suction biopsies.

5. **H - Umbilical hernia**

This is a common finding in neonates especially premature. The hernia protrudes through a defect in the fascia at the umbilical ring but may only be apparent when the baby cries. Over 90% close spontaneously in the 1st 3 years of life. Hence, only observation is needed. Persistence beyond 3 years necessitates surgical closure.

## 44. THEME: PAEDIATRIC GASTROINTESTINAL DISORDERS

OPTIONS

A. Intussusception
B. Hypertrophic pyloric stenosis
C. Meckel's diverticulum
D. Appendicitis
E. Congenital hernia
F. Mesenteric adenitis
G. Acute gastroenteritis
H. Intestinal obstruction

*For each of the patients described below, select the most likely diagnosis from the list of options above. Each option may be used once, more than once, or not at all.*

1. A 9-year-old boy presents with short attacks of central abdominal pain associated with circumoral pallor. He had been treated by his GP for a viral illness a fortnight ago. On examination, the child is pyrexial at 38.7°C. He has diffuse abdominal tenderness though most of it is found in the right iliac fossa.

2. A 6-year-old boy is sent to hospital having developed abdominal pain, bilious vomiting and bleeding per rectum.

3. A 9-year-old boy presents with central abdominal pain radiating to the right iliac fossa. He has low grade pyrexia with the presence of guarding and tenderness in the right iliac fossa.

4. A 6-month-old boy develops sudden onset of screaming associated with drawing up of the legs in cycles. His parents have noticed that he has been passing stools mixed with blood and mucus.

5. A 12-year-old boy is referred with acute abdominal pain associated with diarrhoea and vomiting. On examination, the child is dehydrated with the presence of generalized abdominal tenderness.

## 44. ANSWERS

### 1. F - Mesenteric adenitis

This classically affects school children. Association of attacks of central abdominal pain associated with circumoral pallor is characteristic. Clues may include the presence of prodromal viral illness in 25% of children, presence of extremely high temperature in a few and the presence of abdominal tenderness along the line of the mesentery. When present, shifting tenderness is a valuable sign for differentiating this condition from appendicitis. After laying the patient on the left side for a few minutes, the maximum tenderness moves to the left of the original site. A lymphocytosis is more common than neutrophilia, which again can be an important clue.

### 2. C - Meckel's diverticulum

In 20% of cases the mucosa contains heterotopic epithelium namely gastric, colonic or sometimes pancreatic tissue. This ectopic gastric mucosa may give rise to rectal bleeding.

### 3. D - Appendicitis

Fever is low grade usually in appendicitis unless the appendix has ruptured and an abscess or more general peritonitis has developed. The history may however be vague in infants and very young children.

### 4. A - Intussusception

History again is classical of intussusception. Clues may include the passage of 'red currant jelly' stools, the presence of a sausage shaped lump which may harden with palpation and an associated feeling of emptiness in the right iliac fossa (sign de Dance). Per rectal examination may reveal blood stained mucus on the examining finger. A classical 'claw sign' may be seen on barium enema in an ileo-colic or colocolic intussusception.

### 5. G - Acute gastroenteritis

Acute gastroenteritis is an important differential and is often mistaken for acute appendicitis. Localized tenderness does not usually occur in acute gastroenteritis.

## 45. THEME: PAEDIATRIC CONDITIONS

OPTIONS

A. Nephroblastoma
B. Intussusception
C. Congenital hernia
D. Hypertrophic pyloric stenosis
E. Cystic hygroma
F. Hirschsprung's disease
G. Meconium ileus
H. Hypernephroma
I. Thyroglossal cyst
J. Chronic mesenteric ischaemia

*For each of the patients described below, select the most likely diagnosis from the list of options above. Each option may be used once, more than once, or not at all.*

1. A 6-week-old baby boy is brought to A&E with projectile vomiting for 2 days duration. An episode of vomiting is witnessed in A&E. The vomitus contains milk and is abilious.

2. An infant is brought with a vague lump in the neck on the right side. The lump is ill-defined, nontender, cystic, fluctuant and illuminant.

3. A 3-year-old boy is referred to your clinic with a rapidly growing large abdominal mass felt by the parents. In addition to a large non-tender abdominal lump, examination reveals pyrexia and hypertension.

4. A 4-week-old baby boy presents with gross abdominal distention, constipation since birth and failure to thrive.

5. A 14-year-old boy is referred to your clinic with chronic constipation. Barium enema reveals an area of coning.

## 45. ANSWERS

1. **D - Hypertrophic pyloric stenosis**

Presence of abilious projectile vomiting between 3–7 weeks of birth is classical. Other clues may include the presence of a lump on the right side of the abdomen. In doubtful cases, a test feed is diagnostic. Characteristic peristaltic waves can then be 'induced' and at the same time palpation may reveal a lump. Another important clue may be the presence of hypokalaemic hypochloraemic metabolic alkalosis.

2. **E - Cystic hygroma**

The history is classical of cystic hygroma. Though complete surgical excision is the optimal treatment of a cystic hygroma, this is often technically difficult. Newer modalities include injecting the lesions with OK432.

3. **A - Nephroblastoma**

Wilms tumour is the commonest solid tumour of childhood. Three quarters present before the age of 5 years. The usual presentation is that of an abdominal mass which grows rapidly while the general well being of the child deteriorates. Frank haematuria is rare though microscopic haematuria may occur in up to 40% of cases. Pyrexia is seen in half of these patients and disappears when the tumour is removed. Anorexia and vomiting are also common.

Hypernephroma is renal adenocarcinoma seen in adults.

4. **F - Hirschsprung's disease**

5. **F - Hirschsprung's disease**

Severe constipation in children and adults may occasionally be due to a short segment or Hirschsprung's disease. Faecal soiling is usually absent.

## 46. THEME: INVESTIGATIONS FOR PAEDIATRIC CONDITIONS

OPTIONS

A. Ultrasound scan
B. Rectal biopsy
C. Anorectal manometry
D. Barium enema
E.. Abdominal X-ray
F. Clinical - No radiological investigations
G. CT scan abdomen
H. Diagnostic laparoscopy

*For each of the patients described below, select the most appropriate investigation from the list of options above. Each option may be used once, more than once, or not at all.*

1. An 8-month-old boy presents with sudden onset screaming with passage of red currant jelly stools. A lump is palpable to the left of the umbilicus.

2. A newborn baby presents with abdominal distention, bilious vomiting and a failure to pass meconium. The baby has strong features to suggest Down's syndrome.

3. A 6-year-old boy presents with right iliac fossa tenderness associated with nausea and vomiting. He has typical Mcburney's point tenderness.

4. A 4-week-old baby boy is brought with a 2-day history of projectile vomiting containing milk only. He is dehydrated and emaciated.

5. A term neonate presents with bilious vomiting immediately after birth. The baby has passed meconium after birth. On examination, the abdomen is scaphoid.

## 46. ANSWERS

**1. A - Ultrasound scan**

An abdominal ultrasound scan is now the main investigative tool used to confirm the diagnosis. A 'target sign' is seen when the intussusception is scanned transversely (the rings of the target represent the various layers of the bowel wall).

**2. B - Rectal biopsy**

Though X-ray and enema are initial investigation, definitive diagnosis rests on histological proof obtained by a suction rectal biopsy. Hence the most appropriate investigation would be a rectal biopsy.

**3. F - Clinical - No radiological investigations**

The diagnosis of acute appendicitis is essentially clinical. Ultrasound examination is useful, especially in children and females, although it is not yet routine practice. When indicated, some authors consider a CT scan as the investigation of choice.

**4. A - Ultrasound scan**

Features suggest hypertrophic pyloric stenosis of infancy. Ultrasound is the investigation of choice. It detects the classical features of hypertrophy involving the pyloric canal.

**5. E - Abdominal X-ray**

This is a picture of duodenal atresia. An X-ray would show a 'double-bubble' sign.

## 47. THEME: CHOICE OF SURGERY

OPTIONS

A. Ramstedt's operation
B. Duodenoduodenostomy
C. Staged closure using a silastic silo
D. Duhamel operation
E. Appendicectomy
F. Laparoscopy
G. Laparotomy
H. No intervention

*For each of the patients described below, select the most appropriate treatment from the list of options above. Each option may be used once, more than once, or not at all.*

1. A 16-year-old girl presents with lower vague abdominal pain. She also complains of vaginal discharge. On examination, she has tenderness mainly in the right iliac fossa.

2. A 16-year-old male presents with right lower quadrant abdominal pain, which is exacerbated by coughing and sudden movement. Examination reveals guarding and rebound tenderness maximal over the Mcburney's point.

3. Ultrasonography confirms the presence of pyloric muscle thickening with pyloric canal lengthening in a 4-week-old baby.

4. A neonate presenting with an acute abdomen is seen to have a 'double bubble' shadow on the abdominal X-ray.

5. An antenatal observation of intestine and liver outside the foetal abdomen.

6. A 4-week baby boy presents with a swelling in the umbilical region, which increases in prominence when he cries.

## 47. ANSWERS

1. **F - Laparoscopy**

This is invaluable in teenaged girls and women of childbearing age where there are a number of different causes of right lower quadrant pain and tenderness.

2. **E - Appendicectomy**

3. **A - Ramstedt's operation**

History is typical of hypertrophic pyloric stenosis of infancy and Ramstedt's operation is the treatment of choice.

4. **B - Duodenoduodenostomy**

This is classically duodenal atresia. An end-to-end duodeno-duodenostomy is fashioned by an anastomosis between a transversely opened proximal duodenum and a vertically opened distal duodenum.

5. **C - Staged closure using a silastic silo**

History is typical of an exomphalos major. Staged closure using the above may be possible for a moderate sized lesion.

6. **H - No intervention**

History is typical of umbilical hernia. 90% of these close spontaneously by the age of 3 years. Hence a 'masterly inactivity' is needed at this presentation.

## 48. THEME: PAEDIATRIC INVESTIGATIONS

OPTIONS

A. 'Double-bubble' sign on abdominal X-ray
B. Target lesion on abdominal ultrasound
C. Hypokalaemic hypochloraemic metabolic alkalosis
D. Intramural gas on abdominal X-ray
E. A cone on contrast enema
F. The string sign of Cantor on imaging
G. Classical haustral markings seen on abdominal X-ray

*For each of the patients described below, select the most appropriate feature on investigation from the list of options above. Each option may be used once, more than once, or not at all.*

1. A 6-month-old infant presents with intermittent screaming, drawing up of legs and bleeding per rectum.

2. A premature 6-day-old baby presents with bilious vomiting, abdominal distention and bloody diarrhoea.

3. A 4-week-old baby boy is brought into resus with dehydration due to persisting non bilious vomiting. He is listless and emaciated. On examination a lump is palpable in the right side of the abdomen.

4. A term baby presents with persistent bilious vomiting in the first few hours after birth. Abdomen is soft to palpation and the baby has passed meconium.

5. A 6-week-old baby boy is brought with chronic constipation since birth and failure to thrive.

## 48. ANSWERS

1. **B - Target lesion on abdominal ultrasound**
This is classically a presentation of intussusception.

2. **D - Intramural gas on abdominal X-ray**
Plain abdominal X-rays initially show generalized bowel dilatation with multiple fluid levels. Later, gas shadows may be seen in the bowel wall indicating bowel wall necrosis.

3. **C - Hypokalaemic hypochloraemic metabolic alkalosis**
This is classically hypertrophic pyloric stenosis of infancy.

4. **A - 'Double-bubble' sign on abdominal X-ray**
This is typical of duodenal atresia.

5. **E - A cone on contrast enema**
This is most likely to be Hirschsprung's disease. A cone on contrast enema examination is the best available option.

## 49. THEME: PAEDIATRIC TUMOURS

OPTIONS

A. Nephroblastoma
B. Neuroblastoma
C. Hepatocellular carcinoma
D. Hepatoblastoma
E. Rhabdomyosarcoma
F. Ewing's sarcoma
G. Osteosarcoma
H. Nasopharyngeal carcinoma
I. Sacrococcygeal teratoma
J. Osteoid osteoma
K. Familial adenomatous polyposis (FAP)
L. Osteomyelitis

*For each of the patients described below, select the most appropriate diagnosis from the list of options above. Each option may be used once, more than once, or not at all.*

1. A 2-year-old baby boy is referred to your fast track clinic by the GP for failure to thrive.

   Examination reveals a palpable lump in the right upper quadrant. The kid's father is known to have familial adenomatous polyposis.

2. A 10-year-old girl presents with fever, pain and swelling affecting her left thigh. Examination reveals a tender irregular swelling affecting the mid femur. X-ray shows a typical onion skin periosteal pattern.

3. A 2-month baby girl presents with a solitary mass over the right buttock.

4. A 12-year-old is referred by his GP with pain affecting the right tibia, which has been severe for the last 2 months. On examination, he has an antalgic gait and there is asymmetrical swelling affecting the proximal tibia. X-ray reveals periosteal lifting (Codman's triangle) and 'sun-ray' spicules of new bone within the tumour.

5. A 2-year-old baby boy is brought in with a history of failure to thrive. Examination reveals a large abdominal mass. The child appears flushed, irritable and is found to be hypertensive.

## 49. ANSWERS

1. **D - Hepatoblastoma**

This is the most common malignant liver tumour in early childhood. FAP is associated and so is Beckwith-Weidman syndrome. (This is an important exam question.)

2. **F - Ewing's sarcoma**

This tumour is commonest in childhood. It arises in the midshaft or metaphysis of long bones. Presence of fever complicates the picture. 'Onion skin' arrangement is typical and so is the presence in biopsy of 'small round cells'.

3. **I - Sacrococcygeal teratoma**

Although rare, sacrococcygeal teratoma is amongst the most common of the large tumours seen during the first 3 months of life.

4. **G - Osteosarcoma**

Though primary malignant bone tumours are a rare group in themselves, osteosarcoma is the commonest tumour in this group. In the elderly it occurs secondary to Paget's disease (an important question for the exam). Typical features are as described. It affects the metaphyses of long bones and hence usually affects the tibia or the femur around the knee joint.

5. **B - Neuroblastoma**

Approximately 70% have metastases at the time of diagnosis. Bones are involved more commonly than liver. Excessive catecholamine production may cause hypertension, flushing, sweating and general irritability. Watery diarrhoea and hypokalaemia is seen occasionally. Acute cerebellar ataxia characterized by opsomyoclonus and chaotic nystagmus or the 'dancing eye' syndrome is an unusual manifestation of neuroblastoma of unknown cause. (This is a favorite question with the examiners.)

## 50. THEME: ABDOMINAL DISEASES OF CHILDHOOD

OPTIONS

A. Wilson's disease
B. Psoas haematoma
C. Thalassaemia
D. Reye's syndrome
E. Lactose intolerance
F. Gilbert's syndrome
G. Alpha-1-antitrypsin deficiency
H. Hepatitis A

*For each of the patients described below, select the most appropriate diagnosis from the list of options above. Each option may be used once, more than once, or not at all.*

1. Liver disease is the most common symptom in children; neurological disease is most common in young adults. Characteristic feature is the presence of 'Kayser-Fleischer ring'.

2. A 5-year-old boy presents with nausea, vomiting, lethargy and indifference. Examination reveals a palpable liver. Mom gives a history of viral illness that had persisted the whole of the week before.

3. A 12-year-old haemophiliac presents with right lower abdominal pain and a limp. Attempts to straighten the right leg result in severe pain.

## 50. ANSWERS

1. **A - Wilson's disease**

It is also known as hepatolenticular degeneration. Wilson's disease is a rare autosomal recessive disorder of copper transport, resulting in copper accumulation and toxicity to the liver and brain.. The cornea of the eye can also be affected: the 'Kayser-Fleischer ring' is a deep copper-coloured ring at the periphery of the cornea, and is thought to represent copper deposits.

2. **D - Reye's syndrome**

The presence of a preceding viral illness treated with aspirin is an important clue.

3. **B - Psoas haematoma**

## 51. THEME: PAEDIATRIC NECK LUMPS

OPTIONS

A. Thyroid nodule
B. Thyroglossal cyst
C. Dermoid cyst
D. Cystic hygroma
E. Haemangioma
F. Laryngocele
G. Sternomastoid tumour
H. Carotid tumour

*For each scenario described below, select the most likely diagnosis from the list above. Each option may be used once, more than once, or not at all.*

1. A 4-year-old boy presents with a small cystic midline swelling in the upper neck (just beneath the hyoid bone) which rises with swallowing and protrusion of the tongue.

2. A 7-day infant presents with a large transilluminant fluctuant mass in the posterior triangle of the neck.

3. A week old infant is noted to keep her head to the left. Examination reveals a palpable firm lump in the left side of the neck.

## 51. ANSWERS

### 1. B - Thyroglossal cyst

A thyroglossal cyst may be present in any part of the thyroglossal tract. Common situations include beneath the hyoid (most frequent), in the region of the thyroid cartilage and above the hyoid bone. These swellings move upwards with swallowing and tongue protrusion due to attachment to the foramen caecum. A thyroglossal cyst should be excised because infection is inevitable.

### 2. D - Cystic hygroma

The history is classical of cystic hygroma. Though complete surgical excision is the optimal treatment of a cystic hygroma, this is often technically difficult. Newer modalities include injecting the lesions with OK432.

### 3. G - Sternomastoid tumour

A palpable firm lump in the sternomastoid on the left with decreased head movements to the contralateral side indicates a sternomastoid tumour. They respond to stretching exercises.

## 52. THEME: SCROTAL SWELLINGS

OPTIONS

A. Primary hydrocele
B. Testicular teratoma
C. Lymph varix
D. Testicular torsion
E. Encysted hydrocele of cord
F. Inguinoscrotal hernia
G. Testicular seminoma
H. Epididymo-orchitis
I. Varicocele
J. Inguinal hernia

*For each of the patients described below, select the most likely diagnosis from the list of options above. Each option may be used once, more than once, or not at all.*

1. A 22-year-old man presents with left scrotal swelling which he believes came on after he was hit by a cricket ball a week earlier. On examination, the testis on the left is nontender, smooth, firm and twice the size on the right.

2. A 42-year-old male of south Asian origin presents with a long standing left scrotal swelling. On examination, the testis is not separately palpable and it is possible to get above the swelling. Fluctuation test is positive.

3. A 22-year-old male presents with left scrotal swelling of 1 day duration associated with left scrotal pain. He gave a history of dysuria of a week's duration. On examination the patient was pyrexial & the scrotum red. The testis and epididymis were swollen and very tender.

4. A 22-year-old tall and lean immigrant from Saharan Africa presents with a left sided scrotal swelling and a vague and dragging discomfort of his left scrotum which is characteristically relieved by lying down. On examination, the affected scrotum hangs down, cough impulse is positive and the swelling reduces on lying down.

5. A 22-year-old male presents with a left sided scrotal swelling of a few weeks duration associated with dull aching pain. On examination, the testis is felt separately. Cough impulse is positive. It is not possible to get above the swelling.

## 52. ANSWERS

1. **B - Testicular teratoma.** About 99% of testicular neoplasms are malignant and they are one of the commonest forms of cancer in the young male. Teratomas tend to occur in a younger age group, the peak incidence being between 20 and 35 years of age. Seminomas occur in the middle age group classically between the ages of 35–45.

Clues in this case are a young patient presenting with a history of trauma (history of trauma is present in 10% and is included to mislead), and a non-tender testicular lump (testicular sensations are lost very early in the disease). The trauma in this case most probably drew attention to the presence of the large testis.

2. **A - Primary hydrocele.** Primary hydrocele is most common in middle aged men particularly in tropical countries. Important clues include: (1) Testis is not separately palpable, (2) Possible to get above the swelling indicating that the swelling is purely scrotal in origin, (3) Positive fluctuation/transillumination, (4) Cough impulse is absent.

3. **H - Epididymo-orchitis.** The history is characteristic of epididymo-orchitis. Important clues include: (1) A preceding history of dysuria or prostatitis, (2) Pyrexia on presentation, (3) Raised inflammatory markers (raised white cell count and CRP).

In young men, the most common sexually transmitted infection causing epididymitis is now Chlamydia. Though doxycycline (100 mg bd) is the treatment of choice in young men with chlamydial infection, most urologists in UK would be happy to start empirical treatment with trimethoprim.

4. **I - Varicocele.** The history is characteristic of varicocele. Important clues may include: (1) Vague, dragging discomfort which is worse if testis is unsupported by underwear, (2) 'Bag of worms' feel of the scrotum, (3) Lower than normal position of the scrotum on the affected side, (4) Smaller testis on the affected side, (5) Self reducibility and (6) History of infertility (though this has never been proven conclusively).

95% of varicoceles are seen on the left side. It is also important to remember the association of left sided varicoceles with left renal cancer.

5. **F - Inguinoscrotal hernia.** Features include a positive cough impulse and an inability to get above the swelling.

Points differentiating this from a hydrocele include (1) Ability to feel testis separately, (2) Inability to get above the swelling, (3) Positive cough impulse and (3) Absence of fluctuation and transillumination.

## 53. THEME: SCROTAL SWELLINGS/PAIN

OPTIONS

A. Torsion of the testicular appendage
B. Epididymal cyst
C. Encysted hydrocele of cord
D. Seminoma of testis
E. Sebaceous cysts
F. Teratoma of testis
G. Torsion of the testis
H. Scrotal cancer
I. Acute epididymo-orchitis
J. Haematocele

*For each of the patients described below, select the most likely diagnosis from the list of options above. Each option may be used once, more than once, or not at all.*

1. A 12-year-old boy presents with a sudden onset agonizing pain in his left groin and lower abdomen associated with vomiting. On examination, the left testis has a high lie and the cord above it is tender and twisted.
2. A 38-year-old male presents with a swelling in the right scrotum. The swelling is separate from the testis, non tender, gives a bunch of grapes feel on palpation and brilliantly transilluminant.
3. A 42-year-old male presents with a sudden onset pain and acute enlargement of his left testis. On examination, the testis is normal in position, enlarged, smooth, firm and mildly tender.
4. A 41-year-man presents with a swelling in the left supraclavicular region. Examination of external genitalia reveals a lax hydrocele on the right side.
5. A 32-year man presents with multiple swellings in his scrotum. On examination he has multiple, small, nontender swellings in his scrotum which are attached to the skin.
6. A 9-year-old boy presents with pain in his left scrotum. He is crying and appears to be in a lot of pain. Examination reveals tenderness localized to the upper pole of this testicle. The 'blue dot' sign is positive.

## 53. ANSWERS

1. **G - Torsion of the testis.** Important clues: (1) Though most common in 10–25 year olds, important in under 10 year olds as well, (2) Sudden agonizing pain in groin and lower abdomen, (3) High lie of testis and thickening of the tender twisted cord which can be palpated above it.

It is important to remember that elevation of the testis reduces the pain of epididymo-orchitis and makes it worse in torsion.

2. **B - Epididymal cyst.** They are very common, usually multiple and often bilateral.

Important clues would include: (1) Brilliantly transilluminant cystic lump separate from the testis, (2) Bunch of grapes feel on palpation, (3) Chinese lantern pattern on illumination.

3. **D - Seminoma of testis.** Though this is an atypical presentation, all testicular swellings should be treated with suspicion. The age of the patient, the lie of the testis and the presentation are inconsistent with torsion.

4. **D - Seminoma of testis.** Presence of supraclavicular nodes should alert the clinician to a possibility of testicular tumour (10% of patients can have a lax secondary hydrocele).

5. **E - Sebaceous cysts.** Most sebaceous cysts are found in the hairy parts of the body. Scrotum is a common site. Due to the absence of sebaceous glands on the palms of the hand and the soles of the feet, the sebaceous cysts never occur in these regions.

Important clues are (1) Small, multiple, tense, spherical swellings, (2) Attachment to skin and (3) Presence of punctum.

6. **A - Torsion of testicular appendage (torsion of the hydatid of morgagni).** Important clues include: (1) Localized tenderness and (2) Blue dot sign (only visible early in the course, prior to hydrocele formation and onset of scrotal oedema).

In most cases—and certainly in equivocal cases—immediate scrotal exploration and removal of the infarcted appendage is required to rule out testicular torsion. Although the appendage is often bilateral, appendiceal torsion is usually unilateral; thus, removal of the opposite appendage is not indicated.

## 54. THEME: INVESTIGATIONS FOR SCROTAL CONDITIONS

OPTIONS

A. Scrotal Doppler
B. Tumour makers
C. Aspiration
D. No investigations-Surgery
E. On table Doppler USS-Surgery
F. Scrotal ultrasound
G. Renal ultrasound
H. Urgent radionuclide studies
I. FNA-tumour
J. Herniogram

*For each of the patients described below, select the most appropriate initial investigation from the list of options above. Each option may be used once, more than once, or not at all.*

1. A 10-year-old boy presents with a sudden onset pain in his left scrotum. On examination the left testis has a high lie and the cord above it is tender and twisted.

2. A 26-year-old male presents with a right sided inguino-scrotal swelling of a few weeks duration. On examination, the testis is felt separately. Cough impulse is positive. It is not possible to get above the swelling.

3. A 45-year-old male presents with a left sided scrotal swelling and a vague and dragging discomfort of his left scrotum of a week's duration. On examination, there is a 'bag of worms' feeling in his left scrotum.

4. A 30-year-old male presents with a right testicular swelling and some vague abdominal swelling. He has a history of undescended testes as a child.

## 54. ANSWERS

1. **D - No Investigations-Surgery**

Features are highly suggestive of testicular torsion. Surgical exploration is mandatory. Investigations are of little value: both radionuclide studies and Doppler ultrasound may be employed to show testicular blood flow, but results can be misleading. If seen early, it may be possible to untwist the testis without operation. In most cases, urgent operation is imperative as delay leads to testicular torsion after about 8 hours. If the testis is black and fails to recover its colour, it is necrotic and should be removed to prevent it inducing a sympathetic contralateral orchiopathy. The other testis should be fixed at an early date.

2. **D - No investigations-Surgery**

Features are suggestive of an inguinoscrotal hernia. This is a clinical diagnosis and the patient can be subjected to surgery on clinical grounds alone.

3. **G - Renal ultrasound**

Features clearly suggest a varicocele. If the history is short, particularly in the elderly, or if it is on the right side, then ultrasound investigation for renal adenocarcinoma may be the most appropriate first step.

4. **F - Scrotal ultrasound**

Features are suggestive of a testicular tumour. The first investigation is ultrasonography of the scrotal contents.

## 55. THEME: TREATMENT FOR TESTICULAR TUMOURS

OPTIONS

A. Chemotherapy
B. Retroperitoneal lymph node dissection
C. Radiotherapy
D. Anti androgen therapy
E. Testicular biopsy
F. F/U with serial CT scans
G. Tumor markers/CT scan surveillance
H. Radical orchidectomy

*For each of the patients below, select the most appropriate subsequent treatment from the above list. Each option may be used once, more than once or not at all.*

1. A 40-year-old male presents with a right sided testicular mass which is diagnosed as a seminoma. He undergoes a radical orchidectomy. This is confirmed as stage 1.

2. A 22-year-old male presents with a non seminatous germ cell tumour on the right. He undergoes a radical orchidectomy. This is confirmed as stage 1.

3. A 26-year-old male presents with a left testicular tumour. He undergoes radical orchidectomy. Staging suggests the presence of a 3 cm mass of para-aortic nodes.

4. A 22-year-old man undergoes an orchidectomy for a teratoma of the left testis. Postoperative staging confirms the presence of a 9 cm mass of para-aortic nodes. After a course of chemotherapy the tumour markers normalize and CT scan shows a reduction of the size of nodal mass to 4 cm.

5. A 26-year-old male presents with a supraclavicular lymph node swelling. Examination confirms a left testicular mass. The patient's GP has already arranged for some tumour marker examination, which are highly suggestive of teratoma.

## 55. ANSWERS

**1. C - Radiotherapy**

Seminomas are radiosensitive. After radical orchidectomy, prophylactic irradiation is employed for stage 1 tumours. Stage 2 tumours are also treated with radiotherapy. Patients with metastasis need treatment with cisplatin or carboplatin.

**2. G - Tumour markers/CT scan surveillance**

Teratomas are less sensitive to radiotherapy. Stage 1 tumours are managed by watching the level of serum markers and by repeated computed tomography. Some authors however advocate prophylactic adjuvant chemotherapy for these tumours on the grounds that they are less inconvenient for the patient.

**3. A - Chemotherapy**

Teratoma stage 2 is the likely diagnosis in this case. Stages 2–4 are managed by chemotherapy. Cisplatin, methotrexate, bleomycin and vincristine have been used in various combinations.

**4. B - Retroperitoneal lymph node dissection (RPLND)**

RPLND is indicated in the presence of residual nodes after chemotherapy and normalization of tumour markers. Most often the tissue removed contains only necrotic tissue, but a proportion of patients have foci of mature teratoma or active malignancy.

**5. H - Radical orchidectomy**

The most appropriate subsequent is radical orchidectomy. Staging here subsequently will most likely suggest a stage 3/4 teratoma. Treatment is subsequently with chemotherapy.

## 56. THEME: TREATMENT FOR TESTICULAR SWELLINGS

OPTIONS

A. Surgical aspiration
B. Surgical exploration
C. Orchidectomy
D. Injection of sclerosant
E. Bed rest and antibiotics
F. No treatment
G. Radical orchidectomy with chemotherapy
H. Surgical removal of cyst
I. Herniotomy

*For each of the patients below, select the most appropriate subsequent treatment from the above list. Each option may be used once, more than once or not at all.*

1. A 26-year-old male presents with right scrotal swelling of 2 day duration associated with pain. He gave a history of dysuria of a week's duration. The testis and epididymis were swollen and very tender.

2. A 12-year-old boy presents with an acutely swollen and painful testes on the left side. On examination, the testis lies high in the scrotum.

3. A middle-aged man presents with a discomforting fluctuant swelling in his left scrotum. The testis is felt separately from the swelling. Transillumination is positive.

4. An 8-month-old male infant is brought by his mother with a right scrotal swelling for 2 months duration. The swelling has gradually increased in size. The infant appears generally asymptomatic. The swelling does not reduce on lying down and is transilluminant.

5. A 22-year-old man presents with a right testicular mass that is markedly cystic in consistency. Abdominal examination reveals some vague retroperitoneal lumps.

## 56. ANSWERS

1. **E - Bed rest & antibiotics**
Features are suggestive of epididymo-orchitis. Treatment involves bed rest and appropriate antibiotics as per culture and sensitivity.

2. **B - Surgical exploration**
Please see answer 1 in Theme 54 for explanation.

3. **H - Surgical removal of cyst**
Features suggest an epididymal cyst. Aspiration is futile since the cyst is multilocular. If causing discomfort they should be excised.

4. **I - Herniotomy**
Features suggest a congenital hydrocele. The processus vaginalis is patent and connects with the general peritoneal cavity. They are a special form of indirect inguinal hernia and are treated by herniotomy.

5. **G - Radical orchidectomy with chemotherapy**
Cystic testicular swelling in a young person most likely suggests teratoma. Suspect seminoma in solid swellings in the middle aged patients. This is most likely stage 2 and treatment includes chemotherapy after radical orchidectomy.

## 57. THEME: DIAGNOSIS OF PENILE CONDITIONS

OPTIONS

A. Phimosis
B. Paraphimosis
C. Fracture of shaft of penis
D. Balanoposthitis
E. Peyronie's disease
F. Carcinoma of penis
G. Leukoplakia
H. Paget's disease
I. Balanitis xerotica obliterans
J. Priapism
K. Impotence
L. Genital warts
M. Hypospadias
N. Herpes genitalis
O. Epispadias
P. Urethral calculus

*For each of the patients described below, select the most likely diagnosis from the list of options above. Each option may be used once, more than once, or not at all.*

1. A young male presents to the outpatient clinic with a complaint of whitish appearance of his glans for a month's duration. Examination reveals painless patches of grey-white paint on his glans.
2. A young Afro-Caribbean male presents with a painful penis. He gives a history of sickle-cell disease. On examination, the penis is persistently erect.
3. A young male presents with a red lesion over his glans penis, which occasionally oozes and then crusts over. On examination, a red oozing eczematous lesion is visible on the glans.
4. A 6-year-old kid is brought by his mother because she is concerned his penis balloons up during micturition. On examination the opening of the foreskin is pinhole in size.
5. The staff nurse in ITU is concerned that a patient has developed sudden onset swelling in his penis following a catheterization performed last night. On examination, the glans penis is swollen and oedematous. There is a deep groove just below the corona.

## 57. ANSWERS

1. **G - Leukoplakia**

Leukoplakia is used to describe areas of white, boggy epithelium which is identical to leukoplakia on tongue, vulva and vagina. This is a pre-malignant condition.

Clues include painless whitish paint appearance.

2. **J - Priapism**

Priapism is persistent erection. There are two mechanisms which can cause it: persistent spasm of the venous smooth muscle sphincter and the thrombosis of veins draining the erectile tissue.

Clues in this case include persistently erected painful penis and the history of sickle cell disease. It can also be associated with leukaemia, other blood disorder associated with thrombotic tendencies, renal failure, spinal cord diseases and local prostatic and pelvic disease.

3. **H - Paget's disease**

This is a rare but a well known premalignant condition of the penis. Chronic red eczematous lesions which alternately ooze and crust over are characteristic.

4. **A - Phimosis**

5. **B - Paraphimosis**

It commonly occurs in young men between the ages of 15–30. It is due to the fact that the prepuce is sufficiently tight to get stuck behind the glans penis after an erection. It impedes venous blood and causes oedema and congestion of the glans. It is also seen after catheterization if the foreskin is not pulled forwards over the glans penis after completion of the procedure.

## 58. THEME: DIAGNOSIS OF PENILE CONDITIONS

OPTIONS

A. Phimosis
B. Paraphimosis
C. Fracture of shaft of penis
D. Balanoposthitis
E. Peyronie's disease
F. Carcinoma of penis
G. Leukoplakia
H. Paget's disease
I. Balanitis xerotica obliterans
J. Priapism
K. Impotence
L. Genital warts
M. Hypospadias
N. Herpes genitalis
O. Epispadias
P. Urethral calculus

*For each of the patients described below, select the most likely diagnosis from the list of options above. Each option may be used once, more than once, or not at all.*

1. A 3-month-old baby is brought to your clinic by his mother because she is concerned he has a curved penis. On examination the urethral opening is situated proximally on the ventral surface of the penis.

2. A middle-aged insulin-dependent diabetic presents with itching and pain in his penile foreskin. On examination a whitish discharge is obvious from the subpreputial skin with difficulty in retracting the foreskin.

3. A 42-year-old male presents with a history of difficult intercourse. He complains of a deformity of his erect penis. On examination, hard plaques of fibrosis are palpable in the penis. One of his fingers shows contracture.

4. A 22-year-old male presents in A&E with acute onset pain and swelling in his penis which started acutely during his first intercourse. He can pinpoint the onset of pain to bending his penis during intercourse.

5. A 23-year-old male presents with multiple lesions over his preputial skin. On examination many soft, moist and pedunculated lesions are seen under the prepuce.

## 58. ANSWERS

1. **M - Hypospadias**

The urethra opens on the ventral surface of the penis in hypospadias. Chordee, which is a descriptive term for a curved penis, is commonly associated with hypospadias. The opposite of this is epispadias where the urethral opening is on the dorsal surface of the glans penis.

2. **D - Balanoposthitis**

This condition is commonly associated with diabetes, phimosis and penile cancer.

3. **E - Peyronie's disease**

This is a relatively common cause of deformity of the erect penis. On examination, hard plaques of fibrosis can be palpated in the tunica of one or both corpora cavernosa. It may be due to trauma and is associated with Dupuytren's contracture. Nesbitt's operation is a surgical treatment option in severe cases. Occasionally the plaque may become calcified and visible on the X-ray.

4. **C - Fracture of shaft of penis**

This condition is rare and occurs when the erect penis is bent violently downwards during intercourse.

5. **L - Genital warts**

## 59. THEME: DIAGNOSIS OF PENILE CONDITIONS

OPTIONS

A. Phimosis
B. Paraphimosis
C. Fracture of shaft of penis
D. Balanoposthitis
E. Peyronie's disease
F. Carcinoma of penis
G. Leukoplakia
H. Paget's disease
I. Balanitis xerotica obliterans
J. Priapism
K. Impotence
L. Genital warts
M. Hypospadias
N. Herpes genitalis
O. Epispadias
P. Urethral calculus

*For each of the patients described below, select the most likely diagnosis from the list of options above. Each option may be used once, more than once, or not at all.*

1. A 29-year-old male presents with an ulcer on the glans penis for a few weeks duration. On examination, a classical ulcer with a raised everted edge and necrotic base is seen. A sanguinous discharge was evident.
2. A young male presents with painful, itchy, recurrent lesions on his glans. On examination there were multiple vesicles over the glans.
3. A 49-year-old insulin dependent diabetic complains of an inability to obtain full erection.
4. A 35-year-old male presents with straining at micturition. On examination, the foreskin is thickened, fibrosed, white and tightly adherent to the glans.
5. A young male presents with a sudden onset pain in his penis and haematuria for a few hours duration. He gives a history of left loin pain for a day's duration 2 days earlier. On examination, a hard lump is palpable in the urethra.

## 59. ANSWERS

1. **F - Carcinoma of penis**

Forty percent of patients are under 40 years of age. In uncircumcised males, the lesion may be hidden by the foreskin. Surgical excision usually requires at least partial amputation of the penis, and block dissection of the inguinal lymph nodes if they are involved. Radiotherapy can be used in stage 1 disease if the urethra is not involved and for palliation in stage 4 disease.

2. **N - Herpes genitalis**

Classically this is recurrent. The initial multiple itchy vesicles are soon replaced by painful erosions.

3. **K - Impotence**

Atherosclerosis is responsible for the majority of cases of erectile dysfunction in men over 60 years of age. Diabetes is the second most important cause of erectile dysfunction and impotence is known to occur 10–15 years prior to the general population.

4. **I - Balanitis xerotica obliterans**

This condition is analogous to lichen sclerosis of the vulva in females. Circumcision solves the problem, but if causing meatal stenosis as in the present case, a meatotomy or meatoplasty will also be required.

5. **P - Urethral calculus**

This is a classical presentation. Migratory calculi cause sudden pain in the urethra soon after an attack of ureteric colic. These can be very painful due to mucosal erosion. Haematuria is sometimes seen. It is sometimes possible to feel the calculus as a hard lump in the urethra.

## 60. THEME: DIAGNOSIS OF MALE INFERTILITY

OPTIONS

A. Auto antibodies
B. Beta blocker medication
C. Depression
D. Varicocele
E. Hernia
F. Testicular injury
G. Peripheral vascular disease
H. Psychogenic
I. Retrograde ejaculation
J. Injury to penile nerve supply
K. Post-traumatic stress disorder
L. Hydrocele

*For each scenario listed below, select the most appropriate diagnosis from the above list. Each option may be used once, more than once, or not at all.*

1. A young 28-year-old male presents with infertility of 3 years duration. He complains of a dull aching pain in the left scrotum. Examination confirms oligospermia and the presence of a swelling in the left scrotum which disappears on lying down.

2. A 45-year-old male presents with a history of erectile impotence for the past few months. He feels that this is severely affecting his relationship which has already been strained by his inability to give up his smoking habit of 30 years.

3. A 45-year-old male presents with a history of erectile impotence for the past few months. Past medical history includes a 'hole in the heart' as a baby, asthma, epilepsy, hypertension, jaundice, tuberculosis and cholecystectomy.

4. A 26-year-old male is admitted to hospital following a severe road traffic accident. He has an open book type of pelvic fracture and bleeding from the urethral meatus. He subsequently undergoes a suprapubic cystostomy. He is seen in the outpatients a year from discharge when he complains of erectile impotence.

## 60. ANSWERS

1. **D - Varicocele**

The presence of a varicocele is presumed to interfere with the temperature control of the scrotum which is normally 2.5°C less than rectal temperature. However, many authors believe that varicocele is just a coincidental finding in these patients.

2. **G - Peripheral vascular disease**

Smoking is an important clue in this case. Leriche's syndrome is a well known entity comprising buttock claudication and impotence and is due to an occlusion in the region of the bifurcation of the aorta and the internal iliac arteries.

3. **B - Beta blocker medication**

Drugs such as atenolol are an important cause of erectile dysfunction.

4. **J - Injury to penile nerve supply**

Erectile impotence is common after pelvic fractures with urethral injury and is presumed to be due to injury to the penile nerve supply.

## 61. THEME: PERIOPERATIVE MANAGEMENT

OPTIONS

A. Monitor warfarin-INR
B. Nothing required
C. Antibiotic prophylaxis
D. Monitor regular BM
E. Sliding scale insulin infusion
F. Perioperative heparin
G. Proton pump inhibitors
H. TED stocking

*For each scenario listed below, select the most appropriate option from the above list. Each option may be used once, more than once, or not at all.*

1. A 65-year-old lady is admitted for an elective excision of a large swelling over her thigh. The swelling was initially assumed to be a soft tissue sarcoma, but later confirmed as a lipoma on biopsy. She is known to have had a metallic heart valve replacement and is on life long warfarin for the same.

2. A 65-year-old male is due to undergo a fem-pop bypass. He is known to be insulin dependent.

3. A 22-year-old girl is seen in the day surgery unit for an elective arthroscopy. She has medial knee pain due to a presumed medial meniscal tear.

4. A 65-year-old female is undergoing a total knee replacement. She is known to have had a deep vein thrombosis after a hysterectomy last year.

## 61. ANSWERS

1. **F - Perioperative heparin**

This patient is on warfarin for a metallic valve replacement. So she needs to be switched onto an intravenous heparin infusion to facilitate control perioperatively.

2. **E - Sliding scale insulin infusion**

3. **B - Nothing required**

4. **H - TED stocking**

In view of her past history, in addition to her TED stockings, she will require low molecular weight heparin for thromboprophylaxis post operatively.

## 62. THEME: PROPHYLAXIS OF WOUND INFECTION

OPTIONS

A. Laminar flow in operating theatres
B. 1 week course of antibiotics
C. Appropriate blood glucose control
D. Universal precautions
E. Routine sterile technique only
F. Topical antibiotics
G. 2 sachets of sodium picosulphate 24 hours preoperative

*For each scenario listed below, select the most appropriate option from the above list. Each option may be used once, more than once, or not at all.*

1. An 83-year-old nursing home resident is admitted with an acute abdomen. He undergoes a Hartmann's resection for perforated diverticular disease.

2. A 45-year-old generally fit and well male undergoes a partial medical menisectomy as an arthroscopic day case procedure.

3. A 45-year-old insulin dependent diabetic undergoes a partial medical menisectomy as an arthroscopic day case procedure.

4. A 66-year-old lady undergoes a total knee replacement for osteoarthritis.

5. A 65-year-old diabetic is admitted electively for a low anterior resection of the rectum for a rectal malignancy.

## 62. ANSWERS

1. **B - 1 week course of antibiotics**
2. **E - Routine sterile technique only**
3. **E - Routine sterile technique only**
4. **A - Laminar air flow in operating theatres**
5. **G - 2 sachets of sodium picosulphate 24 hours preoperative**

## 63. THEME: TRAUMA IN YOUNG CHILDREN

OPTIONS

A. Osteopetrosis
B. Osteoporosis
C. Rickets
D. Non accidental injury
E. Accidental fracture
F. Metabolic bone disease of prematurity
G. Hypoparathyroidism
H. Pseudohypoparathyroidism

*For each of the patients described below, select the most appropriate diagnosis from the above list. Each option may be used once, more than once, or not at all.*

1. A 2-year-old baby boy is brought to A&E by his mother with a complaint of swelling of his left thigh for 24 hours duration. His mom tells you that the child had a small trip and fall in his bath tub, but that he had been well initially. X-rays reveals a spiral fracture of his left femur.

2. A 21-month-old baby boy is brought to A&E by his concerned parents after a fall at the child minder's house. The child minder has been kind enough to describe the exact fall and sends a letter to A&E with the parents. She describes a trip and fall in his bath tub. Suspecting a right ankle sprain, she has also given him some cold compress. X-rays confirm a transverse fracture of his right tibia.

## 63. ANSWERS

1. **D - Non accidental injury (NAI)**

It is very important to keep a high index of suspicion for NAI in any child who has a delay in presentation and where the history is not compatible with the findings. A spiral fracture usually indicates a twisting injury rather than a trip and fall.

2. **E - Accidental fracture**

A history consistent with the injury, lack of delay in presentation and the fact that the child minder has described the whole story in a letter makes it more likely for it to be an accidental fracture. Where doubts persist, it is standard practice in UK to fill a cause for concern form.

## 64. THEME: CHILDREN'S ORTHOPAEDICS

OPTIONS

A. Osteopetrosis
B. Osteoporosis
C. Rickets
D. Non accidental injury (NAI)
E. Accidental fracture
F. Osteogenesis imperfecta
G. Hypoparathyroidism
H. Achondroplasia

*For each of the patients described below, select the most appropriate diagnosis from the above list. Each option may be used once, more than once, or not at all.*

1. A 21-month-old baby boy is brought to A&E with what looks like a femur fracture after a history of trivial fall. His mom is single, poorly supported and survives on state benefits. The baby has a blue sclera. Radiology confirms Wormian bones in the skull.

2. This is the commonest cause of short limbed dwarfism. Most cases are autosomal dominant. The limbs are short and there is a lumbar lordosis.

3. A 13-month-old baby boy is brought to A&E with swelling involving the right arm. His mom's boyfriend tells you that an hour ago he lifted the baby boy out of his bunker bed and lost grip of his right hand. The baby apparently twisted around his right arm.

## 64. ANSWERS

1. **F - Osteogenesis imperfecta**

This relatively common dysplasia is caused by an abnormality of collagen type 1 and therefore all connective tissue is involved. The joints are loose, bones fracture and bend (green stick), teeth can be abnormal and there may be neurological and gastrointestinal problems. The classic form (type 1a) is autosomal dominant. Type 3, which is severely deforming, is autosomal recessive. Classical radiological features include osteopenia, deformities, vertebral collapse and Wormian bones in the skull.

2. **H - Achondroplasia**

Features are as described. Trunk height is maintained in this condition, but spinal stenosis is common.

3. **E - Accidental fracture**

Don't be distracted by the story about the mom's boyfriend. Though social history is important in NAI, a consistent history in this case should go against a diagnosis of NAI.

## 65. THEME: SWELLINGS IN THE NECK

OPTIONS

A. Anaplastic carcinoma of thyroid
B. Lymphoma of thyroid
C. Branchial cyst
D. Thyroglossal cyst
E. Submandibular calculus
F. Ranula
G. Sublingual calculus
H. Carcinoma of apex of lung
I. Virchow's node
J. Solitary thyroid nodule

*For each of the patients described below, select the most appropriate diagnosis from the above list. Each option may be used once, more than once, or not at all.*

1. A teenager presents with a slowly enlarging painless swelling in the left side of her neck. Examination reveals a 5 cm smooth fluctuant swelling arising from beneath the anterior aspect of the junction of the upper third and middle third of the sternomastoid muscle.

2. A 70-year-old gentleman presents with anorexia, weight loss and melaena. He has a palpable firm lump in the left supraclavicular fossa.

3. A 55-year-old lady presents with a swelling in her jaw on the left side. The swelling is classically intermittent. It is related to food intake. It increases in size and becomes painful while eating.

4. A 60-year-old lady presents with a small swelling that lies slightly to one side of the midline. The lump moves upwards with swallowing and quite surprisingly on tongue protrusion.

## 65. ANSWERS

1. **C - Branchial cyst**

The most important clue is the typical position. A branchial cyst develops from the vestigial remnants of the 2nd branchial cleft. Though it is fluctuant and may transilluminate in the early stages, if infection supervenes, it may become markedly erythematous and tender.

2. **I - Virchow's node**

This patient in all probability has gastric cancer. This is a classical description for Virchow's node and indicates inoperability.

3. **E - Submandibular calculus**

This is again a typical history. Majority of stones occur in the submandibular glands because their secretions contain mucus, the viscosity is higher and the duct drains antigravity. 80% of stones in the submandibular gland are radiopaque and can be identified using plain radiographs.

4. **D - Thyroglossal cyst**

I make no apologies for the 'incorrect' age. While they mostly occur in children, late onset thyroglossal cysts can occur up to the seventh decade of life.

## 66. THEME: CHEMOTHERAPY

OPTIONS

A. Actinomycin D
B. Asparaginase
C. Cisplatin
D. Cyclophosphamide
E. Doxorubicin
F. Methotrexate
G. Vincristine
H. Cytosine arabinoside
I. Bleomycin

*For each of the descriptions below, select the most appropriate chemotherapeutic agent from the above list. Each option may be used once, more than once, or not at all.*

1. An alkylating agent resulting in haemorrhagic cystitis.

2. An anthracycline with a serious risk of cardiotoxicity.

3. A drug resulting in dose related lung damage.

4. A drug inhibiting initiation of DNA synthesis resulting in conjunctivitis and cerebellar toxicity.

## 66. ANSWERS

1. **D - Cyclophosphamide**

2. **E - Doxorubicin**

3. **I - Bleomycin**

4. **H - Cytosine arabinoside**

All cytotoxic agents have general side effects which include nausea, vomiting, alopecia, bone marrow suppression and stomatitis. Specific side effects are as listed.

## 67. THEME: TUMOUR SYNDROMES/ASSOCIATIONS

OPTIONS

A. MEN 1
B. Gardner's syndrome
C. Meigs syndrome
D. Peutz-Jeghers syndrome
E. Struma ovarii
F. Von-Hippel Lindau syndrome
G. Von Recklinghausen's disease
H. Familial polyposis coli

*For each of the patients described below, select the most appropriate diagnosis from the above list. Each option may be used once, more than once, or not at all.*

1. A 60-year-old lady known to have a family history of ovarian carcinoma presents with fatigue, shortness of breath, increasing abdominal distention, and weight loss. Abdominal examination reveals a vaguely palpable pelvic lump on the left with the presence of ascites.

2. A 60-year-old lady presents with abdominal distention, weight loss, tremors and a feeling of heat intolerance for a month's duration. A thyroid is not palpable and is ruled out as a cause of symptoms. Abdominal examination reveals a 15 cm lower abdominal lump on the right. It is not possible to 'get below the swelling'.

3. A 25-year-old male presents with headaches, problems with balance and walking, dizziness, weakness of the limbs and vision problems. He has also noticed haematuria in recent days. Examination reveals a palpable renal swelling on the right side. He is found to have high blood pressure. Fundoscopy reveals retinal haemangiomas.

4. A 40-year-old male presents with bleeding per rectum. He has melanosis of the oral mucous membrane and the lips.

## 67. ANSWERS

1. **C - Meigs syndrome**

Meigs syndrome is defined as the triad of benign ovarian tumour with ascites and pleural effusion that resolves after resection of the tumour. The ovarian tumour in Meigs syndrome is a fibroma. The history of fatigue and shortness of breath in this question most probably suggests a pleural effusion.

2. **E - Struma ovarii**

The abdominal findings suggest an ovarian tumour. Since the thyroid has been excluded as the origin of the patient's symptoms, struma ovarii is the most likely diagnosis. It is an ovarian tumour which contains thyroid tissue and can cause thyrotoxicosis.

3. **F - Von Hippel Lindau syndrome**

The most common manifestations of VHL are retinal, cerebellar, spinal and medullary haemangioblastomas, renal cysts and carcinoma, pancreatic cysts, phaeochromocytoma and papillary cystadenoma of the epididymis.

4. **D - Peutz-Jeghers syndrome**

This syndrome consists of familial intestinal hamartomatous polyposis affecting the jejunum, where it is a cause of haemorrhage, and often intussusception. The pigmentation of the lips is the *sine qua non*.

## 68. THEME: TUMOUR SYNDROMES/ASSOCIATIONS

OPTIONS

A. MEN 1
B. Gardner's syndrome
C. Meigs syndrome
D. Peutz-Jeghers syndrome
E. Struma ovarii
F. Von-Hippel Lindau syndrome
G. Von Recklinghausen's disease
H. MEN 2

*For each of the patients described below, select the most appropriate diagnosis from the above list. Each option may be used once, more than once, or not at all.*

1. A 40-year-old with a past history of parathyroidectomy for hyperparathyroidism presents with Zollinger-Ellison syndrome.

2. A 40-year-old with a past history of parathyroidectomy for hyperparathyroidism presents with a thyroid cancer and hypertension.

3. A rare autosomal dominant disease characterized by GI polyps, multiple osteomas and soft tissue tumours.

## 68. ANSWERS

1. **A - MEN 1**

2. **H - MEN 2**

These are important questions for the exam. Don't get confused. The aim of this question was to highlight the fact that parathyroid is common for both. MEN 1 include pituitary and pancreatic lesions in addition to parathyroid. MEN 2 include medullary thyroid and phaeochromocytoma in addition to parathyroid.

3. **B - Gardner's syndrome**

Typical features are as described. Onset is in early puberty. Polyps of colon ultimately change into adenocarcinoma by the fourth decade of life. Osteomas most often develop within the angle of the mandible first. Abnormality of the retina may coexist.

## 69. THEME: BIOCHEMISTRY

OPTIONS

A. Hypercalcaemia
B. Hypocalcaemia
C. Hypernatraemia
D. Hyponatraemia
E. Hyperkalaemia
F. Hypokalaemia
G. Hyperglycaemia
H. Hypoglycaemia

*For each of the patients described below, select the most appropriate biochemical finding from the above list. Each option may be used once, more than once, or not at all.*

1. A 65-year-old lady is on tamoxifen for advanced breast cancer. She presents with increasing lethargy, polyuria and polydipsia.

2. A 78-year-old is admitted with acute retention of urine, urinary tract infection and increasing confusion. He is catheterized and treated with intravenous antibiotics. He is also started on intravenous infusion and advised to drink plenty of fluids orally. The following day he becomes increasingly drowsy.

3. A 66-year-old male on the 'water tablet' is scheduled for a right total knee replacement. ECG shows U waves.

4. A 60-year-old male presents to A&E with a 2-hour history of colicky right loin to groin pain. He has 2+ blood in his urine.

5. A 79-year-old residential home inmate is brought to A&E with vomiting, diarrhoea, increasing confusion and oliguria. His ECG shows tall tented T waves.

## 69. ANSWERS

**1. A - Hypercalcaemia**

Hypercalcaemia associated with tumours is commonly due to direct bone involvement in metastatic carcinomas. It is rarely due to elaboration of ectopic PTHrp by squamous cell carcinoma of the lung.

**2. D - Hyponatraemia**

This is most likely due to water intoxication as well as a combination of SIADH and infection.

**3. F - Hypokalaemia**

Most patients in the UK would refer to a diuretic as a water tablet. It is possible that this patient is on a thiazide diuretic (most commonly bendroflumethiazide). U waves suggest hypokalaemia.

**4. A - Hypercalcaemia**

A ureteric colic in this age group may be associated with hyperparathyroidism and hence associated hypercalcaemia and hypercalciuria.

**5. E - Hyperkalaemia**

Diarrhoea and vomiting with associated dehydration may have caused acute renal failure in this patient. Hyperkalaemia can occur and is demonstrated as tall tented T waves on the ECG.

## 70. THEME: HYPONATRAEMIA

OPTIONS

A. Addison's disease
B. Water intoxication
C. Congestive cardiac failure
D. Nephrotic syndrome
E. Diuretic therapy
F. Cirrhosis

*For each of the patients described below, select the most appropriate cause of hyponatraemia from the above list. Each option may be used once, more than once, or not at all.*

1. A 65-year-old male presents to his GP with tiredness, fatigue and lethargy. Examination is normal with a well controlled blood pressure recording. He is known to be hypertensive and his serum sodium values stand at 128 mmol/L.

2. A 35-year-old female presents with weakness and dizziness. She has irregular dusky pigmentation of the skin. She is noted to have pigmentation of the mouth. She is known to have pernicious anaemia. Her blood pressure is 98/62 mm Hg while her serum sodium values stand at 128 mmol/L.

## 70. ANSWERS

1. **E - Diuretic therapy**

Bendroflumethiazide, a first choice antihypertensive, causes hyponatraemia as a well recongnized complication. Options include stopping the antihypertensive for a few days or switching over to an alternative antihypertensive.

2. **A - Addison's disease**

In about 60% of cases, the condition is believed to be due to an autoimmune disease, sometimes in association with autoimmune thyroiditis and pernicious anaemia. Tuberculosis, metastatic carcinoma and amyloidosis account for the remaining 40%. Treatment is medical. Most patients require hydrocortisone daily with fludrocortisone as mineralocorticoid replacement.

## 71. THEME: ECG CHANGES

OPTIONS

A. Concave upwards ST elevation
B. Convex upwards ST elevation
C. ST depression
D. Q waves
E. U waves
F. Sinus tachycardia
G. Shortened PR interval
H. Prolonged PR interval
I. Shortened QT interval
J. Prolonged QT interval
K. J waves
L. Delta waves

*For each of the scenarios described below, select the most appropriate ECG change from the above list. Each option may be used once, more than once, or not at all.*

1. Hypocalcaemia

2. Sotalol

3. WPW syndrome

4. Pericarditis

5. Hypothermia

6. Pulmonary embolism

## 71. ANSWERS

1. **J - Prolonged QT interval**

2. **J - Prolonged QT interval**
Other causes include hypomagnesaemia and amiodarone therapy.

3. **L - Delta waves**

4. **A - Concave upwards ST elevation**
Myocardial infarction causes convex upwards ST elevation.

5. **K - J waves**

6. **F - Sinus tachycardia**
Other features include right axis deviation. A typical $S_1Q_1T_3$ pattern is seen very occasionally.

## 72. THEME: MEDICATIONS IN GI DISORDERS

OPTIONS

A. Nifedipine
B. Hyoscine butylbromide
C. Metoclopramide
D. Infliximab
E. Glyceryl trinitrate
F. Mesalazine
G. Ranitidine
H. Omeprazole
I. Botulinum toxin
J. Nystatin lozenges

*For each of the patients described below, select the most appropriate drug therapy from the above list. Each option may be used once, more than once, or not at all.*

1. A 5-ASA derivative that can induce a remission in mild attacks of ulcerative colitis.

2. Useful in the treatment of diffuse oesophageal spasm.

3. This may be given by endoscopic injection in this motility disorder.

4. Useful in the treatment of candidal oesophagitis.

5. Useful as an ointment in anal fissures.

6. An anti-TNF-α antibody that is given as a single infusion which can produce clinical improvement in patients with steroid resistant Crohn's disease.

## 72. ANSWERS

1. **F - Mesalazine**

2. **A - Nifedipine**

Nifedipine is a calcium channel blocker. It inhibits smooth muscle contraction and may provide symptomatic relief in this disorder. Sublingual nifedipine may be useful for transient relief of symptoms in achalasia cardia.

3. **I - Botulinum toxin**

This may be given by endoscopic injection into the LOS in achalasia cardia. It acts by interfering with cholinergic excitatory neural activity at the LOS.

4. **J - Nystatin lozenges**

5. **E - Glyceryl trinitrate**

6. **D - Infliximab**

GTN is a nitric acid donor and 0.2% ointment when applied to the anal canal produces sufficient relaxation of the sphincter to allow the fissure to heal in up to two-thirds of patients. In addition, blood flow to the area improves which promotes healing. A major side effect is headache.

## 73. THEME: SIDE EFFECTS OF ANTIBIOTICS

OPTIONS

A. Ciprofloxacin
B. Vancomycin
C. Cephradine
D. Erythromycin
E. Gentamicin
F. Metronidazole
G. Tetracycline
H. Chloramphenicol

*For the side effects mentioned below, match the drugs above. Each option may be used once, more than once, or not at all.*

1. Associated with arthropathy in experimental animal studies and is therefore contraindicated in children less than 16 years of age.

2. Well known commonly used antibiotic associated with ototoxicity and nephrotoxicity.

3. Causes brownish discolouration of growing teeth and hence is contraindicated in children and pregnant women.

4. Hated by patients for its metallic taste which is a common side effect. Rarely, it can cause peripheral neuropathy.

5. Can cause gray baby syndrome when given to newborn babies (especially premature infants).

6. Associated with allergic red man syndrome characterized by exfoliative dermatitis, Stevens-Johnson syndrome, toxic epidermal necrolysis and vasculitis.

## 73. ANSWERS

1. **A - Ciprofloxacin**
2. **E - Gentamicin**
3. **G - Tetracycline**
4. **F - Metronidazole**
5. **H - Chloramphenicol**
6. **B - Vancomycin**

## 74. THEME: ANALGESICS IN SURGERY

OPTIONS

A. Fentanyl
B. Pethidine
C. Buprenorphine
D. Morphine
E. Paracetamol
F. Codeine
G. Tramadol
H. Diclofenac

*For the descriptions below, select the most appropriate answer from the list above. Each option may be used once, more than once, or not at all.*

1. This is used in breakthrough pain in patients already receiving opioid therapy for chronic pain.

2. It produces analgesia by two mechanisms—an opioid effect and an enhancement of serotonergic and adrenergic pathways.

3. It is used in obstetric analgesia. It produces prompt but short lasting analgesia. It is a less potent analgesic even in high doses.

## 74. ANSWERS

1. **A - Fentanyl**

2. **G - Tramadol**

3. **B - Pethidine**

## 75. THEME: CYTOTOXIC DRUGS

OPTIONS

A. Doxorubicin
B. 5-Fluorouracil
C. Methotrexate
D. Cisplatin
E. Cyclophosphamide
F. Mercaptopurine
G. Irinotecan
H. Oxaliplatin

*For each mechanism of action/description of cytotoxic drugs mentioned below, select the most appropriate drug from the list of options above. Each option may be used once, more than once, or not at all.*

1. A cytotoxic drug with a folic acid antagonist action used in the treatment of neoplastic diseases, severe psoriasis and adult rheumatoid arthritis.

2. An antimetabolite that acts as a pyrimidine antagonist.

3. Prevents DNA repair by acting as a topoisomerase I inhibitor.

4. A DNA damaging alkylating agent which uses free radical to perform its task.

5. The basis of nearly all regimens of adjuvant and palliative treatments of colorectal cancer.

6. A cytotoxic alkylating agent used to downsize liver metastasis in colorectal cancer.

## 75. ANSWERS

1. **C - Methotrexate**

2. **B - 5-Fluorouracil**

It is used in chemotherapeutic regimens in a wide range of cancers of the stomach, oesophagus, bowel and breast. It is usually used in combination with folinic acid (Leucovorin). Regimens may also include irinotecan and oxaliplatin. The oral form, capecitabine, is also being used now.

3. **A - Doxorubicin**

It is also known as adriamycin. It has marked cardiotoxity. It is used in acute leukaemias, lymphomas and a variety of solid tumours.

4. **E - Cyclophosphamide**

A well known complication is haemorrhagic cystitis. It is commonly used in the treatment of lymphomas; cancers of the ovary, breast and bladder and chronic lymphocytic leukaemia. It is also used in rheumatoid arthritis. Adjuvant chemotherapy in breast cancer results in an approximately 25% decrease in breast cancer mortality.

5. **B - 5-Fluorouracil**

6. **H - Oxaliplatin**

It belongs to a new class of platinum agents. Preclinical studies have shown oxaliplatin to be synergistic with 5-fluorouracil. Paraesthesia is seen in nearly all patients receiving oxaliplatin plus 5-FU, with residual paraesthesia seen in some patients following completion of therapy.

## 76. THEME: HORMONE SECRETING TUMOURS

OPTIONS

A. ADH
B. Calcitonin
C. Erythropoeitin
D. Growth hormone
E. α- Fetoprotein
F. 5-Hydroxytryptamine

*For each of the tumours listed below, select the most likely hormone that is secreted from the list of options mentioned above. Each option may be used once, more than once, or not at all.*

1. Medullary thyroid carcinoma
2. Carcinoid tumour
3. Renal tumour
4. Testicular teratoma
5. Bronchial carcinoma

## 76. ANSWERS

1. **B - Calcitonin**

2. **F - 5-Hydroxytryptamine**

3. **C - Erythropoeitin**

4. **E - α-Fetoprotein**

5. **A - ADH**

Bronchial carcinomas may secrete a variety of hormones including ACTH, ADH, cortisol and parathormone. Medullary thyroid carcinoma is known to secrete calcitonin which is used as a tumour marker and can be used in follow up to screen for recurrence. Renal carcinoma can present with anaemia or in the extreme end of the picture in polycythaemia (due to erythropoeitin release—seen in 4% of patients). Other hormones like renin and calcitonin may be produced by the tumour. Hypercalcaemia is common.

## 77. THEME: PALLIATIVE CARE

OPTIONS

A. Morphine
B. Codeine
C. Tramadol
D. Ibuprofen
E. Hyoscine
F. Radiotherapy
G. Senna
H. Paracetamol
I. Steroids

*For each of the scenarios listed below, select the next likely palliative intervention from the list of options mentioned above. Each option may be used once, more than once, or not at all.*

1. A 55-year-old smoker with features suggesting a superior vena cava (SVC) obstruction from a known non small cell lung carcinoma.

2. A 55-year-old smoker with a known advanced bronchial carcinoma presents with difficulty in breathing due to secretions.

3. A 55-year-old smoker with a known metastatic bronchial carcinoma continues to be in considerable bone pain despite taking full strength codeine.

4. A 55-year-old smoker with a known metastatic bronchial carcinoma is troubled with a severe constipation that he has had since being started on codeine.

5. A 55-year-old female known to have breast cancer presents with headache, nausea and vomiting. She is noted to have papilloedema.

## 77. ANSWERS

### 1. I - Steroids

Note that the next likely intervention is being asked. SVC obstruction is commonly from lung carcinoma or lymphoma. Features include dyspnoea, orthopnoea, facial and upper limb swelling, cough, plethora, cyanosis and venous engorgement. Dexamethasone is given first. Subsequently, urgent radiotherapy is needed for non small cell lung cancer, while chemotherapy is needed for lymphoma and small cell lung cancer.

### 2. E - Hyoscine

This is an antimuscarinic and plays a useful role in helping dry secretions.

### 3. D - Ibuprofen

Since the patient is on codeine, a combination non steroidal analgesic should be tried first. It is important to keep the analgesic ladder in mind, both for exams and for your own practice.

### 4. G - Senna

Opioids cause constipation. Laxatives should be routinely prescribed in these patients.

### 5. I - Steroids

This is most likely to suggest cerebral metastasis. Dexamethasone 4 mg every 6 hours is the recommended dose. This may be followed with radiotherapy or surgery for isolated metastasis.

## 78. THEME: EMBRYOLOGY

OPTIONS

A. 1st branchial pouch
B. 2nd branchial pouch
C. 3rd branchial pouch
D. 4th branchial pouch
E. 5th branchial pouch
F. 6th branchial pouch

*For each of the structures listed below, select the appropriate branchial pouch of origin from the list of options mentioned above. Each option may be used once, more than once, or not at all.*

1. Thymus

2. Superior parathyroid glands

3. Palatine tonsil

4. Eustachian tube

## 78. ANSWERS

1. **C - 3rd branchial pouch**

2. **D - 4th branchial pouch**

3. **B - 2nd branchial pouch**

4. **A - 1st branchial pouch**

The branchial apparatus consists of a series of six mesodermal arches formed during early gestation, separated externally by ectodermally lined branchial clefts and internally by endodermally lined pharyngeal pouches. Specific adult structures are derivated from each branchial arch and the related cleft and pouch. The first branchial cleft persists as the epithelium of the external auditory canal; the other branchial clefts are obliterated as the sinus of His disappears. From each mesodermal branchial arch, specific osseous, cartilaginous and vascular structures develop.

The first branchial arch contributes to facial development; the other arches also contribute to facial development, and are involved in the formation of the pharynx and larynx.

The first branchial pouch results in the eustachian tube. The second branchial pouch is involved in the formation of the palatine tonsil. The third branchial pouch forms the thymus and inferior parathyroid glands, while the fourth branchial pouch forms the superior parathyroid glands.

## 79. THEME: SKIN GRAFTING IN BURNS

OPTIONS

A. Tangential excision and grafting
B. Local steroid injection
C. Escharotomy
D. Wide excision and skin grafting
E. Silver sulfadiazine dressings

*For each of the scenarios described below, select the appropriate management option from the list mentioned above. Each option may be used once, more than once, or not at all.*

1. Marjolin's ulcer – right leg

2. Superficial burns to hand

3. Hypertrophic scar to right forearm

4. Deep dermal burns to thigh

## 79. ANSWERS

1. **D - Wide excision and skin grafting**

A Marjolin's ulcer is a squamous cell carcinoma that develops in an old scar often many years after the original injury. It requires a wide local excision and skin grafting.

2. **E - Silver sulfadiazine dressings**

It has antibacterial properties and can be applied as a coating to affected areas.

3. **B - Local steroid injection**

These are more common in children. Steroid injections are more effective in small raised scars.

4. **A - Tangential excision and grafting**

This is carried out 5–10 days after the burn injury and involves serial shaving of the burn wound until bleeding occurs from the surface.

## 80. THEME: ANTIPLATELET THERAPY

OPTIONS

A. Aspirin
B. Warfarin
C. Clopidogrel
D. Heparin
E. No treatment
F. Antistatin

*For each of the scenarios described below, select the most appropriate treatment option from the list of options mentioned above. Each option may be used once, more than once, or not at all.*

1. A 60-year-old male is seen by the GP for an ear infection. He complains of increasingly severe headaches and weakness in recent days. His blood pressure is recorded as 156/88 mm Hg. He also has a strong family history of ischaemic heart disease.

2. A 60-year-old driving instructor presents with bilateral calf claudication. The claudication distance is about 200 meters. He is a chronic smoker. He has weak foot pulses bilaterally. General and systemic examination is normal.

## 80. ANSWERS

1. **A - Aspirin**

This patient has hypertension and a family history of IHD. He therefore merits an antiplatelet as per the British Hypertensive Society guidelines.

2. **A - Aspirin**

This patient has peripheral vascular disease. He therefore also merits antiplatelet therapy.

## 81. THEME: TREATMENT OF BURNS

OPTIONS

A. Anaesthetize and intubate
B. Conservative management
C. Emollient cream
D. Referral to specialist burns unit
E. Intravenous fluids
F. Strong analgesia
G. Sedation

*For each of the burn scenarios described below, select the most appropriate option from the list of options above. Each option may be used once, more than once or not at all.*

1. A 25-year-old girl is admitted with 20% partial thickness burns over her chest, abdomen and back.

2. A 25-year-old girl is admitted with 7% full thickness burns over her abdomen.

3. A 25-year-old electrician is admitted with 2% full thickness burns over his right hand.

4. A 25-year-old male is admitted following a fire in his workplace. He complains of throat pain. He is conscious and oriented. He has signed nostrils on examination.

5. A 25-year-old boy is admitted with a 2% partial thickness burns involving his non dominant left hand.

## 81. ANSWERS

1. **E - Intravenous fluids**

2. **D - Referral to specialist burns unit**

3. **D - Referral to specialist burns unit**

4. **A - Anaesthetize and intubate**

5. **D - Referral to specialist burns unit**

Burns more than 10% in a child and more than 15% in adults requires intravenous fluid resuscitation. Parkland formula is most commonly used (4 X weight (kg) X % burns=mL crystalloid in 24 hours, half given within the first 8 hours). Full thickness burns more than 5% of body area and full/partial thickness burns involving face, hands, eyes or perineum need specialist attention. Remember that due to a larger surface area, volume ratio and few thermoregulatory compensatory mechanisms, there is a greater tendency in children to hypothermia. Remember non accidental injury.

## 82. THEME: PATHOLOGIES OF THE GROIN

OPTIONS

A. Psuedoaneurysm of femoral artery
B. Saphena varix
C. Strangulated femoral hernia
D. Strangulated obturator hernia
E. Psoas abscess
F. Strangulated inguinal hernia
G. Lymph varix
H. Sliding hernia
I. Aneurysm of femoral artery
J. Inguinal abscess

*For each of the patients described below, select the most likely diagnosis from the list of options above. Each option may be used once, more than once, or not at all.*

1. A middle aged immigrant presents with a swelling in the region of the right groin with a dull aching pain in his spine. Examination reveals a fluctuant, nontender swelling in the upper medial thigh. He is tender over the lower thoracic spine.

2. A young intravenous drug abuser presents with a swelling in the right groin. On examination, needle marks are visible in the groin. Palpation reveals a mildly tender pulsatile swelling in the right femoral triangle.

3. An 80-year-old lady is referred by the out of hours GP, with abdominal pain, distention and vomiting of 2 days duration. The patient is dehydrated, pale and hypotensive. On examination, she has a tense and tender swelling below and lateral to the pubic tubercle, with absent cough impulse.

4. An 80-year-old lady is referred by the out of hours GP, with abdominal pain, distention and vomiting of 2 days duration with the presence of a painful lump in the left groin. The patient also complains of left knee pain. The patient is dehydrated, pale and hypotensive. On examination, a tense lump is palpable below the pubic ramus. It is also felt on vaginal examination.

5. A middle aged lady is concerned she has noticed a lump in the region of the left groin. She is well otherwise. Examination reveals a soft, nontender swelling in the medial side of her left thigh which is below and lateral to the pubic tubercle. She has dilated veins in the left leg.

## 82. ANSWERS

1. **E - Psoas abscess.** Tuberculosis osteomyelitis is rare in UK. It is however occasionally seen in Asian immigrants. Involvements of the spine (Pott's disease) in lower thoracic and lumbar vertebrae may allow a cold abscess to track down the psoas muscle from its origin to its insertion in the lesser trochanter of the femur. It may then track through the subcutaneous fat and discharge through the skin. There is little inflammation and hence it is a 'cold' abscess.

Clues may include an Asian immigrant, raised ESR, a past history of tuberculosis and spinal tenderness.

2. **A - Psuedoaneurysm of femoral artery.** A false aneurysm of the artery may occur due to an accidental puncture of the femoral artery when attempting femoral vein injection. This injury leads to a local haematoma which becomes contained. A local bruit may be audible. An important feature is the presence of expansile pulsation in the femoral region.

3. **C - Strangulated femoral hernia.** A strangulated hernia is characterized by pain, irreducibility and absent cough impulse. In addition, features of obstruction and strangulation would usually give away the answer. Femoral hernia is differentiated from an inguinal hernia as it lies lateral and inferior to the pubic tubercle, while the inguinal hernia lies medial and above the pubic tubercle.

4. **D - Strangulated obturator hernia** An obturator hernia is 6 times more common in women and seen most frequently beyond 60 years of age. It seldom causes a swelling in the Scarpa's triangle, but if the limb is flexed, abducted and externally rotated, it becomes prominent. The patient may hold the ipsilateral leg in semi flexion to limit pain. In more than half of the cases with strangulation, pain is referred along the obturator nerve by its geniculate branch to the knee. Rectal/vaginal examination may occasionally confirm the presence of a tender swelling in the region of the obturator foramen.

5. **B - Saphena varix.** This is typically a saphena varix. It is a saccular, soft and compressible dilatation at the top of the saphenous vein. It often has a bluish tinge. It has an expansile cough impulse and reduces on lying down. A fluid thrill will be felt when the saphenous vein lower down is tapped (percussion or tap test).

## 83. THEME: LUMP IN THE GROIN

OPTIONS

A. Inguinal hernia
B. Ectopic testis
C. Lymph nodes
D. Incompletely descended testis
E. Encysted hydrocele of the cord
F. Saphena varix
G. Psoas abscess
H. Hydrocele of the canal of Nuck

*For each of the patients described below, select the most likely diagnosis from the list of options above. Each option may be used once, more than once, or not at all.*

1. A young male presents with an incidentally discovered swelling in his left groin. Examination reveals a smooth, oval, well defined nontender swelling in the left inguinal region. Cough impulse is negative. The swelling was incidentally observed to move downwards and become less mobile with downward testicular traction.

2. A 28-year-old male presents with a swelling in the left groin. On examination there is an indistinct mass across the groin, down the thigh along the long saphenous vein. He is also noted to have an infiltrating ulcer over his penile skin.

3. A 16-year-old boy presents with a swelling in the right groin. Examination reveals a smooth, oval, slightly tender, firm lump in the inguinal region just above and lateral to the pubic tubercle. The scrotum on that side is underdeveloped and empty.

4. A 45-year-old male presents with a lump in the left groin. Examination reveals a soft, nontender swelling in the left inguinal region above and medial to the pubic tubercle. Cough impulse is positive and the swelling reduces spontaneously on lying down.

## 83. ANSWERS

1. **E - Encysted hydrocele of the cord**

The picture is typical. A typical feature is that it is in continuity with the spermatic cord which enables downward movement when the testis is pulled downwards. The female counterpart of this condition is the hydrocele of the canal of Nuck. Here, the cyst lies in relation to the round ligament.

2. **C - Lymph nodes**

This patient most probably has a carcinoma involving his penis. It is important to remember the general rule that skin lymphatics follow the superficial veins whereas deep lymphatics follow the arteries. Lymph from the skin of the penis and the scrotum drains to the inguinal glands. Lymph from the testicular and spermatic coverings drains to the internal and, then, to the common iliac nodes. Lymph from the testis proper drains to the para-aortic glands.

3. **B - Ectopic testis**

The history is typical. Ectopic testis occurs in one of 4 different sites; superficial inguinal pouch (as in this case), femoral triangle, base of the penis and perineum.

4. **A - Inguinal hernia**

The typical location and features are suggestive of an inguinal hernia.

## 84. THEME: HERNIA

OPTIONS

A. Inguinal hernia
B. Epigastric hernia
C. Femoral hernia
D. Obturator hernia
E. Perineal hernia
F. Spigelian hernia
G. Lumbar hernia
H. Gluteal hernia

*For each hernial site listed below, select the most likely hernial type from the above list. Each answer may be used once, more than once, or not at all.*

1. Pelvic floor
2. Obturator canal
3. Linea alba
4. Hesselbach's triangle

## 84. ANSWERS

1. **E - Perineal hernia**

2. **D - Obturator hernia**

3. **B - Epigastric hernia**

4. **A - Inguinal hernia**

## 85. THEME: HERNIA

OPTIONS

A. Sciatic hernia
B. Paraumbilical hernia
C. Femoral hernia
D. Obturator hernia
E. Perineal hernia
F. Spigelian hernia
G. Lumbar hernia
H. Gluteal hernia

*For each hernial site listed below, select the most likely hernial type from the above list. Each answer may be used once, more than once, or not at all.*

1. Greater sciatic foramen

2. Lesser sciatic foramen

3. Linea semilunaris

4. Triangle of Petit

5. Linea alba

## 85. ANSWERS

1. **H - Gluteal hernia**

2. **A - Sciatic hernia**

3. **F - Spigelian hernia**

4. **G - Lumbar hernia**

5. **B - Paraumbilical hernia**

A gluteal hernia passes through the greater sciatic foramen, either above or below the piriformis. A sciatic hernia passes through the lesser sciatic foramen.

A paraumbilical hernia (syn. supraumbilical or infraumbilical hernia) does not occur through the umbilical scar. It is a protrusion through the linea alba just above or sometimes just below the umbilicus.

Most primary lumbar hernias occur through the inferior lumbar triangle of Petit. Less commonly, they occur through the superior lumbar triangle. Most lumbar hernias are secondary to renal surgery and a large incision is characteristic.

An obturator hernia passes through the obturator canal.

Spigelian hernias are a variant of interparietal or interstitial hernia occurring at the level of the arcuate line. Typically, a soft, reducible mass will be encountered in the infraumbilical region lateral to the rectus muscle. Diagnosis is confirmed by CT scan or ultrasound scan.

An epigastric hernia occurs through the linea alba anywhere between the xiphoid process and the umbilicus. Clinical features range from the symptomless to painful to referred pain (pain suggestive of peptic ulcer). Surgery should be undertaken for symptomatic cases.

Perineal hernia again is very rare. Of special interest to colorectal surgeons is the occurrence of postoperative hernia through a perineal scar after excision of the rectum.

## 86. THEME: HERNIA

OPTIONS

A. Sliding hernia
B. Richter's hernia
C. Laugier's hernia
D. Narath's hernia
E. Littre's hernia
F. Maydl's hernia
G. Prevesical hernia
H. Epiplocele

*For each of the descriptions listed below, select the most appropriate hernia from the above list. Each option may be used once, more than once, or not at all.*

1. Presence of Meckel's diverticulum as a content of the sac.

2. Presence of a portion of the circumference of the intestine.

3. Presence of omentum as the content of the sac.

4. Hernia through a gap in the lacunar ligament.

5. The posterior wall of the hernial sac is formed by a portion of the bladder.

## 86. ANSWERS

1. **E - Littre's hernia**

2. **B - Richter's hernia**

3. **H - Epiplocele**

4. **C - Laugier's hernia**
This is herniation through a gap in the Gimbernat's (lacunar) ligament.

5. **A - Sliding hernia**
The posterior wall of the sac is not formed of peritoneum alone, but by the sigmoid colon and its mesentery on the left, the caecum on the right and sometimes, on either side by a portion of the bladder.

## 87. THEME: HERNIA

OPTIONS

A. Ventral hernia
B. Inflamed hernia
C. Laugier's hernia
D. Narath's hernia
E. Littre's hernia
F. Maydl's hernia
G. Prevesical hernia
H. Pantaloon hernia

*For each of the descriptions listed below, select the most appropriate hernia from the above list. Each option may be used once, more than once, or not at all.*

1. Presence of two separate loops of bowel as the content.

2. Two sacs straddling the inferior epigastric artery one on either side.

3. Presence of a large scar atop a midline hernia.

4. Occurrence of a hernia in congenital dislocation of the hip due to lateral displacement of the psoas muscle.

## 87. ANSWERS

1. **F - Maydl's hernia**

2. **H - Pantaloon hernia**

3. **A - Ventral hernia**

4. **D - Narath's hernia**

Narath's hernia occurs only in patients with CDH. The hernia lies hidden behind the femoral vessels.

Pantaloon hernia is an important cause of immediate postoperative recurrence, one of the sacs having been overlooked at surgery. It is also an important fallacy of the deep ring occlusion test in hernia examination.

## 88. THEME: HERNIA

OPTIONS

A. Paraumbilical hernia
B. Inflamed hernia
C. Laugier's hernia
D. Lumbar hernia
E. Cloquet's hernia
F. Maydl's hernia
G. Prevesical hernia
H. Omphalocele

*For each of the descriptions listed below, select the most appropriate hernia from the above list. Each option may be used once, more than once, or not at all.*

1. Protrusion of prevesical fat and a portion of the bladder that protrude through a small defect in the conjoined muscle.

2. Presence of liver, spleen, stomach outside the abdomen through a defect.

3. Presence of a sac under the fascia covering the pectineus muscle.

4. Presence of acute salpingitis within the hernial sac.

5. Large red, hot trophic ulcers in the dependent aspect of a large umbilical hernia.

## 88. ANSWERS

1. **G - Prevesical hernia**

2. **H - Omphalocele**

3. **E - Cloquet's hernia**

4. **B - Inflamed hernia**

5. **B - Inflamed hernia**

Prevesical hernia is different from a sliding hernia involving the bladder. A portion of the bladder may form the posterior wall of the hernia constituting a sliding hernia. In a prevesical hernia, however, a portion of the bladder and prevesical fat protrude through a small defect in the medial part of the conjoined muscle just above the pubic tubercle.

Inflammations of the contents of the sac (e.g., acute appendicitis, salpingitis) or from external causes (e.g., the trophic ulcers which develop in the dependent areas of a large umbilical or incisional hernia) constitute an inflamed hernia.

## 89. THEME: INDIRECT HERNIA

OPTIONS

A. Infantile
B. Congenital
C. Bubonocele
D. Funicular
E. Scrotal
F. Vaginal

*For each of the descriptions listed below, select the most appropriate variant of indirect hernia from the above list. Each option may be used once, more than once, or not at all.*

1. Hernia limited to the inguinal canal.

2. A complete hernia.

3. The processus vaginalis is closed just above the epididymis.

## 89. ANSWERS

1. **C - Bubonocele**

2. **E - Scrotal**

The testis appears to lie within the lower part of the hernia.

3. **D - Funicular**

The testis lies below the hernia. The testis is felt separately from the hernia.

## 90. THEME: REPAIR OF HERNIA

OPTIONS

A. Herniotomy
B. Bassini repair
C. Shouldice repair
D. Gilbert's repair
E. Lichtenstein tension free mesh hernioplasty
F. Mass closure
G. Laparoscopic repair
H. McEvedy repair
I. Lothiessen repair
J. Abrahamson's darning
K. Laparotomy

*For each of the descriptions listed below, select the most appropriate method of hernia repair from the above list. Each option may be used once, more than once, or not at all.*

1. A 2-year-old baby boy is seen with a congenital hernia on the right side.

2. A 45-year-old male is referred with painful recurrent right inguinal hernia. He has had 2 repairs in the past.

3. A 65-year-old male is seen for follow up in your clinic with a 6 cm midline incisional hernia after emergency laparotomy he underwent for a perforated duodenal ulcer 6 months ago.

4. A 65-year-old male presents to A&E with features suggestive of obstruction. An irreducible lump is palpable in the right groin below and lateral to the pubic tubercle.

## 90. ANSWERS

1. **A - Herniotomy**

Congenital hernias are more common in males with a high incidence in preterm infants. Repair should be undertaken immediately after diagnosis due to the high chance of incarceration.

2. **G - Laparoscopic repair**

The best method of repairing recurrent inguinal hernia is laparoscopic with the advantage being approach and repair through virgin previously unexplored tissue.

3. **G - Laparoscopic repair**

Laparoscopy is now making big inroads in incisional hernia repair and is considered the treatment of choice in many institutions where technical expertise is available.

4. **H - McEvedy repair**

McEvedy repair involving a transverse (unilateral Pfannenstiel) incision is preferred in the emergency setting. The Lockwood (low approach) should only be preferred in the elective setting.

## 91. THEME: SKIN LESIONS

OPTIONS

A. Squamous cell carcinoma
B. Bowen's disease
C. Superficial spreading malignant melanoma
D. Nodular melanoma
E. Basal cell carcinoma
F. Acral lentiginous malignant melanoma
G. Keratoacanthoma
H. Ganglion
I. Chloasma

*For each of the patients described below, select the most likely diagnosis from the list of options above. Each option may be used once, more than once, or not at all.*

1. A 70-year-old residential home resident presents with a lesion on her cheek that had been increasing in size rapidly over the past 2 months. On examination she has a 7 mm hemispherical nodule that has a rolled edge and a central horny plug.

2. A 70-year-old residential home resident presents with a lesion on her cheek which is hyperkeratotic and ulcerated. The nodular area on the edge has been noted to be growing rapidly.

3. A 70-year-old residential home resident presents with a progressively increasing flat, red scaly plaque on the trunk. The GP has been treating the patient for a solar keratosis with topical steroid application with no benefit.

4. A 25-year-old pregnant girl presents with increasing pigmentation on her face.

5. A 70-year-old residential home resident presents with a spot on the face. Examination reveals a nodular swelling with pearly rolled edge and telangiectatic vessels.

## 91. ANSWERS

### 1. G - Keratoacanthoma

This is a benign condition resulting from a rapidly growing collection of hair follicles. It often regresses spontaneously for which reason treatment is usually conservative. Indications for removal include (1) Doubtful cases where malignancy cannot be excluded, and (2) Cosmetic reasons. It is important to remember that clinically there is never any extension into local tissues and local lymph nodes should not be involved.

### 2. A - Squamous cell carcinoma

This is a typical presentation. These tumours appear more red, indurated and ulcerate sooner compared to basal cell carcinoma. Sunlight/ ultraviolet light is known aetiological factor. Occasionally they arise as a complication of long standing chronic granulomas like syphilis, lupus vulgaris and leprosy, chronic ulcers, osteomyelitis, and long standing burn scars or venous scars (the last two are a favorite with the examiners). Histological features include invasive nests of cells showing variable central keratinisation and horn cell formation.

### 3. B - Bowen's disease

Treatment options for large lesions include radiotherapy and chemotherapy. For smaller lesions surgical excision remains the best treatment option.

### 4. I - Chloasma

### 5. E - Basal cell carcinoma

85% of these tumours occur in the head and neck region. Commonest histological variant is the nodular form. Surgery is the treatment of choice. For small superficial lesions electrodessication and curettage can be tried. Importantly, these tumours are radiosensitive. This can be attempted in elderly patients unsuitable for surgery or for specialized anatomical sites.

## 92. THEME: SOFT TISSUE SWELLINGS

OPTIONS

A. Neuroma
B. Lipoma
C. Ganglion
D. Desmoid tumour
E. Rhabdomyosarcoma
F. Glomus tumour
G. Pyogenic granuloma
H. Oral cancer
I. Schwannoma

*For each of the patients described below, select the most likely diagnosis from the list of options above. Each option may be used once, more than once, or not at all.*

1. A 40-year-old male presents with a lump on his lower lip which has appeared and rapidly increased in size over the past week following a minor injury. Examination reveals a red, soft 5 mm pedunculated nodule that looks like a haemangioma.

2. A 40-year-old male presents with a lump on the dorsal aspect of his right wrist joint that disappears on extension of the joint.

3. These lumps arise following trauma. They are very painful and are characteristically described as a complication of amputation stump formation.

4. This tumour is commonly found in the nail bed and causes pain that is out of proportion to the size of the tumour which is only a few millimeters.

5. These lobulated and encapsulated tumours arise from the neurilemmal cells. They are soft and whitish in appearance.

6. These non malignant tumours are composed of highly vascular connective tissue containing multinucleated plasmodial masses resembling foreign body giant cells. An intraperitoneal form is associated with familial adenomatous polyposis.

## 92. ANSWERS

1. **G - Pyogenic granuloma**

These are commonly acquired reactive, proliferative vascular lesions of the skin and mucous membranes. They arise after minor trauma. They are most commonly seen on the face, lips, the fingers and toes. Treatment is excision.

2. **C - Ganglion**

A ganglion is a cystic, myxomatous degeneration of fibrous tissue found most commonly over the dorsum of the hand over the scapulolunate ligament.

3. **A - Neuroma**

The description is classically one of a false neuroma. It arises from the connective tissue of the nerve sheath after injury to a nerve (laceration or amputation). They consist of fibrous tissue and coiled nerve fibres. In contrast, true neuromas are rare tumours and include ganglioneuroma, neuroblastoma and myelinic neuroma.

4. **F - Glomus tumour**

This tumour arises from a cutaneous glomus which is a specialized organ that regulates the temperature of the skin. In addition to the points already mentioned, it is important to remember that this tumour causes pain that is burning in nature and radiates peripherally. It is more often noticeable when the limb is exposed to sudden changes in temperature.

5. **I - Schwannoma**

This is synonymous with neurilemmoma.

6. **D - Desmoid tumour**

A desmoid tumour arises in the musculoaponeurotic structures of the abdominal wall below the level of the umbilicus. It is a completely unencapsulated fibroma and creaks when cut. They can also occur in cases of familial polyposis coli (Gardner's syndrome).

## 93. THEME: SKIN LESIONS

OPTIONS

A. Basal cell carcinoma
B. Squamous cell carcinoma
C. Keratoacanthoma
D. Dermoid cyst
E. Dermatofibroma
F. Malignant melanoma

*For each of the patients described below, select the most likely diagnosis from the list of options above. Each option may be used once, more than once, or not at all.*

1. A 5-year-old boy is brought by parents with a small midline swelling in the neck.

2. A 5-year-old boy is brought in by concerned parents with a lump at the outer orbit of the left eye. Examination reveals a 2 cm ovoid, smooth, soft cystic lump.

3. A 30-year-old male presents with a 2 cm lump in the right leg. It appears brownish and looks more like a mole. Biopsy suggests a benign neoplasm of the fibroblasts of the dermis.

## 93. ANSWERS

1. **D - Dermoid cyst**

2. **D - Dermoid cyst**

They are found at the sites of closure of embryonal fissures. They may be found at the inner or outer angles of the orbit, the midline of the neck or the scalp.

3. **E - Dermatofibroma**

These are fixed to the epidermis and are mobile. They are more common on the lower limbs and result from minor trauma or an insect bite which causes a reactive proliferation of histiocytes (it is also known as hystiocytoma or sclerosing angioma). Biopsy is characteristic.

## 94. THEME: MANAGEMENT OF SKIN CANCERS

OPTIONS

A. Radiotherapy
B. Local excision with 3 mm margin
C. Local excision with 6 mm margin
D. Local excision with 10 mm margin
E. Local excision with 30 mm margin
F. Local excision with 50 mm margin

*For each description of skin cancer below, select the most likely management from the list of options above. Each option may be used once, more than once, or not at all.*

1. A cystic basal cell carcinoma lesion at the inner canthus of the eye.

2. Sclerosing basal cell carcinoma over the cheek.

3. Superficial spreading melanoma less than 1 mm thick.

4. Basal cell carcinoma fixed to bone.

## 94. ANSWERS

1. **B - Local excision with 3 mm margin**
This should be sufficient in a cystic basal cell carcinoma especially at this location which is cosmetically important. Radiotherapy is contraindicated as it may produce scarring or radiation dermatitis.

2. **C - Local excision with 6 mm margin**
This variant does not have a clearly defined edge and hence a wider margin of excision is needed to prevent local recurrence.

3. **D - Local excision with a 10 mm margin**
Remember, as a general rule, a margin of 1 cm for each mm Breslow thickness is appropriate.

4. **A - Radiotherapy**
Fixation to bone is an indication for radiotherapy.

## 95. THEME: UPPER GASTROINTESTINAL HAEMORRHAGE

OPTIONS

A. Mallory-Weiss tear
B. Oesophageal varices
C. Gastric tumour
D. Gastric ulcer
E. Angiodysplasia
F. Stress ulceration
G. Aortic enteric fistula
H. Dieulafoy's disease

*For each of the patients described below, select the most appropriate diagnosis from the above list. Each option may be used once, more than once, or not at all.*

1. A 76-year-old male presents with an episode of small, fresh bright red haematemesis. On examination the patient is quite pale. His blood pressure is 110/60 mm Hg with a pulse rate 86/min. He is quite pale. There is a history of anorexia and weight loss for the last 6 months.

2. A middle aged heavily drunk man presents with an episode of small, fresh bright red haematemesis. There is no obvious pallor. His blood pressure is 118/70 mm Hg with a pulse rate of 94/min. He gives a history of a forceful vomiting immediately after consumption of alcohol an hour earlier.

3. A 60-year-old known alcoholic presents with sudden onset painless vomiting of copious volumes of dark-red blood. Cachexia and gross pallor are evident on examination. His blood pressure is 70 mm Hg systolic and his pulse is 134/min. He has ascites.

4. A 76-year-old lady presents to A&E with a large painless 'coffee ground' vomitus. Her blood pressure is 98/60 mm Hg. She gives a history of dyspepsia related to ingestion of food.

5. A 33-year-old male in the intensive care unit for the last 13 days following neurosurgery after a RTA is seen to bring up some coffee ground vomitus. His observations are stable.

## 95. ANSWERS

1. **C - Gastric tumour**
Bleeding is usually not torrential but may be unremitting. The presence of anorexia and weight loss should raise the possibility of a tumour. Oesophageal carcinoma is a rare cause of upper GI bleeding.

2. **A - Mallory-Weiss tear**
Bright red bloody vomit usually preceded by forceful vomiting without blood usually clinches the diagnosis (for the purpose of the exam). Vigorous vomiting produces a vertical split which is in the gastric mucosa immediately below the squamocolumnar junction at the cardia in 90% of cases. It involves the oesophagus in 10% of cases.

3. **B - Oesophageal varices**
Clues which might be included in the exam include any of the signs of liver failure, encephalopathy, ascites or other signs of portal hypertension.

4. **D - Gastric ulcer**
History suggestive of peptic ulceration in the past should clinch this diagnosis. Ingestion of NSAIDs may be an important clue. NSAIDs can also cause erosive gastritis.

5. **F - Stress ulceration**
This is seen in patients with major injury/illness, following major surgery or those who have major co-morbidity.

## 96. THEME: GASTROINTESTINAL HAEMORRHAGE

OPTIONS

A. Mallory-Weiss tear
B. Oesophageal varices
C. Gastric tumour
D. Posterior duodenal ulcer
E. Angiodysplasia
F. Stress ulceration
G. Aortic enteric fistula
H. Dieulafoy's disease
I. Caecal carcinoma
J. Anterior duodenal ulcer

*For each of the patients described below, select the most appropriate diagnosis from the above list. Each option may be used once, more than once, or not at all.*

1. A 65-year-old is referred by the GP with a 2-month history of anorexia, weight loss, tiredness and weakness. Examination reveals pallor. He also demonstrates a palpable mass in the right iliac fossa.

2. A 55-year-old lady known to have severe rheumatoid arthritis and atrial fibrillation is admitted with acute onset abdominal pain, pallor and melaena. While in hospital she throws up huge amounts of blood in the vomitus.

3. A 65-year-old chronic alcoholic presents with malaena. On examination the patient is drowsy. Abdominal examination confirms the presence of ascites and splenomegaly.

4. A 65-year-old male known to have aortic stenosis presents with acute onset painless bleeding per rectum. He requires transfusion of a few units of blood. He is not known to have diverticular disease. A barium enema examination is normal. Colonoscopy is subsequently undertaken and it shows a reddish raised area in the ascending colon.

## 96. ANSWERS

1. **I - Caecal carcinoma**

That was a simple question. Chronic blood loss due to the mass is the most likely cause of anaemia resulting in tiredness and weakness.

2. **D - Posterior duodenal ulcer**

This is the most likely answer from the list of options enlisted above. Bleeding is usually a feature of posterior duodenal ulcers due to erosion of the gastroduodenal artery.

3. **B - Oesophageal varices**

Clues which might be included in the exam include any of the signs of liver failure, encephalopathy, ascites or other signs of portal hypertension.

4. **E - Angiodysplasia**

This is another favorite with the examiners. There is an association with aortic stenosis as mentioned in the question. It is seen in elderly patients over the age of 60 years and the characteristic sites include the ascending colon and caecum. If the bleeding is not too brisk, a colonoscopy may show the characteristic lesion. Selective superior and inferior mesenteric angiography shows the site and extent of the lesion by a blush. If this fails, a radioactive test using technetium-99m labelled red cells may localize the source of haemorrhage.

## 97. THEME: GASTROINTESTINAL HAEMORRHAGE

OPTIONS

A. Barium swallow
B. Barium enema
C. Gastrografin enema
D. Laparoscopy
E. Upper GI endoscopy
F. CT colonography
G. Colonoscopy
H. Technetium-99m scanning

*For each of the patients described below, select the most appropriate investigation from the above list. Each option may be used once, more than once, or not at all.*

1. A 22-year-old male presents with repeated episodes of maroon bleeding per rectum. There is no history of abdominal pain, vomiting or distention. Both upper GI endoscopy and colonoscopy are normal.

2. A 77-year-old lady is admitted with passage of blood per rectum. His blood pressure is 106/68 mm Hg and his pulse rate is 86/min. He has recently been complaining of a change in bowel habits.

3. A 60-year-old known alcoholic presents with sudden onset painless vomiting of copious volumes of dark-red blood. His blood pressure is 70 mm Hg systolic and his pulse is 134/min.

4. A 60-year-old known alcoholic patient is admitted to A&E department with passage of large clots of fresh blood per rectum. There is no history of vomiting or haematemesis. His blood pressure is 70 mm Hg systolic with a pulse rate of 135.

5. A 22-year-old male is referred by the GP with a few episodes of bright red rectal bleeding. Rigid sigmoidoscopy and proctoscopy do not reveal any abnormality.

## 97. ANSWERS

1. **H - Technetium-99m scanning**

Meckel's diverticulum is suspected in this case. In cases of suspected GI haemorrhage, where a Meckel's diverticulum is suspected, the abdomen is imaged with gamma camera after the injection of 30–100 μCi of 99mTc-labelled pertechnetate intravenously.

2. **G - Colonoscopy**

This patient most probably has either a colorectal cancer or diverticular disease. Colonoscopy would be the preferred investigation in this case for the simple reason that it would facilitate biopsy if need be.

3. **E - Upper GI endoscopy**

This patient is probably bleeding from his oesophageal varices. Most centres would employ sclerotherapy using 5% ethanolamine oleate in these cases. Endoscopic banding has shown encouraging early results with a lower incidence of oesophageal ulceration and may replace sclerotherapy in the future.

4. **E - Upper GI endoscopy**

This patient is probably bleeding from a peptic ulcer. As a rule any patient who attends A&E with massive fresh rectal bleeding sufficient to cause a haemodynamic compromise should undergo an upper GI endoscopy to exclude a bleeding peptic ulcer.

5. **G - Colonoscopy**

This patient most probably has a polyp. Colonoscopy is recommended because of its higher sensitivity and specificity and the advantage of being therapeutic when compared to a standard barium enema.

## 98. THEME: RECTAL BLEEDING

OPTIONS

A. Familial adenomatous polyposis
B. Colorectal cancer
C. Diverticular disease
D. Intussusception
E. Juvenile polyp
F. Anal fissure
G. Crohn's disease
H. Anal carcinoma

*For each of the patients described below, select the most likely cause of rectal bleeding from the above list. Each option may be used once, more than once, or not at all.*

1. A 62-year-old male presents with a 6-week history of intermittent bright red rectal bleeding associated with pain, mucus discharge and tenesmus. Examination reveals an area of ulceration at the anal verge with the presence of a mass in the left inguinal region.

2. An 8-year-old boy presents with a 4-week history of pain in the right iliac fossa with intermittent fevers, rectal bleeding, and anaemia and weight loss.

3. A teenager with a family history of colorectal cancer is referred by the GP with a complaint of painless bleeding per rectum.

4. A preschool kid is brought to the GP with painless bleeding, mixed with stool.

5. A 24-year-old postpartum lady presents with a 2-week history of slight bright streaks of blood on the toilet paper. This is associated with mucus discharge, constipation, straining and pain.

## 98. ANSWERS

**1. H - Anal carcinoma**

The presence of bleeding, pain, tenesmus and mucus discharge in a 62-year-old male should arouse suspicion for cancer. The presence of an ulcer at the anal verge with the presence of inguinal lymph nodes most probably represents an anal carcinoma. Additional clues may include: (1) Homosexual male, (2) Association with human papilloma virus type 16 and (3) Presence of an ulcer with typical neoplastic features in the anal canal or verge. Typical clinical features include rectal bleeding, mucus discharge, tenesmus, the sensation of a lump in the anus and a change in bowel habit.

**2. G - Crohn's disease**

The presence of Crohn's disease can be varied. There is often a history of mild diarrhoea extending over many months occurring in bouts accompanied by intestinal colic. There may be pain, particularly in the right iliac fossa with a tender palpable mass. Intermittent fever, secondary anaemia and weight loss is common. An important clue may be the presence of anal conditions (e.g., perianal abscess, fissure or fistulae). Children who develop this illness before puberty exhibit retarded growth and sexual development.

**3. A - Familial adenomatous polyposis**

A family history of colorectal cancer should raise the possibility of FAP as the likely diagnosis. Polyps are usually visible on sigmoidoscopy by the age of 15 years. Carcinoma of the large bowel occurs 10–20 years after the onset of polyposis. If the diagnosis is made during the adolescence, operation is deferred usually till the age of 18 years.

**4. E - Juvenile polyp**

This is a relatively common cause of painless bleeding per rectum. They are classified as hamartomatous polyps and may occur occasionally as multiple lesions in the colon. They are often associated with a congenital defect such as a malrotation or Meckel's diverticulum. They have minimal malignant potential.

**5. F - Anal fissure**

Anal fissure occur in the midline posteriorly in 90% of cases. An anterior anal fissure is much more common in women, particularly in those who have borne children. Symptoms include pain, bleeding, constipation and discharge. Additional clues include the presence of a sentinel tag and a tightly closed, puckered anus on examination.

## 99. THEME: DYSPHAGIA

OPTIONS

A. Oesophageal carcinoma
B. Benign oesophageal stricture
C. Achalasia cardia
D. Diffuse oesophageal spasm
E. Para-oesophageal hernia
F. Pharyngeal pouch
G. Plummer-Vinson syndrome
H. Retrosternal goiter

*For each of the patients described below, select the most likely cause of dysphagia from the above list. Each option may be used once, more than once, or not at all.*

1. A 72-year-old female presents with dysphagia and regurgitation of undigested food. She has seen her GP in recent times for recurrent chest infections. She has noticed a visible swelling in the neck on occasions.

2. A 60-year-old immigrant from Africa presents with dysphagia, lethargy and generalized weakness. She is grossly anaemic on examination with evidence of koilonychias, cheilosis and angular stomatitis.

3. A 54-year-old man presents with dysphagia, odynophagia and substernal midline constricting chest pain. A cardiac cause for pain has been ruled out and barium swallow demonstrates a typical 'corkscrew' oesophagus.

4. A middle aged lady presents with intermittent dysphagia for solids and liquids, which is exacerbated by stress for many years. She has recently noticed regurgitation. Barium swallow shows a typical 'bird's beak' appearance.

5. A 60-year-old smoker presents with a 6-month history of progressive dysphagia, anorexia and weight loss. Examination reveals cervical lymphadenopathy.

## 99. ANSWERS

1. **F - Pharyngeal pouch.** This condition is twice as common in women as in men. Initially the patients present with globus type symptoms of a feeling of something in the throat. As the diverticulum enlarges patients may experience regurgitation of undigested food. Clues may include (1) Waking up in the middle of the night with a feeling of tightness in the chest, (2) Fits of unexplained coughing, (3) Unexplained recurrent chest infections, (4) Gurgling noises from the neck on swallowing and a (5) Visible swelling in the neck which increases with intake of food.

2. **G - Plummer-Vinson syndrome.** This syndrome is associated with prolonged iron deficiency anaemia. It is characterized by microcytic hypochromic anaemia in addition to features already mentioned. There may also be atrophic inflammation of the mucosa of the pharynx and upper oesophagus with areas of hyperkeratosis, ulceration and the formation of high, usually anteriorly placed oesophageal webs. Long term follow up is needed due to the risk of developing upper oesophageal cancer.

3. **D - Diffuse oesophageal spasm.** Presence of retrosternal chest pain with dysphagia is characteristic. Weight loss is not a feature of this condition. Endoscopy is usually unremarkable, where a barium swallow may reveal intense muscle contractions which may appear as a 'cork screw'. Treatment with long-acting nitrates can provide temporary relief of symptoms. Benzodiazepines and psychotropic drugs may be effective in some patients and pneumatic dilatation may help.

4. **C - Achalasia cardia.** This is due to loss of ganglion cells in Auerbach's plexus, which causes a failure of relaxation at the lower end of the oesophagus. There is progressive dysphagia to both solids and liquids. A firm diagnosis can be made by oesophageal manometry which shows a hypertensive lower oesophageal sphincter which does not relax completely on swallowing. Barium meal shows a typical bird beak appearance. There is no gas bubble in the stomach on plain radiography because no bolus with its accompanying normal gas bubble ever passes through the sphincter. The oesophagus becomes dilated and tortuous (mega-oesophagus) which may give an impression of a 'double right heart border'.

5. **A - Oesophageal carcinoma** This is a typical history for oesophageal carcinoma. Complications include cough/pneumonia from overspill, tracheo-oesophageal fistula, aorto-oesophageal fistula and hoarseness of voice due to recurrent laryngeal nerve palsy, all of which are signs of advanced and incurable disease. Palpable lymphadenopathy is likewise a sign of advanced disease.

## 100. THEME: ACUTE ABDOMEN

OPTIONS

A. Acute pancreatitis
B. Biliary colic
C. Perforated peptic ulcer
D. Acute cholecystitis
E. Acute appendicitis
F. Ruptured ectopic pregnancy
G. Ruptured spleen
H. Ruptured AAA

*For each of the patients described below, select the most likely cause of acute abdomen from the above list. Each option may be used once, more than once, or not at all.*

1. A 21-year-old girl presents with a day's history of central abdominal pain followed by the right iliac fossa. She is mildly pyrexial at 38°C with guarding and rebound tenderness in the right iliac fossa.

2. A middle aged female presents with severe colicky upper abdominal pain radiating to the right shoulder. Inflammatory markers are normal.

3. A 55-year-old male, a known case of rheumatoid arthritis, on NSAIDs presents with severe abdominal pain. Abdomen is distended with guarding and rigidity. Erect chest X-ray shows free gas under the dome of the right hemidiaphragm.

4. An 8-weeks pregnant teenaged girl presents to A&E with acute onset of lower abdominal pain radiating to the right shoulder. She is pale and hypotensive on examination.

5. A middle aged male of African origin is brought to A&E after being involved in a RTA. He has upper abdominal pain with guarding. Bruises and palpable rib fractures are evident over the left lower rib cage. He is hypotensive (BP 70/50 mm Hg) with a pulse of 146/min.

## 100. ANSWERS

1. **E - Acute appendicitis**

2. **B - Biliary colic**

Biliary colic is typically caused by a stone in the common bile duct. It is characterized by sudden onset colicky abdominal pain in the right upper quadrant with radiation to the right scapular region or right shoulder. There may be associated nausea and vomiting. Inflammatory markers are usually normal.

3. **C - Perforated peptic ulcer**

Presentation is typical. The patient, who may have a history of peptic ulcer disease or NSAIDs ingestion, develops sudden onset severe generalized pain. The abdomen does not move with respiration. There is a board like rigidity. The commonest site of perforation is the anterior aspect of the duodenum. All patients should have serum amylase performed as distinguishing between peptic ulcer, perforation and pancreatitis may be difficult. The initial priorities in treatment are resuscitation and adequate analgesia. Treatment is principally surgical.

4. **F - Ruptured ectopic pregnancy**

This is the 1st possibility in any sexually active women presenting with abdominal pain or bleeding. Tubal colic causes abdominal pain, which may precede vaginal bleeding. Usually there is a history of a missed menstrual period. Pregnancy test will be positive. Cervical excitation produces pain. Signs of intraperitoneal bleeding become apparent with referred pain to the shoulder. Pelvic ultrasonography is the investigation of choice when an ectopic pregnancy is suspected.

5. **G - Ruptured spleen**

Splenic rupture should be suspected after any trauma, especially a closed injury caused by direct external violence. Even trivial trauma can sometimes rupture a spleen especially in diseased or enlarged spleen, e.g., malaria, infectious mononucleosis and haematological malignancies. Clinical features include shock, upper abdominal guarding, local bruising and abdominal distention. Kehr's sign, which is pain referred to the left shoulder, may be an important clue.

## 101. THEME: ACUTE ABDOMEN

OPTIONS

A. Acute pancreatitis
B. Biliary colic
C. Perforated peptic ulcer
D. Acute cholecystitis
E. Strangulated femoral hernia
F. Mesenteric ischaemia
G. Acute intestinal obstruction
H. Ruptured abdominal aortic aneurysm

*For each of the patients described below, select the most likely cause of acute abdomen from the above list. Each option may be used once, more than once, or not at all.*

1. An 85-year-old male is brought to A&E with sudden onset of abdominal pain radiating to back for a few hours duration. He looks pale. His BP is 80/58 mm Hg and his pulse rate is 125/min.

2. A 55-year-old obese lady presents with sudden onset severe colicky pain in the upper abdomen. She complains of nausea and vomiting. On examination her temperature is 38.1°C. She has guarding in the right upper quadrant on examination.

3. A 76-year-old male presents with severe abdominal pain. On examination, however, the abdomen is soft. His ECG shows atrial fibrillation.

4. A young woman presents with sudden onset severe abdominal pain and some rectal bleeding. She has an Hb of 18 g/dL with leucocytosis and evidence of severe metabolic acidosis on blood gases.

5. An 88-year-old female presents in shock to A&E. She complains of abdominal distention, pain, vomiting and constipation of 2 days duration. On examination she has a tender lump in her right groin.

## 101. ANSWERS

**1. H - Ruptured abdominal aortic aneurysm**

A diagnosis of ruptured or leaking aortic aneurysm should be considered in any elderly male presenting with abdominal pain radiating to the back. Features of shock may be evident. Abdominal signs including distention, guarding and rigidity may also be evident. Immediate surgical intervention is mandatory.

**2. D - Acute cholecystitis**

The patient usually has episodes of right subcostal pain to begin with. As the condition progresses, the patient becomes systemically unwell. Pain becomes continuous, and is associated with nausea, vomiting and pyrexia. The patient will be tender in the right subcostal area and may develop guarding, rigidity and a palpable mass. The main difference from biliary colic is the inflammatory component (local peritonism, fever and raised white cell count and CRP). In more than 90% of cases the symptoms of acute cholecystitis subside with conservative management.

**3. F - Mesenteric ischaemia**

**4. F - Mesenteric ischaemia**

Acute mesenteric ischaemia is caused by sudden occlusion of the SMA due to thrombosis or embolism, or an acute thrombosis of the mesenteric veins. Atrial fibrillation may have been responsible for an embolic event (which accounts for 25–30% of patients) in the first scenario. In the 2nd variant polycythaemia leading to hyperviscosity and thrombosis is the most likely aetiology. Acute mesenteric ischaemia is characterized by severe abdominal pain which is out of proportion to abdominal signs. Later signs of acute abdomen develop with evidence of GI blood loss. Leucocytosis and severe metabolic acidosis will usually clinch the diagnosis.

**5. E - Strangulated femoral hernia**

Additional clues may include the presence of a tense, tender, irreducible hernia with absence of cough impulse.

## 102. THEME: ABDOMINAL PAIN

OPTIONS

A. Ischaemic colitis
B. Biliary colic
C. Perforated peptic ulcer
D. Acute cholecystitis
E. Acute pancreatitis
F. Mesenteric ischaemia
G. Disc prolapse
H. Ruptured abdominal aortic aneurysm

*For each of the patients described below, select the most likely cause of abdominal pain from the above list. Each option may be used once, more than once, or not at all.*

1. A 40-year-old chronic alcoholic presents with severe epigastric pain radiating to the back, associated with several episodes of vomiting. She is tender with guarding in the epigastrium.

2. A 50-year-old male presents with acute onset abdominal pain and vomiting. His BP is 90/76 mm Hg with a pulse rate of 110/min. His abdomen is distended with presence of generalized guarding and rigidity. Percussion reveals a resonant note over the liver.

3. A 40-year-old grossly obese lady with known cholecystitis presents to A&E with abdominal pain, shock and anuria. She has mild icterus on examination.

4. A 30-year-old male on steroids for rheumatoid arthritis presents to A&E with abdominal pain, back pain and some bruising in the flanks. Patient has marked tachypnoea and tachycardia.

5. A 76-year-old male presents with sudden onset severe back pain, which he attributes to lifting heavy weights. His feet are cold. His pulse rate is 122/min with a blood pressure 86 mm Hg systolic.

## 102. ANSWERS

1. **E - Acute pancreatitis**

2. **C - Perforated peptic ulcer**

3. **E - Acute pancreatitis**

4. **E - Acute pancreatitis**

Acute pancreatitis can mimic most causes of the acute abdomen. It should be considered in any patient who develops shock or anuria regardless of whether they have abdominal pain. Patient in scenario 1 is an alcoholic with typical epigastric pain radiating to the back. Patient in scenario 3 most probably has gallstone pancreatitis. Nausea, vomiting and retching are usual accompaniments. Features of shock, tachycardia, and tachypnoea may be evident. Features suggesting a gall stone pancreatitis include mild icterus and a swinging pyrexia suggesting cholangitis. Grey Turner sign (bluish discolouration in flanks) and Cullen's sign (bluish discolouration around umbilicus) may be additional clues.

5. **H - Ruptured abdominal aortic aneurysm**

Back pain with hypotension and tachycardia in anybody more than 55 years is a ruptured AAA unless proven otherwise. The history of lifting heavy weights is misleading.

## 103. THEME: ABDOMINAL CONDITIONS

OPTIONS

A. Crohn's disease
B. Biliary colic
C. Perforated peptic ulcer
D. Ruptured ectopic pregnancy
E. Appendix mass
F. Renal adenocarcinoma
G. Carcinoma of rectum
H. Ruptured abdominal aortic aneurysm

*For each of the patients described below, select the most likely cause from the above list. Each option may be used once, more than once, or not at all.*

1. A 24-year-old girl is brought to A&E with severe generalized lower abdominal pain. She is pale and her BP is 90/60 mm Hg.

2. A teenaged boy presents with right iliac fossa pain for 3 months duration. He also has intermittent fevers, diarrhoea and weight loss. On examination he is pale and wasted with a vague mass palpable in the right iliac fossa.

3. A teenaged girl presents with right iliac fossa pain for 4 days with pyrexia of 37.8°C. On examination she has a well defined palpable mass in the right iliac fossa.

4. A 66-year-old lady is referred by the GP with altered bowel habits, a sense of incomplete evacuation, and blood mixed with her stools.

## 103. ANSWERS

1. **D - Ruptured ectopic pregnancy**

2. **A - Crohn's disease**

A long history of diarrhoea and vomiting with the presence of right iliac fossa signs/symptoms is more suggestive of Crohn's disease. 'Food fear' is well known. On colonoscopy the earliest signs are aphthoid like ulcers surrounded by a rim of erythematous mucosa. The best investigation of the small intestine is small bowel enema. Iron deficiency from haemorrhage may lead to a microcytic anaemia. Terminal ileitis causing vitamin $B_{12}$ malabsorption may occasionally cause a microcytic anaemia.

3. **E - Appendix mass**

4. **G - Carcinoma of rectum**

Colonic malignancy is the second most common cause for cancer deaths in the UK. Clinical presentation reflects the location of the tumour. A carcinoma in the caecum progresses silently, the only manifestation being occult blood in the stools and persistent anaemia due to chronic blood loss. A mass may be palpable in the right iliac fossa. A tumour in the ascending colon may give rise to colicky abdominal pain, though it is more likely to be a feature of transverse/descending colon cancer due to the partial obstruction of an annular constricting lesion. Change in bowel habit is also a feature of transverse/descending colon cancer due to a constricting lesion. Tumours in the rectum secrete mucus and bleed from the ulcerated surface. Tenesmus and 'early morning' bloody diarrhoea are features of rectal cancer.

## 104. THEME: ABDOMINAL DISEASE

OPTIONS

A. Typhoid fever
B. Ulcerative colitis
C. Crohn's disease
D. Familial adenomatous polyps
E. Diverticular disease
F. Juvenile polyps
G. Post cricoid malignancy
H. Gastric cancer
I. Angiodysplasia
J. Annular pancreas

*For each of the following conditions below, select the most likely associated disease from the above list. Each option may be used once, more than once, or not at all.*

1. Osteomas

2. Sacroileitis

3. Ankylosing spondylitis

4. Pyoderma gangrenosum

## 104. ANSWERS

1. **D - Familial adenomatous polyps**

2. **B - Ulcerative colitis**

3. **B - Ulcerative colitis**

4. **B - Ulcerative colitis**

## 105. THEME: ABDOMINAL DISEASE

OPTIONS

A. Typhoid fever
B. Ulcerative colitis
C. Crohn's disease
D. Familial adenomatous polyps
E. Diverticular disease
F. Juvenile polyps
G. Post cricoid malignancy
H. Gastric cancer
I. Angiodysplasia
J. Annular pancreas

*For each of the following conditions below, select the most likely associated disease from the above list. Each option may be used once, more than once, or not at all.*

1. Iritis

2. Sclerosing cholangitis

3. Desmoids

4. Enteroenteric fistula

## 105. ANSWERS

1. **B - Ulcerative colitis**

2. **B - Ulcerative colitis**

3. **D - Familial adenomatous polyps**

4. **C - Crohn's disease**

## 106. THEME: ABDOMINAL DISEASE

OPTIONS

A. Typhoid fever
B. Ulcerative colitis
C. Crohn's disease
D. Familial adenomatous polyps
E. Diverticular disease
F. Juvenile polyps
G. Post cricoid malignancy
H. Gastric cancer
I. Angiodysplasia
J. Annular pancreas

*For each of the following conditions below, select the most likely associated disease from the above list. Each option may be used once, more than once, or not at all.*

1. Cholecystitis

2. Enterovesical fistula

3. Sideropenic dysphagia

4. Colovesical fistula

## 106. ANSWERS

1. **A - Typhoid fever**

2. **C - Crohn's disease**

3. **G - Post cricoid malignancy**

4. **E - Diverticular disease**

## 107. THEME: ABDOMINAL DISEASE

OPTIONS

A. Typhoid fever
B. Ulcerative colitis
C. Crohn's disease
D. Familial adenomatous polyps
E. Diverticular disease
F. Juvenile polyps
G. Post cricoid malignancy
H. Gastric cancer
I. Angiodysplasia
J. Annular pancreas

*For each of the following conditions below, select the most likely associated disease from the above list. Each option may be used once, more than once, or not at all.*

1. Perianal abscess

2. Phlebitis

3. Aortic stenosis

4. Down's syndrome

## 107. ANSWERS

1. **C - Crohn's disease**

2. **A - Typhoid fever**

3. **I - Angiodysplasia**

4. **J - Annular pancreas**

Enteroenteric fistulas are more likely to complicate Crohn's disease than diverticular disease. Contrarily, Colovesical fistulas are more likely to complicate diverticular disease. Anal pathology is much more prevalent in Crohn's disease.

Venous thrombosis, particularly of the left common iliac vein, is an occasional complication of typhoid fever. Acute typhoid cholecystitis may occasionally occur and can cause perforation.

## 108. THEME: INVESTIGATIONS FOR ABDOMINAL PAIN

OPTIONS

A. FBC
B. Diagnostic laparoscopy
C. X-ray abdomen
D. Beta HCG
E. Ultrasound scan of abdomen
F. Erect chest X-ray
G. Immediate laparotomy
H. Serum amylase

*For each of the patients described below, select the most likely specific diagnostic investigation from the above list. Each option may be used once, more than once, or not at all.*

1. An 8-year-old boy presents with a 12 hour history of central abdominal pain which has now shifted to the right iliac fossa.

2. A 22-year-old girl presents to A&E in a state of shock. She complains of lower abdominal pain. She is pale with a BP of 82/50 mm Hg and a pulse of 128/min.

3. A 64-year-old alcoholic presents with acute onset abdominal pain radiating to the back associated with vomiting. On examination the patient is tachycardic but otherwise normotensive. There is discolouration of the flanks.

4. A 50-year-old female, on large doses of analgesics for rheumatoid arthritis, presents with acute onset epigastric pain and vomiting. On examination the abdomen is distended. The pain is made worse by movement and the patient lies still.

5. A 72-year-old male presents to A&E in shock. He is complaining of central abdominal pain radiating to his back. On examination, he is pale with abdominal distention and rigidity. The lower extremities are cold and clammy.

## 108. ANSWERS

1. **E - Ultrasound scan of abdomen**
This boy most likely has acute appendicitis. Though the diagnosis is essentially clinical, abdominal ultrasound examination is a useful diagnostic tool particularly in children with an accuracy of over 90%. Many centres, however, employ a CT scan.

2. **D - Beta HCG**
This is a typical history for a ruptured ectopic pregnancy. A pregnancy test is indicated as the first step.

3. **H - Serum amylase**
The history is typical of acute pancreatitis. A serum amylase 4 times above normal is indicative of the disease. Plain abdominal X-ray findings may include a generalized or local ileus (sentinel loop), a colon 'cut off' sign and a renal 'halo' sign.

4. **F - Erect chest X-ray**
The history again is typical of a perforated peptic ulcer most likely due to NSAID use. An erect chest X-ray will demonstrate the presence of pneumoperitoneum and clinch the diagnosis.

5. **G - Immediate laparotomy**
This patient most probably has a ruptured AAA. This is a grave surgical emergency. Anterior rupture into the peritoneum is usually fatal since the patient quickly exsanguinates. A clue may be the presence of a pulsatile mass in the abdomen. Urgent laparotomy is the gold standard for any patient suspected to have a ruptured AAA.

## 109. THEME: INVESTIGATIONS FOR ABDOMINAL PAIN

OPTIONS

A. FBC
B. Diagnostic laparoscopy
C. Supine X-ray abdomen
D. Mesenteric angiography
E. Ultrasound scan of abdomen
F. Erect chest X-ray
G. Immediate laparotomy
H. Barium meal-small bowel follow through

*For each of the patients described below, select the most likely specific diagnostic investigation from the above list. Each option may be used once, more than once, or not at all.*

1. An 80-year-old male presents with severe abdominal pain associated with fresh red rectal blood. There are no signs on abdominal examination. Patient is in shock with a fast irregular pulse.

2. A 40-year-old male is brought to A&E following a road traffic accident. He is pale, tachycardic and in shock. Abdomen is distended with guarding and rigidity. He has visible bruising over his left lower rib cage with palpable fractures underneath.

3. A 90-year-old male of African origin presents with an increasingly painful and swollen abdomen over the last 2 days associated with absolute constipation. He gives a history of persisting chronic constipation for quite some time.

4. A 38-year-old lady is admitted with vomiting, colicky abdominal pain and a distended abdomen. Her past history includes an open cholecystectomy, an open appendicectomy, two caesarean sections, a Nissen fundoplication and repair of incisional hernia.

5. A 16-year-old presents with a year's history of vague right iliac fossa pain, diarrhoea, vomiting and weight loss.

## 109. ANSWERS

1. **D - Mesenteric angiography**

This patient most likely has an embolic occlusion in his mesenteric circulation due to atrial fibrillation. Mesenteric angiography followed by embolectomy or bypass surgery with a laparotomy and bowel resection may be needed depending on the clinical course.

2. **G - Immediate laparotomy**

The history is typical for splenic rupture. Urgent laparotomy, with splenectomy/spleen preservation where possible, is the correct management.

3. **C - Supine X-ray abdomen**

Sigmoid volvulus is the most probable diagnosis here. Predisposing factors include a high residue diet and chronic constipation. It is the commonest cause of large bowel obstruction in indigenous black Africans. A plain radiograph shows massive colonic distention. The classic appearance is of a dilated loop of bowel running diagonally across the abdomen from right to left with two fluid levels seen, one within each loop of bowel. This is called the 'omega loop' or the 'bent inner tube' sign. Flexible sigmoidoscopy or rigid sigmoidoscopy with insertion of a flatus tube should be carried out to allow deflation of the gut.

4. **C - Supine X-ray abdomen**

This is likely to be acute intestinal obstruction due to adhesions. A supine abdominal X-ray is indicated.

5. **H - Barium meal-small bowel follow through**

History is suggestive of Crohn's disease. A barium meal followed by a follow through would be the ideal investigation.

## 110. THEME: INVESTIGATIONS OF THE GASTROINTESTINAL TRACT

OPTIONS

A. FBC
B. Diagnostic laparoscopy
C. Surgery
D. Ultrasound of abdomen
E. Barium enema
F. CT scan of abdomen
G. Flexible sigmoidoscopy
H. Colonoscopy

*For each of the patients described below, select the most likely specific diagnostic investigation from the above list. Each option may be used once, more than once, or not at all.*

1. A 22-year-old man presents with a 12-hour history of central abdominal pain, which is now localizing to the right iliac fossa. Examination reveals tenderness, guarding and rebound tenderness in the right iliac fossa.

2. An 80-year-old male living in the mental asylum presents with abdominal distention, vomiting and constipation for a few days duration. His medical records reveal a long history of constipation.

3. A 20-year-old boy presents with a history of a few episodes of bright red rectal bleeding without any change in bowel habits.

4. A 96-year-old nursing home resident presents with alternating diarrhoea and constipation and passing blood per rectum.

## 110. ANSWERS

1. **C - Surgery**
History is typical of acute appendicitis. The diagnosis here is clinical and radiological investigations are not needed.

2. **G - Flexible sigmoidoscopy**
History is typical of sigmoid volvulus. A flexible sigmoidoscopy or rigid sigmoidoscopy with insertion of a flatus tube should be carried out to allow deflation of the gut. Alternatively, if this is not mentioned in the options, colonoscopy may be selected.

3. **G - Flexible sigmoidoscopy**
From the history, the source of bleeding is in all probabilities in the left colon.

4. **F - CT scan of abdomen**
The age of the patient decides the answer here. Many centres use a CT scan to identify colorectal cancers in the above-80 age group.

## 111. THEME: ABDOMINAL LUMPS

OPTIONS

A. Gallbladder mass
B. Renal adenocarcinoma
C. Pancreatic cancer
D. Mesenteric cyst
E. Caecal carcinoma
F. Appendicular mass
G. Acute diverticulitis
H. Crohn's disease

*For each of the patients described below choose the single most likely diagnosis from the above list of options. Each option may be used once, more than once or not at all.*

1. A 45-year-old chronic alcoholic presents with epigastric discomfort, anorexia and jaundice. On examination, the gallbladder is palpable.

2. A 60-year-old lady presents with abdominal pain, lethargy, weakness and pallor for 6 months. On examination, she has a palpable minimally tender mobile lump in the right iliac fossa. Stool examination reveals occult blood.

3. An 18-year-old budding model presents with an incidentally discovered abdominal lump. She has no symptoms otherwise. Examination reveals a fluctuant swelling in the umbilical region, which moves freely in one direction.

4. A 60-year-old lady presents with left abdominal pain, nausea, anorexia and constipation. Patient is flushed and feverish. Examination reveals a tender left iliac fossa with a palpable sausage shaped mass.

5. A 50-year-old male presents with general debility, loss of energy, weight loss and bone pain. On examination, a lump is palpable in the left lumbar region. It is ballotable and bimanually palpable.

## 111. ANSWERS

1. **C - Pancreatic cancer**

Most frequent symptoms of pancreatic cancer are non specific. Jaundice is the commonest sign and neariy 85% of patients present with this. Pain is a common feature of pancreatic cancer. Typically, it is epigastric pain radiating to the back. Migratory thrombophlebitis (Trousseau sign) and venous thrombosis may be important clues. Courvoisier's law is another important clue.

2. **E - Caecal carcinoma**

A carcinoma in the caecum progresses silently, the only manifestation being occult blood in the stools and persistent anaemia due to chronic blood loss. A mass may be palpable in the right iliac fossa.

3. **D - Mesenteric cyst**

Chylolymphatic cyst is the commonest variant of mesenteric cyst. They are classically seen in the 2nd decade of life. They may present as a painless fluctuant swelling which moves freely in a plane at right angles to the attachment of the mesentery. Other presentation include recurrent attacks of abdominal pain due to recurring temporary impaction of food bolus in a segment of bowel narrowed by the cyst, or possibly from torsion of the mesentery. Occasionally an acute abdominal presentation may be seen from torsion of the mesentery, rupture of the cyst, haemorrhage into the cyst and infection. Chylolymphatic cysts can be enucleated *in toto*.

4. **G - Acute diverticulitis**

The clinical diagnoses rest solely on the site of the pain, the tenderness, and, when present, the mass. Complications include recurrent inflammation and pain, perforation, intestinal obstruction, haemorrhage and fistula formation (vesicocolic, vaginocolic, enterocolic, colocutaneous). Vesicocolic fistula is most common.

5. **B - Renal adenocarcinoma**

Haematuria is the commonest mode of presentation of a renal carcinoma. Three other common modes of presentation include general debility (as in this case), pain in the loin or a mass. Rarer presentations include ureteric colic (clot colic), bone pain, pathological fractures, pyrexia of unknown origin, hypertension and features of erythrocythaemia. Presentation with a varicocele is a favourite with many examiners.

## 112. THEME: ABDOMINAL LUMPS

OPTIONS

A. Carcinoma caecum
B. Carcinoma ascending colon
C. Carcinoma sigmoid
D. Carcinoma rectum
E. Gall stone ileus
F. Pseudo obstruction
G. Acute diverticulitis
H. Sigmoid volvulus

*For each of the patients described below choose the single most likely diagnosis from the above list of options. Each option may be used once, more than once or not at all.*

1. A 74-year-old obese women presents with severe abdominal pain, vomiting and abdominal distention. Supine abdominal and erect chest films confirm the presence of multiple central fluid levels, an air fluid level in the biliary tree with absence of air under the right dome of the diaphragm.

2. A 74-year-old woman presents with severe abdominal pain, vomiting and abdominal distention. She was seen by her GP recently for anorexia and weight loss. Clinical examination reveals visible peristalsis in the mid abdomen. An ill-defined mass is palpable in the right iliac fossa. Supine abdominal and erect films confirm the presence of multiple central fluid levels with absence of air under the right dome of the diaphragm.

3. You are the RSO (resident surgeon on call). You receive a bleep from the spinal unit in the middle of the night about a 65-year-old gentleman who underwent a surgery on his vertebrae 4 days ago. He has had progressively increasing abdominal distention with constipation. He looks relatively well for his distention. Abdominal radiographs confirm gross colonic distention down to the pelvic brim with marked caecal distention.

4. A 78-year-old black nursing home resident presents with abdominal distention, hiccough, wretching and absolute constipation. Examination reveals a non tender grossly distended abdomen. Supine abdominal films show massive colonic distention.

## 112. ANSWERS

### 1. E - Gall stone ileus

The history suggests small bowel obstruction. It occurs in the elderly and is due to erosion of a large gallstone through the gallbladder into the duodenum (choledochoduodenal fistula). Classically, there is impaction about 60 cm proximal to the ileocaecal valve. The stone may not always be visible (remember that 90% of gall stones are radiolucent). Presencc of air or an air-fluid level in the biliary tree with intestinal obstruction clinches the diagnosis.

### 2. A - Carcinoma caecum

This is a classical presentation again. Clues include the patient's age, her recent symptoms of anorexia and weight loss, a palpable mass in the right iliac fossa and features predominantly suggesting a small bowel obstruction.

### 3. F - Pseudo obstruction

Pseudo obstruction describes an obstruction, usually of the colon, in the absence of a mechanical cause or acute intra-abdominal disease. This may occur in an acute or chronic form. The acute form of colonic pseudo-obstruction is known as Ogilvie syndrome and presents as acute large bowel obstruction. Marked caecal distention on the X-ray is a characteristic feature. For this reason, caecal perforation is a well recognized complication.

### 4. H - Sigmoid volvulus

It is the commonest cause of large bowel obstruction in indigenous black Africans. Important clues could include old age, history of chronic constipation, and history of dementia, nursing home resident status and a classic radiological appearance. Classic appearance is of a dilated loop of bowel running diagonally across the abdomen from right to left with two fluid levels seen, one within each loop of bowel.

## 113. THEME: POSTOPERATIVE PYREXIA

OPTIONS

A. Deep vein thrombosis
B. Urinary tract infection
C. Respiratory tract infection
D. Basal atelectasis
E. Wound infection
F. Clostridium difficile infection
G. Anastomotic leak
H. Pelvic abscess

*For each of the situations below, select the most likely cause of post operative pyrexia from the above list. Each option may be used once, more than once, or not at all.*

1. A 58-year-old lady underwent a left total knee replacement 4 days ago. Her temperature is 37.9°C. Her knee is minimally swollen, but the wound looks healthy. Her left calf is markedly swollen and tender.

2. An 88-year-old nursing home resident underwent a laparotomy for a small duodenal perforation 2 weeks ago. Postoperative recovery was delayed by a prolonged period of hypotension and renal failure for which she was catheterized. Review of observation charts reveal blood pressure of 118/70 mm Hg, catheter output of 1400 mL/24 hours, and temperature of 38.1°C. There is no cough and chest X-ray from morning is normal.

3. A 68-year-old lady undergoes emergency abdominal surgery for a diverticular perforation and abscess. 7 days after surgery she develops diarrhoea with passage of mucus in the stools. She has pyrexia of 38°C. Rectal examination reveals tenderness.

4. An elderly lady undergoes left hemicolectomy for carcinoma of the colon. On the 5th postoperative day, her observations show a temperature of 38.2°C, blood pressure of 100/62 mm Hg and a low urine output. She has distention, tenderness and guarding in the abdomen.

## 113. ANSWERS

1. **A - Deep vein thrombosis**

Unilateral pitting oedema may be an additional clue. When suspected, an urgent Doppler ultrasound should be arranged.

2. **B - Urinary tract infection**

Urinary tract infection should be considered in any patient with a catheter in situ for more than 5 days.

3. **H - Pelvic abscess**

Pelvic abscess is a common sequel to any case with diffuse peritonitis as well as anastomotic leakage after bowel and rectal surgery. The most characteristic symptoms of a pelvic abscess are diarrhoea and the passage of mucus in the stools. In fact, passage of mucus, for the first time in a patient who has, or is, recovering from peritonitis is pathognomonic of pelvic abscess. Rectal examination may reveal tenderness and bulging of the anterior rectal wall.

4. **G - Anastomotic leak**

Any failure to recover in a predictable manner should alert one to a possibility of an anastomotic leak.

## 114. THEME: POSTOPERATIVE COMPLICATIONS

OPTIONS

A. Pulmonary embolism
B. Wound dehiscence
C. Respiratory tract infection
D. Basal atelectasis
E. Wound infection
F. Clostridium difficile infection
G. Anastomotic leak
H. Subphrenic abscess

*For each of the situations below, select the most likely postoperative complication from the above list. Each option may be used once, more than once, or not at all.*

1. An 80-year-old lady undergoes a laparotomy for a perforated duodenal ulcer that she developed from NSAID ingestion for rheumatoid arthritis. On day 6 of surgery, she develops pyrexia of 38.2°C. She is tender in the right upper quadrant of the abdomen. Coarse crackles are heard on the right lung base.

2. A 60-year-old man undergoes a laparotomy for a perforated duodenal ulcer with gross peritonitis. You are called to examine his wound for large serosanguinous discharge on day 8.

3. A 55-year-old man undergoes a left total hip replacement. On post operative day 5 while awaiting an ambulance to go home, he suddenly develops tachypnoea and chest discomfort. His saturations drop to 86% on air. Urgent ECG is normal.

## 114. ANSWERS

1. **H - Subphrenic abscess**

This is a classical complication following repair of a perforated duodenal ulcer.

2. **B - Wound dehiscence**

A serosanguinous (pink) discharge is the most pathognomonic sign of impending wound disruption and implies that intraperitoneal contents are lying extraperitoneal. It classically develops between days 6 to 8. Return to the operating theatre with closure is needed.

3. **A - Pulmonary embolism**

This is a typical presentation of pulmonary embolism which is a medical emergency. Full immediate anticoagulation with heparin is needed in addition to standard resuscitation. Massive embolism may be treated by infusion of fibrinolytic drugs.

## 115. THEME: INVESTIGATION OF POSTOPERATIVE COMPLICATIONS

OPTIONS

A. Chest X-ray
B. MRI
C. Venography
D. Doppler ultrasound
E. Calcium
F. Pulmonary angiogram
G. FBC
H. Abdominal X-ray

*For each of the patients described below choose the single most likely investigation from the above list of options. Each option may be used once, more than once, or not at all.*

1. A 70-year-old patient presents with left calf pain and tenderness on day 5 after a left total knee replacement.

2. A 70-year-old patient presents with sudden breathlessness and collapses on day 8 after a left total knee replacement. He has a tender and swollen left calf.

3. A 66-year-old post-thyroidectomy patient presents with tetany. The facial muscles twitch on tapping the preauricular region.

4. A 60-year-old patient in the ICU with a severe head injury develops abdominal distention and rigidity.

## 115. ANSWERS

1. **D - Doppler ultrasound examination**
This patient most likely has a deep vein thrombosis (DVT).

2. **F - Pulmonary angiogram**
A V/Q scan is the preferred initial investigation in suspected cases of pulmonary embolism. Its role is however limited in patients with chronic obstructive airways disease. Spiral CT is the next best option. Pulmonary angiogram is the gold standard investigation of choice.

3. **E - Calcium**
Chvostek's sign is described here. Hypocalcaemia is due to hypoparathyroidism which is a complication of thyroidectomy. It is characterized by muscle twitches, cramps and spasms.

4. **A - Chest X-ray**
This patient most probably has developed a perforation. In the majority of cases, a past history of peptic ulcer disease will be present. However, a silent ulcer may perforate in a minority. Chest X-ray will show the presence of free gas under the right dome of the diaphragm.

## 116. THEME: SURGICAL INVESTIGATIONS

OPTIONS

A. ERCP
B. Small bowel enema
C. Abdominal ultrasound
D. Rectal biopsy
E. Laparoscopy
F. Double contrast barium enema
G. Spiral CT scan

*For each of the following scenarios, select the most appropriate investigation from the above list. Each option may be used once, more than once or not at all.*

1. Hirschsprung's disease
2. Meckel's diverticulum
3. Small bowel Crohn's disease
4. Pancreatic cancer
5. Sclerosing cholangitis
6. Biliary ductal stones
7. Diverticular disease of colon

## 116. ANSWERS

1. **D - Rectal biopsy**

2. **B - Small bowel enema**

3. **B - Small bowel enema**

4. **G - Spiral CT scan**

5. **A - ERCP**

6. **A - ERCP**

7. **F - Double contrast barium enema**

ERCP may reveal the 'chain of lakes' appearance of sclerosing cholangitis.

## 117. THEME: SURGICAL INVESTIGATIONS

OPTIONS

A. Endoscopy
B. Endoscopic biopsy
C. Abdominal ultrasound
D. MRI
E. Laparoscopy
F. USG
G. CT scan
H. Colonoscopy

*For each of the following scenarios, select the most appropriate investigation from the above list. Each option may be used once, more than once or not at all.*

1. Uncomplicated angiodysplasia of the colon

2. Hypertrophic pyloric stenosis of infants

3. Aorto enteric fistula

4. Gastric lymphoma

5. Trichobezoar

6. Secondaries in the liver

7. Gall stones

8. Pelvic spread of rectal cancer

9. Screening for family history of colon cancer

10. Subphrenic abscess

## 117. ANSWERS

1. **H - Colonoscopy**

Colonoscopy can be attempted in suspected cases providing the bleeding is not too brisk. Selective superior and inferior mesenteric angiography shows the site and extent of the lesion by a blush. If this fails, a radioactive test using technetium-99m ($^{99m}$Tc)-labelled red cells may confirm and localize the source of haemorrhage.

2. **F - USG**

3. **G - CT scan**

4. **B - Endoscopic biopsy**

Gastric lymphoma is seldom diagnosed on endoscopy alone which is non specific.

5. **A - Endoscopy**

6. **G - CT scan**

7. **C - Abdominal ultrasound**

8. **D - MRI**

A MRI gives the best contrast resolution and hence is the preferred investigation here. It is helpful in predicting a role for neoadjuvant chemotherapy.

9. **H - Colonoscopy**

10. **F - USG**

This is an early complication of biliary surgery. This must be considered if a patient develops an unexplained swinging fever a few days after surgery. Diagnosis is best made with an ultrasound. Treatment is by percutaneous needle drainage under ultrasound guidance or occasionally by open operation.

## 118. THEME: SURGICAL INVESTIGATIONS

OPTIONS

A. Small bowel follow through
B. Gastrografin enema
C. Abdominal ultrasound
D. MRI
E. Double contrast barium enema
F. USG
G. CT scan
H. Colonoscopy

*For each of the following scenarios, select the most appropriate investigation from the above list. Each option may be used once, more than once or not at all.*

1. Mucocele of the gallbladder

2. Empyema of the gallbladder

3. Pancreatic necrosis

4. Colonic anastomotic repair

5. Insulinoma

6. Ileal tumour

7. Colovesical tumour

## 118. ANSWERS

1. **C - Ultrasound**

2. **C - Ultrasound**

3. **G - CT scan**

4. **B - Gastrografin enema**

5. **G - CT scan**

6. **A - Small bowel follow through**

7. **E - Double contrast barium enema**

Acute and chronic gallbladder pathologies are best seen on the ultrasound. Suspected colonic anastomotic leaks are best assessed using a water soluble Gastrografin enema. Colovesical fistulas are best assessed using a double contrast barium enema.

## 119. THEME: PANCREATIC TUMOURS

OPTIONS

A. HPPomas
B. VIPoma
C. Insulinoma
D. Glucagonoma
E. Somatostatinomas
F. Zollinger-Ellison syndrome

*For each of the patients described below, select the most likely pancreatic tumour from the list of options below. Each option may be used once, more than once, or not at all.*

1. A high school teacher presents with episodes of aggressive behaviour, headache and visual disturbance typically brought on by a missed lunch. He has noticed that he is all right on days he has his lunch.

2. A 45-year-old male is referred to your consultant clinic with severe peptic ulcer disease refractory to medical therapy. Upper GI endoscopy reveals ulcers in distal duodenum.

3. A 42-year-old lady is brought to A&E with abdominal pain, diarrhoea, lethargy and weakness. She is dehydrated. She has hypokalaemia and acidosis on blood investigations.

4. A 45-year-old lady is referred with weight loss, lethargy and a skin rash. On examination, the skin rash consists of symmetrical erythematous lesions that have crusted erosions and involve the perineum, groin, thighs, buttocks and lower limbs.

## 119. ANSWERS

### 1. C - Insulinoma

Insulinoma is the most common endocrine tumour in the adults. The excess circulating insulin manifests as symptomatic hypoglycaemia. Most of the symptoms are the result of adrenergic hyperactivity consequent on episodes of hypoglycaemia, e.g., weakness, sweating, hunger, palpitations and tremor. The hypoglycaemia has direct cerebral effects leading to headaches, visual disturbances, dizziness, confusion, aggressive behaviour, seizures and coma. An important clue is the relationship of symptoms to fasting with relief of symptoms on eating.

### 2. F - Zollinger-Ellison syndrome

Suspect this in any patient with (1) severe peptic ulcer disease refractory to medical therapy, (2) multiple peptic ulcers or ulcers in unusual locations, (3) recurrent peptic ulcer disease following acid reducing surgery, (4) peptic ulcer disease in association with a strong family history of ulcer disease. The diagnosis is confirmed if basal gastrin level is more than 100 pg/mL.

### 3. B - VIPoma

Patients with this condition develop profuse secretory diarrhoea, which is an important clue. The diagnosis is confirmed by assay of plasma levels of VIP which exceeds 190 pg/mL.

### 4. D - Glucagonoma

An important clue here is the presence of necrolytic migratory erythema with features as enlisted in the question. The diagnosis is confirmed by finding elevated plasma glucagons concentration.

## 120. THEME: POSTOPERATIVE RESPIRATORY COMPLICATIONS

OPTIONS

A. Adult respiratory distress syndrome
B. Narcotic overdose
C. Pulmonary embolism
D. Chest infection
E. Pneumothorax
F. Aspiration pneumonia
G. Empyema
H. Pleural effusion

*For each of the following scenarios, select the most appropriate complication from the above list. Each option may be used once, more than once or not at all.*

1. An 80-year-old lady undergoes an urgent laparotomy for a left perforated colonic tumour. Observations on day 2 stand as temperature-39.1°C, BP-130/78 mm Hg, pulse 108/min. Examination reveals reduced air entry and percussion dullness in right lower chest.

2. A morbidly obese 67-year-old lady undergoes a left total knee replacement. She is progressing well after surgery, when the nurses call you on day 6 after surgery because she looks cyanosed and has blood stained sputum.

3. A 46-year-old year old male undergoes a unicompartmental left total knee replacement. He is found drowsy and unresponsive by the nursing staff. On examination his respiratory rate is 12/min.

## 120. ANSWERS

1. **F - Aspiration pneumonia**

Risk of regurgitation of gastric contents in the perioperative period is very high for any emergency laparotomy. The right lung is more susceptible because the anatomy of the right main bronchus will direct aspirated material preferentially into that lung field.

2. **C - Pulmonary embolism**

The presentation is typical of pulmonary embolism.

3. **B - Narcotic overdose**

Clues in this case include the drowsiness and decreased responsiveness associated with a depressed respiratory effort. Other important clues may be the presence of pinpoint pupils.

## 121. THEME: TIMING OF SURGICAL PROCEDURES

OPTIONS

A. Operate at next available list
B. Operate after 2 weeks
C. Urgent surgery
D. Operate after 6 weeks
E. Operate after 6 months
F. Repeat investigation after 6 months and reassess
G. Wait some years and then operate

*For each of the following scenarios, select the most appropriate timing for a surgical procedure from the list of options mentioned above. Each option may be used once, more than once, or not at all.*

1. A 67-year-old male with relatively mild symptoms of prostatism, a reasonably good flow rate of 11 mL/sec and a borderline bladder emptying (residual urine 110 mL).

2. A 66-year-old male presents with vague lower abdominal pain. On examination a suprapubic swelling is palpable, which is confirmed as a 1400 mL bladder with bilateral hydronephrosis. Renal functions are normal.

3. A 45-year-old insulin dependent diabetic presents with a day's history of upper abdominal pain. Investigations reveal the presence of gas in a distended gallbladder with marked pericholecystic fluid.

4. A young lady undergoes a laparotomy for Crohn's disease. This is complicated by the development of a controlled enterocutaneous fistula 10 days from surgery.

5. A 14-year-old child presents with central colicky abdominal pain radiating to the right iliac fossa for 4 days. He is mildly pyrexial. Rest of the observations are stable. Palpation after adequate analgesia reveals a well-defined mass in the right iliac fossa.

6. A 6-month-old baby girl is brought with a swelling in the belly button region which increases in size when the baby cries. It assumes a classical conical shape.

## 121. ANSWERS

1. **F - Repeat investigation after 6 months and reassess**
In men with mild symptoms, reasonable flow rates (>10 mL/sec) and good bladder emptying (residual urine <100 mL), careful discussion over the merits and side effects of operative treatment is warranted. Waiting for 6 months is indicated. After this, a repeat assessment is indicated.

2. **A - Operate at next available list**
With no evidence of infection or uraemic symptoms catheterization is not indicated. For those who are uraemic, urgent catheterization is indicated to allow the renal function to recover.

3. **C - Urgent surgery**
Indications for emergency surgical intervention in acute cholecystitis include: (1) progression of disease during conservative management, (2) presence of an inflammatory mass in the right hypochondrium, (3) established generalized peritonitis, (4) presence of gas in the gall bladder/biliary tract, (5) development of intestinal obstruction.

4. **E - Operate after 6 months**
After week 1 of surgery, a re-laparotomy is technically very difficult. Since this is a controlled fistula, the aim would be to ensure proper nutrition and wound management.

5. **D - Operate after 6 weeks**
If an appendix mass is present and the condition of the patient is stable, the standard treatment is conservative (Ochsner-Sherren regimen). Criteria for stopping conservative treatment include: a rising pulse rate, increasing abdominal pain, increasing size of the mass and vomiting or copious gastric aspirate. Clinical improvement is usually evident within 24–48 hours. Failure of a mass to resolve should raise the suspicion of a carcinoma or Crohn's disease. Using this regimen about 90% will resolve without any incident in which case an elective appendicectomy should be arranged in 6–8 weeks time.

6. **G - Wait some years and then operate**
This is an umbilical hernia of infancy. Most will disappear spontaneously by the age of 2 years (some authors mention 3 years). Hence conservative treatment is needed in this case. If the hernia persists at 2 years of age, it is unlikely to resolve and herniorrhaphy is indicated.

## 122. THEME: JAUNDICE

OPTIONS

A. Choledochal cyst
B. Pancreatic cancer
C. Duodenal carcinoma
D. Acute cholangitis
E. Bile duct calculi
F. Acute cholecystitis
G. Empyema of the gallbladder
H. Chronic pancreatitis
I. Extra hepatic biliary atresia

*For each scenario listed below, select the most appropriate diagnosis from the above list. Each option may be used once, more than once, or not at all.*

1. A week-old baby is brought with jaundice, pale stools, dark urine and severe pruritus.

2. A 45-year-old chronic alcoholic presents with epigastric discomfort radiating to back, and jaundice. On examination, the gallbladder is palpable.

3. A 34-year-old man is under surveillance for familial adenomatous polyposis. He underwent a total colectomy and ilio-rectal anastomosis for the same 2 years ago. He presents with complaints of vague abdominal pain and jaundice.

4. A 1-year-old Japanese baby girl is brought with jaundice and episodes of frequent crying. Examination reveals a vague mass in the right hypochondrium.

5. An obese 56-year-old lady presents with abdominal pain, fever, rigors and jaundice. She has a tender hepatomegaly on palpation.

6. An obese 56-year-old lady undergoes an open cholecystectomy. She presents with jaundice 3 days after surgery.

## 122. ANSWERS

1. **I - Extra hepatic biliary atresia**

In about a third of cases, jaundice is present at birth. Differential includes any jaundice in the neonate giving a cholestatic picture. Neonatal hepatitis is the most difficult to differentiate. Both extrahepatic biliary atresia and neonatal hepatitis are associated with giant cell transformation of the hepatocytes.

2. **B - Pancreatic cancer**

3. **C - Duodenal cancer**

The commonest extraintestinal manifestation of FAP is a duodenal carcinoma.

4. **A - Choledochal cyst**

There is a strong female predominance. It is commoner in Japan than in western populations. Symptoms can be vague and as enlisted in the question. Complications include recurrent cholangitis, pancreatitis, hepatic abscess, calculus disease, cyst rupture and portal vein thrombosis. There is an increased risk of cholangiocarcinoma.

5. **D - Acute cholangitis**

Fever, pain and rigors classically constitute the Charcot's triad. The diagnosis is confirmed on ultrasound, which shows dilated ducts. Blood culture may identify the causative organism. This is a medical emergency and delay can cause organ failure secondary to septicaemia. Treatment consists of third generation cephalosporins, rehydration, and endoscopic drainage with extraction of causative ductal stones.

6. **E - Bile duct calculi**

Obstructive jaundice after a cholecystectomy should alert one to bile duct calculi that were missed at the time of surgery.

## 123. THEME: SURGICAL PRINCIPLES – NUTRITION

OPTIONS

A. Elemental/low residue diet
B. Feeding jejunostomy
C. Feeding gastrostomy
D. Nasogastric tube feeding
E. High protein enteral diet
F. Total parenteral nutrition

*For each scenario listed below, select the most appropriate option from the above list. Each option may be used once, more than once, or not at all.*

1. A 24-year-old girl with known Crohn's disease develops a fistula in the right iliac fossa. Investigations confirm a low output distal small bowel fistula.

2. A 24-year-old girl is brought in unconscious after a RTA in a drowsy state. She is admitted to the neurosurgical intensive therapy unit. It is judged that she may need nutritional support for a week.

3. A 24-year-old girl is brought in unconscious after a RTA in a drowsy state. She is admitted to the neurosurgical intensive therapy unit and is on the ventilator. Her head injuries are quite significant and she is likely to follow a long protracted course on the ventilator.

4. A 65-year-old male undergoes a radical total gastrectomy. There are some concerns with reconstruction intraoperatively.

5. A 65-year-old male develops a leak from his neck anastomosis site after a transhiatal oesophagectomy.

## 123. ANSWERS

1. **A - Elemental/low residue diet**

Enteral nutrition should be employed as far as possible. An elemental/low residue diet gets completely absorbed by the time it reaches the terminal small intestine. This should promote healing of the fistula.

2. **D - Nasogastric tube feeding**

As per the principle highlighted above, enteral nutrition should be employed here. Since she needs only temporary nutritional support, a nasogastric tube feeding is ideal.

3. **C - Feeding gastrostomy**

This is indicated when the passage of a fine bore nasogastric tube is not possible or when more than 4 weeks of enteral feeding is anticipated as in this case. The contraindications to feeding gastrostomy include gastric disease, impaired gastric emptying, significant gastro-oesophageal reflux and a loss of gag reflux.

4. **B - Feeding jejunostomy**

An intraoperatively performed feeding jejunostomy is most logical, which would allow early enteral nutrition.

5. **F - Total parenteral nutrition**

Total restriction of all oral intake is mandatory in the management of patients with an oesophageal leak. A nasogastric tube insertion cannot be attempted.

## 124. THEME: POSTOPERATIVE RENAL MANAGEMENT

OPTIONS

A. Administer desmopressin
B. Replace loss with equivalent dextrose
C. Intravenous frusemide
D. Catheterisation
E. Replace loss with equivalent Hartmann's solution

*For each scenario listed below, select the most appropriate option from the above list. Each option may be used once, more than once, or not at all.*

1. An 80-year-old male complains of intense lower abdominal pain 10 hours after an inguinal hernia repair. Review of observation charts reveals anuria. He has a palpable suprapubic lump.

2. A 60-year-old male undergoes emergency laparotomy. Observation chart reads as: Intravenous input 2400 mL/24 hours, nasogastric aspirate 1700 mL/24 hours, urine output 400 mL/24 hours.

3. An 88-year-old male undergoes an emergency laparotomy for a perforated duodenal ulcer with gross peritonitis. You are called by the nurse from HDU to review the patient for oliguria. Observation chart reads as intravenous input of 2.5 liters each over the last 3 days with an output of 200 mL over the last 12 hours. His urine output yesterday was 600 mL/24 hours. He appears breathless and has bilateral basal crepitations on auscultation.

## 124. ANSWERS

1. **D - Catheterisation**

This patient typically has urinary retention. It is commonly seen in elderly patients after hernia repair.

2. **E - Replace loss with equivalent Hartmann's solution**

The intestinal fluid that is lost is rich in electrolytes and should be replaced by an equivalent amount of normal saline or Hartmann's solution. The same applies to high output ileostomy losses in the immediate postoperative period.

3. **C - Intravenous frusemide**

This patient has developed pulmonary oedema secondary to cardiac failure. Initial steps in management would include restricting intravenous fluids and giving intravenous frusemide.

## 125. THEME: MANAGEMENT OF TRAUMA

OPTIONS

A. Immediate laparotomy
B. CT scan abdomen
C. Skull X-ray
D. CT head
E. Diagnostic peritoneal lavage
F. Diagnostic laparoscopy

*For each scenario listed below, select the most appropriate management option from the above list. Each option may be used once, more than once, or not at all.*

1. A young lady is brought to A&E after a road traffic accident involving her car with a motorcycle. She is hypotensive when brought into hospital, but responds to fluid resuscitation. Her BP now is 106/70 mm Hg with a pulse of 106/min. She has a bruising in the region of her left lower chest. Rest of the survey shows no other injury.

2. A 20-year-old male is brought after a RTA following high speed driving. He has a big laceration involving his forehead. His GC scale on admission reads as E2, V3, and M2. No other injuries are apparent on primary survey and he is haemodynamically stable with normal bowel sounds.

3. A 24-year-old male is brought after a violent assault. He has a big stab wound in the paraumbilical region with visible omental prolapse. He is haemodynamically stable. Abdominal examination reveals generalized tenderness with guarding away from the stab wound entry site.

## 125. ANSWERS

1. **B - CT scan abdomen**

Since the patient has responded to fluid resuscitation, an urgent CT scan is indicated to identify the cause of hypotension in the first place. She has bruising over her left lower chest which might indicate a splenic injury. A scan would demonstrate intraperitoneal blood and also identify the cause of bleeding. The findings of the scan coupled with the patient's subsequent progress should help determine the need for laparotomy.

2. **D - CT head**

A major head injury with a GCS of 7 is a criterion for an emergency CT head.

3. **A - Immediate laparotomy**

This patient has omental prolapse with evidence of peritonitis. Immediate laparotomy is mandatory.

## 126. THEME: INVESTIGATION IN LOWER GI SURGERY

OPTIONS

A. Per rectal examination
B. Proctoscopy
C. Examination under anaesthesia
D. Reassure
E. Stool culture and microscopy
F. Colonoscopy
G. CT scan abdomen
H. Sigmoidoscopy
I. Barium enema
J. Faecal occult blood test

*For each scenario listed below, select the most appropriate investigation from the above list. Each option may be used once, more than once, or not at all.*

1. You are a research fellow in surgery and are conducting a survey on knowledge and attitude of first degree relatives of colorectal cancer. One patient from your survey population presents to his GP concerned because both his dad and grand dad died in their 40s from colorectal cancer.

2. A 26-year-old lady presents to you with a 2-month history of occasional bleeding per rectum. Bleeding is slight and consists of streaks on the stools. On further questioning she tells you that she tends to constipate herself for fear of pain that she experiences when she opens her bowels.

3. A 70-year-old lady presents with a 3-month history of bleeding per rectum, which she describes as streaks on the toilet paper. She has had increasing constipation, straining and pain in the back passage when opening her bowels since a 'failed' excision of haemorrhoids 3 years ago. Inspection of the back passage reveals a stenosed anal canal. No fissure is visualized and because of the intense pain, a digital rectal examination is not deemed appropriate.

4. A 20-year-old student from the University of Leeds presents with a bloody diarrhoea after a period of elective tropical medicine attachment in Sri Lanka. She also reports a change in bowel habit.

5. A 64-year-old male presents with a 2-month history of diarrhoea, anorexia and weight loss. Stool culture and sigmoidoscopy are both normal.

## 126. ANSWERS

1. **F - Colonoscopy**

Because of the strong family history, this is the most appropriate screening procedure. In the presence of 2 first degree relatives, this patient would need a colonoscopy at the age of 35 (or 5 years younger than the earliest case in the family) and then every 5 years thereafter along with yearly faecal occult blood testing.

2. **A - Per rectal examination**

This is a typical history for a fissure in ano. Classical clinical features include pain on defaecation, bright red bleeding, mucus discharge and constipation. Direct inspection is all that is needed at this stage. A typical history, a tightly closed, puckered anus and occasionally a sentinel tag are characteristic of this condition. By gently parting the anus, the lower end of the fissure can be seen. Because of the intense pain, a digital examination should be avoided at this stage.

3. **C - Examination under anaesthesia**

This patient may have an anal fissure secondary to an anal stricture as a direct complication of haemorrhoidectomy. At her age she may also have an underlying carcinoma. In the absence of directly visualized pathology, it is important to examine under anaesthesia.

4. **E - Stool culture and microscopy**

This is again typical of tropically acquired diarrhoea and a stool culture and microscopy is indicated for shigellosis and amoebiasis amongst other things.

5. **F - Colonoscopy**

This is colorectal cancer unless proved otherwise. In the presence of normal stool culture and a normal sigmoidoscopy examination, the most appropriate next step would be colonoscopy.

## 127. THEME: PREOPERATIVE INVESTIGATIONS

OPTIONS

A. C-Spine X-ray
B. Full blood count
C. Chest X-ray
D. Coagulation screen
E. Ultrasound-abdomen
F. Echocardiography of heart
G. No investigations
H. ERCP
I. Toxic screen

*For each scenario listed below, select the most appropriate investigation from the above list. Each option may be used once, more than once, or not at all.*

1. A 40-year-old lady is due to undergo a planned laparoscopic cholecystectomy for calculi. On admission, liver function tests show a raised alkaline phosphatase. She had been admitted acutely 6 weeks earlier when her liver function tests were normal and an ultrasound scan had shown the presence of calculi in the gall bladder with normal bile duct diameter.

2. A 65-year-old lady is admitted for an elective excision of a large swelling over her thigh. The swelling was initially assumed to be a soft tissue sarcoma, but later confirmed as a lipoma on biopsy. She is known to have had a metallic heart valve replacement and is on life-long warfarin for the same.

3. A 26-year-old male is admitted for an elective hernia repair. He denies any significant past history. He has recently taken to full time work and admits to smoking about 2 cigarettes per day for the past few weeks. He denies use of any illicit drugs.

4. A 68-year-old lady is admitted for an elective knee replacement surgery. The only significant past history is one of rheumatoid arthritis but she tells you she has been in remission for the last couple of years and has been off immunosuppressants.

5. A 55-year-old male is admitted for an elective hernia repair. He is a life-long smoker and complains of a chronic cough.

## 127. ANSWERS

1. **H - ERCP**

This patient possibly has calculi in the bile duct. Hence most surgeons would perform a preoperative ERCP. Some surgeons would still prefer to perform an intraoperative cholangiogram followed by common bile duct exploration (laparoscopic or open).

2. **D - Coagulation screen**

This patient is on warfarin and hence a coagulation screen is indicated.

3. **G - No investigations**

For those of you who got it right, well done. For those who didn't, focus. The smoking history is not significant and the mention about illicit drugs is only a red herring.

4. **A - C spine X-ray**

5. **C - Chest X-ray**

## 128. THEME: AETIOLOGY OF PERITONITIS

OPTIONS

A. Paralytic ileus
B. Clostridium difficile infection
C. Colonic pseudo-obstruction
D. Pelvic abscess
E. Liver trauma
F. Haemoperitoneum
G. Perforated viscus

*For each scenario listed below, select the most appropriate diagnosis from the above list. Each option may be used once, more than once, or not at all.*

1. An 18-year-old male undergoes an emergency appendicectomy. At surgery the appendix is found to be gangrenous and perforated. 5 days after surgery the patient develops a spiking fever and diarrhoea.

2. An 18-year-old male is brought in following a road traffic accident. He is tachycardic and hypotensive. He is tender in the left lower chest and the left upper hypochondrium.

3. A 65-year-old lady is brought to A&E with severe abdominal pain. She is known to have arthritis and takes non steroidal analgesics.

4. An 84-year-old nursing home resident is admitted under the care of the elderly with a right sided stroke. A week later, he is referred to you for a grossly distended abdomen and absolute constipation for 1 day. Supine abdominal X-ray shows dilated loops of large bowel.

5. A 74-year-old male undergoes resection of part of his small intestine for a local gastrointestinal stromal tumour. 2 days after surgery he develops progressively severe abdominal distention and vomiting. His abdomen is non tender. Percussion reveals a tympanic abdomen. Auscultation reveals absent bowel sounds. The nasogastric tube which had been blocked since the morning is opened and it produces copious amounts of aspirate.

## 128. ANSWERS

1. **D - Pelvic abscess**

The most common presentation is spiking pyrexia. Other symptoms include a feeling of pelvic pressure or discomfort associated with loose stool or tenesmus. Rectal examination reveals a boggy mass in the pelvis anterior to the rectum. Pelvic ultrasound usually suffices for diagnosis. Treatment involves transrectal drainage.

2. **F - Haemoperitoneum**

This patient most probably is a case of ruptured spleen and haemoperitoneum secondary to it.

3. **G - Perforated viscus**

I agree the history is limited. But this is the only likely answer from the list of options provided.

4. **C - Colonic pseudo-obstruction**

Pseudo-obstruction describes an obstruction, usually of the colon, in the absence of a mechanical cause or acute intra-abdominal disease. This may occur in an acute or chronic form. The acute form of colonic pseudo-obstruction is known as Ogilvie syndrome and presents as acute large bowel obstruction. Marked caecal distention on the X-ray is a characteristic feature. For this reason, caecal perforation is a well recognized complication.

5. **A - Paralytic ileus**

This is classical of paralytic ileus. Well-known causes include the post operative state, infection, uraemia and hypokalaemia. Reflex ileus is also well known and occurs following fractures of the spine or ribs, retroperitoneal haemorrhage or even the application of a plaster jacket.

## 129. THEME: DYSPHAGIA/ ODYNOPHAGIA

OPTIONS

A. Carcinoma of oesophagus
B. Achalasia
C. Pharyngeal pouch
D. Motor neurone disease
E. Sideropenic dysphagia
F. Monilial oesophagitis
G. Schatzki's ring

*For each of the patients described below, select the most appropriate diagnosis from the above list. Each option may be used once, more than once, or not at all.*

1. A 45-year-old male is referred to your consultant's outpatient clinic for odynophagia. Past medical history includes asthma for which he takes steroid inhalers. He is allergic to morphine. Endoscopy shows numerous white plaques.

2. A 45-year-old male on chemotherapy for an advanced haematological malignancy presents with retrosternal discomfort and dysphagia for a week's duration.

3. A 45-year-old male presents with a 6-month history of regurgitation of undigested food a few hours after his meals. He has recently noticed some gurgling noises in the neck on swallowing.

## 129. ANSWERS

1. **F - Monilial oesophagitis**

2. **F - Monilial oesophagitis**

Candida albicans is the causative agent. It is seen in immunocompromised patients including patients on steroid inhalers for asthma. The allergy of morphine in the first question is just a red herring. There may be visible thrush in the throat. Endoscopy shows numerous plaques that cannot be moved, unlike food residues. A biopsy is diagnostic.

3. **C - Pharyngeal pouch**

This condition is twice as common in women as in men. Initially the patients present with globus type symptoms of a feeling of something in the throat. As the diverticulum enlarges, patients may experience regurgitation of undigested food. Clues may include (1) waking up in the middle of the night with a feeling of tightness in the chest, (2) fits of unexplained coughing, (3) unexplained recurrent chest infections, (4) gurgling noises from the neck on swallowing and (5) visible swelling in the neck which increases with intake of food. Though the classical presentation is not as common, it is a favourite question with the examiners.

## 130. THEME: PANCREATO-BILIARY DISEASE

OPTIONS

A. Biliary colic
B. Acute pancreatitis
C. Acute cholecystitis
D. Cholangiocarcinoma
E. Carcinoma of gallbladder
F. Empyema of the gallbladder
G. Cholangitis
H. Mucocele of the gallbladder
I. Carcinoma of head of the pancreas

*For each scenario listed below, select the most appropriate diagnosis from the above list. Each option may be used once, more than once, or not at all.*

1. A 45-year-old obese lady presents with flatulent dyspepsia. She has had episodes of intermittent colicky epigastric and right hypochondriac pain for the past few months. Physical examination is however normal.

2. A 45-year-old obese lady known to have gall stones presents with a 1-day history of acute onset severe central abdominal pain radiating to her back. Her pain score is 10/10 and she requires morphine to settle her pain. Examination reveals generalized vague abdominal tenderness.

3. A 45-year-old obese insulin dependent diabetic is admitted with a 4-week history of right upper quadrant abdominal pain which has worsened in the last few days. He has swinging pyrexia. Though he is not clinically jaundiced, he has a palpable and tender gall bladder.

4. An 80-year-old gentleman is admitted from the nursing home with a progressively worsening jaundice over the last 1-week. Abdominal examination reveals a palpable liver. No gallbladder is palpable however.

## 130. ANSWERS

1. **A - Biliary colic**

2. **B - Acute pancreatitis**

Up to 70% of acute pancreatitis in the UK are caused by biliary calculi. Alcohol accounts for only 25% of cases.

3. **F - Empyema of gallbladder**

It may be a sequel of acute cholecystitis or the result of a mucocele getting infected. Emergency percutaneous drainage is indicated with cholecystectomy planned for later.

4. **D - Cholangiocarcinoma**

The palpable liver most probably suggests a metastatic involvement. Local spread is frequent and metastases are common at the time of presentation. The diagnosis is confirmed by biopsy. Note that the classical presentation for a carcinoma of the head of the pancreas is a palpable gallbladder.

## 131. THEME: CUTANEOUS MANIFESTATIONS OF TUMOURS

OPTIONS

A. Pyoderma gangrenosum
B. Café-au-lait spots
C. Circumoral pigmentation
D. Galactorrhoea
E. Hirsuitism
F. Pellagra
G. Acanthosis nigricans
H. Migratory thrombophlebitis

*For each scenario listed below, select the most appropriate cutaneous manifestation from the above list. Each option may be used once, more than once, or not at all.*

1. Ovarian cancer

2. Prolactinoma

3. Gastric adenocarcinoma

4. Pancreatic carcinoma

## 131. ANSWERS

1. **E - Hirsuitism**

2. **D - Galactorrhoea**

3. **G - Acanthosis nigricans**

4. **H - Migratory thrombophlebitis**

## 132. THEME: CUTANEOUS MANIFESTATIONS OF TUMOURS

OPTIONS

A. Pyoderma gangrenosum
B. Café-au-lait spots
C. Circumoral pigmentation
D. Galactorrhoea
E. Hirsuitism
F. Pellagra
G. Acanthosis nigricans
H. Migratory thrombophlebitis
I. Necrolytic migratory erythema

*For each scenario listed below, select the most appropriate cutaneous manifestation from the above list. Each option may be used once, more than once, or not at all.*

1. Carcinoid syndrome

2. Acute myeloid leukaemia

3. Glucagonoma

4. Peutz-Jeghers syndrome

## 132. ANSWERS

1. **F - Pellagra**

2. **A - Pyoderma gangrenosum**

3. **I - Necrolytic migratory erythema**

4. **C - Circumoral pigmentation**

## 133. THEME: TYPES OF POLYPS

OPTIONS

A. Adenomatous
B. Dysplastic
C. Villous
D. Metaplastic
E. Hamartomas
F. Fibroepithelial
G. Inflammatory

*For each of the descriptions below, select the most appropriate variant of polyp from the list of options above. Each option may be used once, more than once, or not at all.*

1. Polyps giving rise to diarrhoea, mucus discharge and hypokalaemia.

2. Ulcerative colitis

3. Polyps found on routine screening. Familial in nature and can number more than a hundred.

4. Associated with Peutz-Jegers syndrome.

## 133. ANSWERS

1. **C - Villous**

Villous adenoma is a type of adenomatous polyp. Characteristic features are mentioned. The risk of malignancy developing in an adenoma increases with increase in size of the tumour.

2. **G - Inflammatory**

Easy to guess! They may occur in 20% of patients and may be numerous. They are also referred to as pseudo polyps. They result from previous episodes of ulceration leaving islands of spared mucosa which will remain prominent when the adjacent mucosa heals.

3. **A - Adenomatous**

These vary from the tubular adenoma to the villous adenoma. In familial adenomatous polyposis, more than 100 adenomas are present.

4. **E - Hamartomas**

They have minimal malignant potential and are only removed if they are causing troublesome pain, bleeding or hypoproteinaemia.

## 134. THEME: SCORING SYSTEMS

OPTIONS

A. Ranson's criteria
B. Child-Pugh's system
C. APACHE 2
D. RTS, ISS

*For each of the patients described below, select the most appropriate scoring system from the list of options described above. Each option may be used once, more than once or not at all.*

1. A 75-year-old undergoes emergency surgery for a ruptured abdominal aortic aneurysm. Postoperatively he is shifted to the intensive care unit.
2. A 55-year-old alcoholic is admitted with severe upper abdominal pain going to the back associated with nausea and vomiting. His blood gases on admission show a picture of metabolic acidosis.
3. A 55-year-old alcoholic is admitted with encephalopathy, jaundice and abdominal distention. He has marked pedal oedema with the presence of a large ascites. His spleen is palpable.
4. A 22-year-old male is admitted after being assaulted with a knife. He has multiple stab wounds over his chest and abdomen.

## 134. ANSWERS

### 1. C - APACHE 2

APACHE stands for acute physiology and chronic health evaluation. It is a physiologically based classification system and is widely used in the ICU. The APACHE classification system can be used to control for case mix, compare outcomes, evaluate new therapies, and study the utilization of ICUs.

### 2. A - Ranson's criteria

This is quite well known and is used to predict prognosis in acute pancreatitis. It is based on variables measured immediately and after 48 hours of admission.

### 3. B - Child-Pugh's system

This classification allows an easy method of describing the severity of liver disease and allows comparison of treatments for patients with chronic liver disease. There are 3 classes (A, B or C) based on five different variables: Bilirubin, albumin, ascites, neurological disorder and nutrition.

### 4. D - RTS, ISS

The Revised Trauma Score (RTS) and the Injury Severity Score (ISS) are tools used to compare severity of injury and outcome of interventions in trauma patients.

## 135. THEME: FISTULA

OPTIONS

A. Fistula in ano
B. High output fistula
C. Low output fistula
D. Gastrocolic fistula
E. Vesicocolic fistula
F. Biliary fistula
G. Aortic enteric fistula
H. Arteriovenous fistula
I. Aortoduodenal fistula
J. Urethral fistula

*For each of the scenarios described below, select the most appropriate type of fistula. Each option may be used once, more than once or not at all.*

1. A 65-year-old male known to have significant peripheral vascular disease presents with haematemesis. He has had multiple surgeries in the past including an aortic graft for ruptured aortic aneurysm, and axillo-bifemoral grafts. Upper GI endoscopy is obscured by the presence of blood. However, no mass or ulcer is visualized.

2. A 34-year-old male presents with a swelling in the left anticubital fossa. Examination reveals a pulsatile swelling with an old healed scar atop it. He tells you that he was stabbed there a few months ago. On palpation, a thrill is detected and auscultation reveals a buzzing continuous bruit. Nicoladoni's sign is positive.

3. A 26-year-old lady has been troubled with persistent foul smelling faeculent discharge through her back passage.

4. A 70-year-old lady presents with a history of pneumaturia and of passing occasional faecal matter in the urine.

## 135. ANSWERS

### 1. G - Aortic enteric fistula

This is usually a diagnosis of exclusion in the early stages. The bleeding may not always be massive. One thing that will be constant in the history is a surgery on the aorta with graft insertion. Only rarely is it seen in patients with an untreated aortic aneurysm.

### 2. H - Arteriovenous fistula

They may be surgically created in patients undergoing renal dialysis or may be acquired after a penetrating wound or sharp blow. Dilated veins will be seen. Pressure on the artery proximal to the fistula causes the swelling to diminish in size, and the thrill and bruit to cease. This is known as the Nicoladoni's sign or Branham's sign.

### 3. A - Fistula in ano

They result from perianal abscesses and treatment requires good understanding of the anatomy of the region. In general, treatment involves laying open the fistula.

### 4. E - Vesicocolic fistula

In patient with diverticulitis any urinary symptom may herald the formation of a vesicocolic fistula. Other types of fistula seen in diverticular disease include vaginocolic, enterocolic and colocutaneous. However, vesicocolic fistula is the commonest.

## 136. THEME: LYMPHATIC DRAINAGE

OPTIONS

A. Superficial inguinal
B. Deep inguinal
C. Para aortic
D. Internal iliac
E. Inferior mesenteric

*For each of the scenarios described below, select the most appropriate option from above. Each option may be used once, more than once or not at all.*

1. Vulva

2. Scrotal skin

3. Upper half of anal canal

4. Rectal

### 136. ANSWERS

1. A - Superficial inguinal

2. A - Superficial inguinal

3. D - Internal iliac

4. D - Internal iliac

## 137. THEME: CAUSES OF SHOCK

OPTIONS

A. Anaphylactic
B. Septic
C. Cardiogenic
D. Hypovolaemic
E. Neurogenic
F. Traumatic

*For each of the scenarios described below, select the most appropriate type of shock from the list of options given above. Each option may be used once, more than once or not at all.*

1. A 70-year-old male is brought to A&E in severe shock. He complained of back pain before collapsing suddenly. On examination, his abdomen is distended. He looks pale and his pulse stands at 140/min with a blood pressure of 60 mm Hg systolic. He improves partly with fast crystalloid infusion.
2. A 75-year-old male is brought to A&E in severe shock. He had been out to celebrate his grand daughter's birthday when he complained of sudden onset shortness of breath and dizziness. His pulse is 35/min with a blood pressure of 65/40 mm Hg.
3. A 78-year-old lady is brought to A&E in severe shock. She has been increasingly confused for a week. The nursing home has noticed extremely foul smelling urine for the last 2 days. She is pyrexial at 39°C with a pulse of 140/min and a blood pressure of 65/40 mm Hg.
4. A 44-year-old business executive is known to be allergic to nuts. He accidentally consumes biscuits containing some nuts and lands in A&E in shock. He requires definitive airway management. His pulse is rapid and thready with a rate of 100/min and a blood pressure of 86/44 mm Hg.
5. A 23-year-old chap is involved in a bad road traffic accident. He comes to A&E in shock. He complains of pain in the back. He is however unable to lift his legs and complains of a heavy sensation in the legs. Chest, abdomen and pelvic examination are normal. No obvious long bone deformity is obvious. However, his pulse is 120/min with a blood pressure of 66 mm Hg systolic. The diastolic blood pressure is not recordable.

## 137. ANSWERS

1. **D - Hypovolaemic**

This is due to loss of intravascular volume by haemorrhage, dehydration, vomiting and diarrhoea. Until 10–15 per cent blood volume is lost, the blood pressure is maintained by tachycardia and vasoconstriction. This patient most probably has a ruptured AAA.

2. **C - Cardiogenic**

Cardiogenic shock occurs when more than 50% of the wall of the left ventricle is damaged by infarction. Acute massive PE from a thrombus originating in a deep vein or an air embolus if obstructing more than 50% of the pulmonary vasculature will cause acute right ventricular failure.

3. **B - Septic**

Hyperdynamic (warm) septic shock occurs in serious Gram-negative infections. At first, the patient has abnormal or increased cardiac output with tachycardia and a warm, dry skin, but the blood is shunted past the tissue cells, which become damaged by anaerobic metabolism (lactic acidosis). A hypovolaemic hypodynamic (cold) septic shock follows if severe sepsis or endotoxaemia is allowed to persist.

4. **A - Anaphylactic**

Penicillin administration is amongst the common causes of anaphylaxis. The antigen combines with immunoglobin E (IgE) on the mast cells and basophils, releasing large amounts of histamine and slow-release substance-anaphylaxis (SRS-A). These cause bronchospasm, laryngeal oedema and respiratory distress with hypoxia, massive vasodilatation, hypotension and shock.

5. **E - Neurogenic**

RTA with inability to lift legs and a heavy sensation are important clues. It is caused by traumatic or pharmacological blockade of the sympathetic nervous system producing dilatation of resistance arterioles and capacitance veins leading to relative hypovolaemia and hypotension. Trauma to the spinal cord and spinal anaesthesia lead to a systolic pressure around 70 mm Hg.

Other forms of shock to remember include vasovagal shock, psychogenic shock, traumatic shock and burns shock. A careful look at the given history should help you clinch the diagnosis.

## 138. THEME: NAIL CHANGES

OPTIONS

A. Clubbing
B. Koilonychia
C. Platynychia
D. Beau's lines
E. Leuconychia
F. Onycholysis
G. Onychogryposis
H. Melanonychia
I. Splinter haemorrhage
J. Yellow nail syndrome

*For each of the scenarios described below, select the most appropriate nail change from the list of options given above. Each option may be used once, more than once or not at all.*

1. Bronchogenic carcinoma

2. Cirrhosis of liver

3. Severe illness/surgery

4. Hyperthyroidism

## 138. ANSWERS

1. **A - Clubbing**

2. **A - Clubbing**

3. **D - Beau's lines**

4. **F - Onycholysis**

Just like the skin, the fingernails tell a lot about a person's state of health. Pitting (the presence of small depressions on the nail surface) is often accompanied with crumbling of the nail. Detachment of the nail can also occur (the nail becomes loose and sometimes even comes off). Ridges (linear elevations) can develop along the nail occurring in a lengthwise or crosswise direction. Beau's lines are linear depressions that occur crosswise (transverse) in the fingernail. They can occur after illness, trauma to the nail, and with malnutrition. Leukonychia describes white streaks or spots on the nails. Koilonychia is an abnormal shape of the fingernail where the nail has raised ridges and is thin and concave. This disorder is associated with iron deficiency anaemia.

## 139. THEME: NAIL CHANGES

OPTIONS

A. Clubbing
B. Koilonychia
C. Platynychia
D. Beau's lines
E. Leuconychia
F. Onycholysis
G. Onychogryposis
H. Melanonychia
I. Splinter haemorrhage
J. Yellow nail syndrome

*For each of the scenarios described below, select the most appropriate nail change from the list of options given above. Each option may be used once, more than once or not at all.*

1. Infective endocarditis

2. Iron deficiency anaemia

3. Psoriasis

4. Lymphoedema

## 139. ANSWERS

1. **I - Splinter haemorrhage**

2. **B - Koilonychia**

3. **F - Onycholysis**

4. **J - Yellow nail syndrome**

## 140. THEME: OCULAR SIGNS

OPTIONS

A. Argyll Robertson pupil
B. Cataract
C. Chemosis
D. Arcus senilis
E. Horner's syndrome
F. Kayser-Fleischer rings

*For each of the scenarios described below, select the most appropriate ocular sign from the list of options given above. Each option may be used once, more than once or not at all.*

1. Graves' disease

2. Wilson's disease

3. Pancoast tumour

4. Atherosclerosis

## 140. ANSWERS

1. **C - Chemosis**

2. **F - Kayser-Fleischer rings**

A Kayser-Fleischer ring is a rim of brownish green pigment seen in the periphery of the cornea. It signifies excessive deposition of copper in Descemet's membrane. The upper pole is affected more frequently than the lower. Kayser-Fleischer rings are noted in 90% of patients with Wilson's disease and occasionally, in patients with prolonged cholestasis or cryptogenic cirrhosis. The ring is noted most easily in patients with blue eyes. In other patients, slit-lamp examination may be required.

3. **E - Horner's syndrome**

Horner's syndrome results from an interruption of the sympathetic nerve supply to the eye, and is characterized by the classic triad of miosis (i.e., constricted pupil), partial ptosis, and loss of hemifacial sweating (i.e., anhidrosis). Horner syndrome may result from a lesion of the primary neuron; brainstem stroke or tumour or syrinx of the preganglionic neuron; trauma to the brachial plexus; tumours (e.g., pancoast) or infection of the lung apex; a lesion of the postganglionic neuron; dissecting carotid aneurysm; carotid artery ischaemia; migraine; or middle cranial fossa neoplasm.

4. **D - Arcus senilis**

## 141. THEME: FAMILIAL CANCER SYNDROMES

OPTIONS

A. Familial adenomatous polyposis
B. Wilms' tumour
C. Xeroderma pigmentosa
D. Hereditary non polyposis colon cancer (HNPCC)
E. Retinoblastoma
F. Von Hippel Lindau
G. Von Recklinghausen's disease
H. Li Fraumeni syndrome

*For each of the scenarios described below, select the most appropriate familial cancer syndrome from the list of options given above. Each option may be used once, more than once or not at all.*

1. This is an autosomal dominant cancer that occurs in early childhood. There are both hereditary and non-hereditary forms. In the hereditary form, multiple tumours are found in both eyes, while in the non-hereditary form only one eye is affected and by only one tumour.

2. An autosomal dominant cancer predisposition syndrome associated with soft-tissue sarcoma, breast cancer, leukaemia, osteosarcoma, melanoma, and cancer of the colon, pancreas, adrenal cortex, and brain. Individuals are at increased risk for developing multiple primary cancers.

3. An autosomal dominant condition characterized by the presence of numerous polyps mainly in the large bowel, but also in the stomach, duodenum and small intestine.

4. Inherited as an autosomal recessive trait associated with a defect in DNA gyrase.

## 141. ANSWERS

1. **E - Retinoblastoma**

In the hereditary form, a gene called Rb is lost from chromosome 13. The tumour develops from the immature retina.

2. **H - Li Fraumeni syndrome**

Two forms of Li-Fraumeni syndrome are recognized: classic Li-Fraumeni syndrome (LFS) and Li-Fraumeni-like syndrome (LFL). Classic LFS is defined by the following criteria:

- A proband with a sarcoma diagnosed before 45 years of age, AND
- A first-degree relative with any cancer under 45 years of age, AND
- A first- or second-degree relative with any cancer under 45 years of age or a sarcoma at any age.

LFL shares some, but not all of the features listed for LFS.

3. **A - Familial adenomatous polyposis (FAP)**

The main risk is the development of large bowel cancer, but duodenal and ampullary tumours have also been reported. FAP can be associated with benign mesodermal tumours such as desmoid tumours and osteomas. Epidermoid cysts can also occur (Gardner's syndrome).

4. **C - Xeroderma pigmentosa**

Those affected are extremely sensitive to the ultraviolet portion of sunlight. Ultraviolet light exposure damages DNA in skin cells.

People with xeroderma pigmentosa cannot repair the damaged DNA and rapidly develop skin atrophy, splotchy pigmentation, spidery blood vessels in the skin (telangiectasia), and skin cancers. Affected people develop increasing disfigurement following any intermittent exposure to sunlight. Malignant skin lesions are often present before the child is 5 years old.

## 142. THEME: ANORECTAL CAUSES OF PAIN

OPTIONS

A. Fissure in ano
B. Diverticulitis
C. Crohn's disease
D. Proctalgia fugax
E. Strangulated piles
F. Rectal cancer
G. External piles

*For each of the scenarios described below, select the most appropriate cause for pain in the rectum from the list of options given above. Each option may be used once, more than once or not at all.*

1. A 45-year-old male is known to have piles for some time. He has recently noticed that they have increased in size and occasionally prolapse. He presents with acute onset pain in his back passage for the past few hours. Examination reveals a dark purple external haemorrhoid which feels solid.

2. A 28-year-old lady presents with a history of chronic constipation for the past few months. She complains of severe pain on defaecation with passage of stools which are blood stained.

3. A 28-year-old lady presents with a cramp like severe intermittent rectal pain occurring most frequently in bed at night which lasts for a few minutes and resolves spontaneously. Past medical history includes an abortion at the age of 16 years of age and anxiety for the past 5 years.

## 142. ANSWERS

1. **E - Strangulated piles**

One or more of the internal haemorrhoids prolapse and become gripped by the external sphincter. This results in increased congestion. 2nd degree haemorrhoids are most prone to this complication. Thrombosis follows strangulation. Although strangulated piles are very painful, fully thrombosed piles are not (they are however tender).

2. **A - Fissure in ano**

Classical clinical features include pain on defaecation, bright red bleeding, mucus discharge and constipation. Direct inspection is all that is needed at this stage. A typical history, a tightly closed, puckered anus and occasionally a sentinel tag are characteristic of this condition. By gently parting the anus, the lower end of the fissure can be seen. Because of the intense pain, a digital examination should be avoided at this stage.

3. **D - Proctalgia fugax**

Classical features have again been mentioned. The past history of anxiety/stress is also a helpful feature. It is possibly due to segmental cramp in the pubococcygeus muscle. A more chronic form of the disease has been termed the 'levator syndrome' and can be associated with severe constipation.

## 143. THEME: STATISTICAL TESTS

OPTIONS

A. Paired T test
B. Unpaired T test
C. Mann-Whitney U test
D. Chi squared test

*For each of the studies described below, select the most appropriate statistical test from the list of options above. Each option may by used once, more than once, or not at all.*

1. A study comparing postoperative morbidity between patients receiving perioperative blood transfusion versus those not receiving any after curative gastric resection for gastric adenocarcinoma.

2. A placebo-controlled trial is conducted for a new drug for benign prostatic hyperplasia. Maximum flow rate achieved after the trial is compared with those at the beginning of the trial. Individual results are compared between the two groups.

## 143. ANSWERS

1. **D - Chi squared test**

This is a non parametric test for comparing two or more proportions from independent groups. It makes no assumption about the underlying population distribution. A *P* value <0.05 is taken to imply a true difference.

2. **C - Mann-Whitney U test**

This is again a non parametric significance test used to compare the distribution of a given variable between two groups.

## 144. THEME: TRIAL DESIGN AND PRINCIPLES

OPTIONS

A. Type I error
B. Type II error
C. Single blinding
D. Double blinding
E. Cross over
F. Null hypothesis
G. Exclusion bias
H. Randomisation
I. Minimisation
J. Exclusion bias

*For each of the descriptions below, select the most appropriate term from the list of options above. Each option may be used once, more than once, or not at all.*

1. The term used to describe a situation in which one fails to reject the null hypothesis when a difference is really present.

2. In a medical experiment, the comparison of treatments may be distorted if the patient, the person administering the treatment and those evaluating it know which treatment is being allocated. It is therefore necessary to ensure that the patient and/or the person administering the treatment and/or the trial evaluators don't know which treatment is allocated to whom.

3. The process by which experimental units are allocated to treatments.

4. A method of allocation in comparative studies that provides treatment groups that are very closely similar for several variables.

## 144. ANSWERS

1. **B - Type II error**

Type I error - benefit is perceived when really there is none (false positive).

Type II error - benefit is missed because study has small numbers (false negatives).

The probability of type I and II errors can be reduced by performing a prior power analysis in which the correct sample size is estimated on the basis of setting $\alpha$ and $\beta$ values which represent the probabilities that a type II and type I error will be committed.

2. **D - Double blinding**

3. **H - Randomisation**

Randomisation is preferred since alternatives may lead to biased results.

The main point is that randomisation tends to produce groups for study that are comparable in unknown as well as known factors likely to influence the outcome, apart from the actual treatment under study. The analysis of variance F tests assume that treatments have been applied randomly.

4. **I - Minimisation**

Simple randomisation is the commonest method used to reduce selection bias. Minimisation is an alternative to simple randomisation.

## 145. THEME: BASIC TERMS IN STATISTICS

OPTIONS

A. Bias
B. Sensitivity
C. Specificity
D. False negative
E. False positive
F. Error
G. Regression
H. Subgroup analysis
I. Likelihood ratio

*For each of the descriptions below, select the most appropriate term from the list of options above. Each option may be used once, more than once, or not at all.*

1. A surgical trial is conducted for a new drug to be used in claudication. At analysis the statistician concludes an incorrect sample size. The trial shows benefit for the new drug when really there is none.

2. A term referring to systematic inaccuracy.

3. Ability to exclude a true negative.

4. A random source of inaccuracy.

5. A possible benefit from a research study is not picked up because the sample size selected for the study is small.

6. It indicates the value of a test for increasing certainty about a positive diagnosis. It is numerically equal to the sensitivity/(1 - specificity).

## 145. ANSWERS

1. **E - False positive**
This is a type I error. An incorrect sample size is probably the most frequent reason for research to be invalid. It is always best to seek advice from an expert statistician before the trial is begun.

2. **A - Bias**
Bias is due to systematic inaccuracy due to either consistent under or over recording. Different types include confirmation bias, publication bias, selection bias, recall bias and response bias.

3. **C - Specificity**
The probability of picking up a genuine positive result is the sensitivity of the test, where the ability to exclude a true negative is the specificity of the test.

4. **F - Error**

5. **D - False negative**
This is a type II error.

6. **I - Likelihood ratio**

## 146. THEME: TYPES OF BIAS

OPTIONS

A. Exclusion bias
B. Confirmation bias
C. Publication bias
D. Selection bias
E. Recall bias
F. Response bias

*For each of the descriptions below, select the most appropriate type of bias from the list of options above. Each option may be used once, more than once, or not at all.*

1. This is a type of statistical bias describing the tendency to search for or interpret information in a way that confirms one's preconceptions.

2. This type of bias, also called the positive outcome bias, is typically the tendency for researchers to publish experimental results that have a positive result, while consequently not publishing findings which have a negative result.

3. An erroneous influence potentially affecting the conclusions of a trial caused by systematic differences in withdrawals form the trial.

4. This is a type of statistical bias which occurs when the way a survey respondent answers a question is affected not just by the correct answer, but also by the respondent's memory.

5. This is a type of statistical bias which can affect the results of a statistical survey if respondents answer questions in the way they think the questioner wants them to answer rather than according to their true beliefs.

## 146. ANSWERS

1. **B - Confirmation bias**

2. **C - Publication bias**

Publication bias may distort meta-analysis of large numbers of studies. The problem is particularly significant when the research is sponsored by entities that may have a financial interest in achieving favourable results.

3. **A - Exclusion bias**

Drop outs from a trial can introduce bias quite easily since the tendency is to exclude participants to favour the outcome of the trial.

4. **E - Recall bias**

5. **F - Response bias**

Selection bias is the error of distorting a statistical analysis by pre- or post-selecting the samples. Typically this causes measures of statistical significance to appear much stronger than they are, but it is also possible to cause completely illusory artifacts. Selection bias can be the result of scientific fraud by manipulating data directly, but more often is either unconscious or due to biases in the instruments used for observation.

## 147. THEME: SCIENTIFIC EVIDENCE

OPTIONS

A. Case report
B. Case series
C. Case control study
D. Cohort study
E. Meta-analysis
F. Randomised controlled trial
G. Cross sectional study
H. Uncontrolled trial

*For each of the descriptions of scientific evidence below, select the most appropriate type of study from the list of options above. Each option may be used once, more than once, or not at all.*

1. A study which involves identifying patients who have the outcome of interest (cases) and control patients who do not have that same outcome, and looking back to see if they had the exposure of interest. The exposure could be some environmental factor, a behavioural factor, or exposure to a drug or other therapeutic intervention.

2. A report on a single patient with an outcome of interest.

3. A statistical synthesis of the numerical result of several trials which all address the same question.

4. Involves identification of two groups of patients: one which received the exposure of interest, and one which did not, and following these groups forward for the outcome of interest.

5. A report on a series of patients with an outcome of interest. No control group is involved.

6. The observation of a defined population at a signal point in time or time interval. Exposure and outcome are determined simultaneously.

## 147. ANSWERS

1. **C - Case control study**
2. **A - Case report**
3. **E - Meta-analysis**
4. **D - Cohort study**
5. **B - Case series**
6. **G - Cross sectional study**

## 148. THEME: STATISTICAL TERMS

OPTIONS

A. Single blinding
B. Double blinding
C. Relative risk
D. Confidence intervals
E. Odds ratio
F. Placebo effect
G. Confounding factor
H. Risk factor

*For each of the descriptions below, select the most appropriate term from the list of options above. Each option may be used once, more than once, or not at all.*

1. It quantifies the uncertainty in measurement.

2. An aspect of a person's condition, lifestyle or environment that increases the probability of occurrence of a disease.

3. A measure of how much a particular risk factor influences the risk of a specified outcome.

4. This is an inactive intervention, received by the participants allocated to the control group in a clinical trial, which is indistinguishable from the active intervention received by patients in the experimental group.

## 148. ANSWERS

1. **D - Confidence intervals**

It is usually reported as 95% CI, which is the range of values within which we can be 95% sure that the true value for the whole population lies. A caveat is that the confidence interval relates to the population sampled. If we have a small sample of part of a population, or a very small sample of the whole population, then the confidence interval that is generated is not necessarily that for the whole population.

2. **H - Risk factor**

3. **C - Relative risk**

4. **F - Placebo effect**

## 149. THEME: NHS ISSUES

OPTIONS

A. Clinical audit
B. Clinical governance
C. NHS trusts
D. Commission for health improvement
E. National service frameworks

*For each of the descriptions below, select the most appropriate term from the list of options above. Each option may be used once, more than once, or not at all.*

1. They promote improvement in the quality of the NHS and independent healthcare. They have a wide range of responsibilities, all aimed at improving the quality of healthcare. They also have a statutory duty to assess the performance of healthcare organisations, award annual performance ratings for the NHS and coordinate reviews of healthcare by others.

2. A framework through which NHS organizations are accountable for continuously improving the quality of their services and safeguarding high standards of care by creating an environment in which excellence in clinical care will flourish.

3. A quality improvement process that seeks to improve patient care and outcomes through systematic review of care against explicit criteria and the implementation of change.

## 149. ANSWERS

1. **D - Commission for health improvement**

2. **B - Clinical governance**

3. **A - Clinical audit**

The definitions for clinical governance and clinical audit have to be learnt. You may not be asked your name in an interview but are sure to be asked on these issues. Audit can assess structure, the process and the outcome. It is important to remember the components of the audit cycle which involve:

- Observation of existing practice
- The setting of standards
- Comparison between observed and set standards
- Implementation of change
- Reaudit of clinical practice

Please refer to any standard textbook or any website for more details (e.g., www.dh.gov.uk).

## 150. THEME: AUDIT TECHNIQUES

OPTIONS

A. Basic clinical audit
B. Incident review
C. Focused audit
D. Criterion audit
E. Global audit
F. National studies

*For each of the descriptions below, select the most appropriate term from the list of options above. Each option may be used once, more than once, or not at all.*

1. Audit on morbidity and mortality in orthopaedics presented in the monthly audit meeting in a district hospital.

2. A retrospective analysis that is judged against chosen criteria.

3. An audit on specific outcomes

4. Audit comparing mortality after ruptured abdominal aortic aneurysm repair between 2 different hospitals.

## 150. ANSWERS

1. **A - Basic clinical audit**

2. **D - Criterion audit**

3. **C - Focused audit**

4. **E - Global audit**

## 151. THEME: COMPONENTS OF CLINICAL GOVERNANCE

OPTIONS

A. Patient and public involvement
B. Clinical risk management
C. Clinical audit
D. Clinical effectiveness
E. Staffing and staff management
F. Education, training and continuing personal and professional development
G. Use of information to support clinical governance and health care delivery

*For each of the descriptions below, select the most appropriate match from the list of components of clinical governance mentioned above. Each option may be used once, more than once, or not at all.*

1. You contact your medical staffing officer. You are told that she is away on an appraisal.

2. You are a surgical house officer. You receive a memorandum that mentions at least 60% compulsory attendance over a period of 6 months in the weekly surgical grand round. A register is to be maintained to record attendance.

3. A patient writes to the clinical director concerned about the fact that her appointment to see a general surgeon has twice been postponed at short notice.

4. A report indicates that 60% of patients had to wait 9 months after a temporary colostomy before having their colostomy reversed, which is much more than international standards.

## 151. ANSWERS

1. **E - Staffing and staff management**
This component entails the NHS trust's approach to human resource management, staff development and performance. Appraisal is one of the tools.

2. **F - Education, training and continuing personal and professional development**
This component includes the trust's strategy and plans for education, training and continuing development, with descriptions of education and training activities.

3. **B - Clinical risk management**
It includes the system for risk management including the way in which the different elements, e.g., incidents and complaints, are brought together and how they link with other governance activity.

4. **C - Clinical audit**
Options A–G are the 7 components of clinical governance. It is important to remember these components.

## 152. THEME: LAW SURROUNDING DEATH

OPTIONS

A. Coroner
B. Procurator Fiscal
C. Coroner's office
D. Any medical practitoner
E. Registrar of birth and deaths
F. Medical pracitioner who attended during previous 14 days

*For each of the statements below, select the most appropriate match from the list of options mentioned above. Each option may be used once, more than once, or not at all.*

1. Calls an inquest
2. Certify death
3. Calls an inquest in Scotland
4. Issue immediate death certificate

## 152. ANSWERS

1. **A - Coroner**

2. **D - Any medical practitioner**

3. **B - Procurator Fiscal**

4. **F - Medical pracitioner who attended during previous 14 days**

Only the coroner is entitled to hold an inquest on any case that is reported to him or her. The coroner is called a Procuratory Fiscal in Scotland.

## 153. THEME: DEATH CERTIFICATES

OPTIONS

A. Issue a death certificate
B. Ask the Patient's GP to issue a death certificate
C. Report to the coroner
D. Order a hospital postmortem

*For each of the scenarios described below, select the most appropriate answer from the list of options mentioned above. Each option may be used once, more than once, or not at all.*

1. A 90-year-old lady is admitted with a fracture neck of femur and a chest infection. She never really recovers while in hospital and progressively deteriorates. Family is informed and she is not for resuscitation in case of arrest. She dies 6 weeks into hospital.

2. A 75-year-old male who lives alone is dashed into A&E resus after being found collapsed on the floor by his carer. Despite resuscitation, he cannot be revived and is pronounced dead. He is known to have a past history of 3 myocardial infarctions.

3. A 64-year-old male is admitted for a Whipple's procedure for a cancinoma involving the head of the pancreas. 6 days after surgery, the patient dies from a severe myocardial infarction.

## 153. ANSWERS

1. **A - Issue a death certificate**

If a doctor has attended the deceased in the preceding fourteen days and is confident that he knows the cause of death, he can issue a death certificate.

2. **C - Report to the coroner**

This patient may have had 3 MI's in the past. However, one is not sure about the cause of death in this case. Informing the coroner is compulsory for all deaths as listed below:

- Violent deaths
- Deaths when a doctor has not attended in the previous 14 days
- Cause of death unknown or uncertain
- Accidental death
- Doubtful stillbirth
- Deaths related to surgery or anaesthetic
- Deaths within 24 hours of admission to hospital

3. **A - Issue a death certificate**

Only deaths that occur during or within 24 hours of surgery/anaesthetic/invasive procedure need to be referred to the coroner by law.

## 154. THEME: BENIGN BREAST DISEASE

OPTIONS

A. Cystosarcoma phyllodes
B. Antibioma
C. Breast cyst
D. Lactational breast abscess
E. Duct ectasia
F. Carcinoma of breast

*For each of the patients described below, select the most appropriate diagnosis from the above list. Each option may be used once, more than once, or not at all.*

1. A 34-year-old female presents with a red, hot, tender lump in her left breast for 2 days. She has been unable to feed her 1 month old baby on that breast.

2. A perimenopausal female presents with a greenish nipple discharge which is occasionally stained with blood. She is noted to have a slit like nipple retraction. A chronic indurated mass is palpable beneath the areola. FNAC shows benign cells. She has some coarse calcification on mammogram.

3. A 48-year-old patient presents with bilateral breast lumps. Aspiration reveals a greenish discharge and the lumps disappear. The patient presents to you a few months later with a history of recurrence on the right side.

4. A 46-year-old lady presents with a large massive tumour involving the whole of the right breast with uneven bosselated surface. There is an ulceration of the overlying skin. Examination reveals that the lump is mobile on the chest wall.

## 154. ANSWERS

### 1. D - Lactational breast abscess

This is a typical presentation. Bacterial mastitis occurring in the lactational period is classical. However, bacterial mastitis may be associated with an infected haematoma or with periductal mastitis. Most cases of lactational mastitis are caused by Staphylococcus aureus and if hospital acquired, are likely to be penicillin resistant. Another favourite question with the examiners is an 'antibioma'. It occurs when antibiotics are used in the presence of undrained abscess.

### 2. E - Duct ectasia

In the presence of a mass or nipple retraction, it is very important to exclude a breast carcinoma. Periductal mastitis and fibrosis may cause the slit like nipple retraction. There may be a single or multi duct discharge. The discharge may be serous, blood stained and grumous. Antibiotic therapy may be tried initially—flucloxacillin and metronidazole. However, surgery (Hadfield's operation) is sometimes the only option left.

### 3. C - Breast cyst

These occur in the 40–50 age group usually and are due to non integrated involution of stroma and epithelium. They are often bilateral and multiple. If the cyst resolves completely on aspiration and if the aspirate is not blood stained, no further treatment is needed. However, it is important to remember that about 30% will recur. If, however, on aspiration a residual lump persists or if the fluid is blood stained, an excision biopsy is advisable. Recurrence is also an indication for an excision biopsy and hence indicated in this patient.

### 4. A - Cystosarcoma phyllodes

This is again a typical presentation of the above mentioned condition. Clues include the large tumour, bosselated surface and the fact that the lump remains mobile despite the size and the overlying skin ulceration. It is important to remember that the overlying skin ulceration is due to pressure rather than a direct infiltration. Despite the name, these tumours are rarely cystic and only very rarely develop features of sarcomatous tumour when they metastasise via the blood stream.

## 155. THEME: THYROID CANCER

OPTIONS

A. Papillary carcinoma
B. Follicular carcinoma
C. Anaplastic carcinoma
D. Medullary carcinoma
E. Malignant lymphoma
F. Thyroid teratoma
G. Sarcoma of thyroid

*For each of the patients described below, select the most appropriate diagnosis from the above list. Each option may be used once, more than once, or not at all.*

1. A 70-year-old lady presents with a rapidly growing, hard, fixed lump in the neck with features of tracheal obstruction which requires urgent tracheal decompression.

2. A middle aged immigrant female previously residing in an endemic goitrous area presents with a thyroid tumour that has spread haematogenously to lung and bone. There is no lymphadenopathy.

3. A 22-year-old girl presents with a few swellings in the neck. Your consultant notes enlarged lymphadenopathy in the anterior triangle of the neck and decides to investigate this further as a thyroid cancer.

4. A 70-year-old lady with a long standing history of Hashimoto's thyroiditis develops a rapidly growing goiter.

5. A middle aged male with a family history of multiple endocrine neoplasia presents with diarrhoea and a palpable thyroid lump.

## 155. ANSWERS

1. **C - Anaplastic carcinoma**
Also known as undifferentiated carcinoma, these occur mainly in elderly womer and have a very poor prognosis. Surgery is justified only if there is no infiltration through the thyroid capsule and no evidence of metastases.

2. **B - Follicular carcinoma**
The incidence of follicular carcinoma is high in endemic goitrous areas due to TSH stimulation. They appear to be macroscopically encapsulated but microscopically there is invasion of the capsule and of the vascular spaces in the capsular region. Blood borne metastasis is the favoured route of spread.

3. **A - Papillary carcinoma**
These are the commonest thyroid tumors and the age of the patient is characteristic. Multiple foci may occur in the same lobe as the primary tumour or less commonly both lobes. Spread to the lymph nodes is common. Histologically, the tumour shows papillary projections and characteristic pale, empty nuclei (orphan Annie-eyed nuclei). When a papillary carcinoma presents as an enlarged lymph node in the jugular chain with no palpable abnormality of the thyroid, it is also known as an occult carcinoma. Prognosis is excellent.

4. **E - Malignant lymphoma**
Malignant lymphoma can present in a patient known to have autoimmune thyroiditis. Hence lymphocytic infiltration in the autoimmune process may be an aetiological factor. Response to radiotherapy is good and radical surgery is unnecessary once the diagnosis is established by biopsy.

5. **D - Medullary carcinoma**
This is a simple question really. Medullary carcinoma arises from parafollicular C cells derived from the neural crest. A high level of serum calcitonin is produced by many medullary tumours. Diarrhoea is seen in 30% and is due to 5-hydroxytryptamine or prostaglandins produced by the tumour cells. Medullary carcinoma may arise in combination with adrenal phaeochromocytoma and hyperparathyroidism (usually due to hyperplasia) in the syndrome known as multiple endocrine neoplasia type 2a (MEN 2a).

## 156. THEME: PROGNOSIS OF THYROID CANCER

OPTIONS

A. Less than 10% survival at 3 years
B. Less than 10% survival at 10 years
C. 20–30% survival at 10 years
D. 70% survival at 10 years
E. 2% mortality at 25 years
F. 46% mortality at 25 years

*For each of the patients described below, select the most appropriate value from the above list. Each option may be used once, more than once, or not at all.*

1. A 75-year-old lady is diagnosed with anaplastic carcinoma.
2. A 35-year-old male is diagnosed with medullary carcinoma which has spread to the cervical lymph nodes.
3. A 48-year-old lady with a small differentiated thyroid cancer without distant metastasis.
4. A 42-year-old male with a 2 cm follicular carcinoma with minor capsular involvement.
5. A 30-year-old female with papillary carcinoma with distant metastasis.

## 156. ANSWERS

1. **A - Less than 10% survival at 3 years**

These are the least common (0.5%–1.5%) and most deadly of all thyroid cancers. In most cases death occurs within months rather than within years.

2. **D - 70% survival at 10 years**

This is the third commonest form of thyroid cancer. Overall, 10 year survival rates are 90% when all the disease is confined to the thyroid gland, 70% with spread to cervical lymph nodes, and 20% when spread to distant sites is present.

3. **E - 2% mortality at 25 years**

4. **E - 2% mortality at 25 years**

5. **F - 46% mortality at 25 years**

Patients with differentiated thyroid cancers can be divided into two groups: high-risk (25 year mortality of 46%) and low-risk (25 year mortality rate of 2%). Low-risk group consists of men 40 years of age and under and women 50 years of age and under without distant metastases. It also includes older patients with intrathyroid papillary carcinoma or follicular carcinoma with minor capsular involvement (tumours less than 5 cm in diameter and no distant metastases). The high-risk group includes all patients with distant metastases, all older patients with extra thyroid papillary carcinoma or follicular carcinoma with major capsular involvement, and tumours 5 cm or more in diameter regardless of extent of disease.

## 157. THEME: GYNAECOMASTIA

OPTIONS

A. XXY trisomy
B. Liver failure
C. Cimetidine
D. Omeprazole
E. Gaviscon
F. Leprosy
G. Teratoma of testis
H. Physiological
I. Bronchial carcinoma
J. Pituitary disease
K. Down's syndrome

*For each of the patients described below, select the most appropriate diagnosis from the above list. Each option may be used once, more than once, or not at all.*

1. A 12-year-old boy is seen for a slightly enlarged right breast. He has normal developmental features and his parents tell you that he is always at the top of his batch. Examination confirms a small gynaecomastia on the right side. He has scanty pubic hair, a developing penis and testicular size that is normal for his age.

2. A 46-year-old chronic alcoholic presents with confusion, ascites and haematemesis. He is noted to have bilateral gynaecomastia.

3. A 48-year-old male is known to have 'indigestion' for some time for which he takes medications. He has presented to you with gynaecomastia involving both breasts.

4. A 17-year-old boy is referred to you with gynaecomastia. He is a school dropout following poor grades, is tall and thin. His penis and testicles are both small for his age. He also demonstrates only scanty pubic hair and no axillary hair.

## 157. ANSWERS

1. **H - Physiological**
2. **B - Liver failure**
3. **C - Cimetidine**
4. **A - XXY trisomy**

## 158. THEME: GYNAECOMASTIA

OPTIONS

A. XXY trisomy
B. Spironolactone
C. Cimetidine
D. Phenytoin
E. Metformin
F. Leprosy
G. Teratoma of testis
H. Insulin
I. Bronchial carcinoma
J. Pituitary disease
K. Diabetes mellitus
L. Digoxin
M. Atenolol
N. Aspirin
O. Metastasis

*For each of the patients described below, select the most appropriate diagnosis from the above list. Each option may be used once, more than once, or not at all.*

1. A 66-year-old male is known to be on digoxin for atrial fibrillation, on insulin and metformin for poorly controlled diabetes and on phenytoin for epilepsy. He presents with gynaecomastia.

2. A 65-year-old male is on spironolactone, atenolol and aspirin. He presents with gynaecomastia.

3. A 65-year-old male is admitted to hospital with cough and haemoptysis. Examination and investigations confirm a mass in the lungs.

## 158. ANSWERS

1. **L - Digoxin**

2. **B - Spironolactone**

3. **I - Bronchial carcinoma**

Hypertrophy of the male breast may be unilateral or bilateral. It is important to remember some of the most important causes. Physiological enlargement around puberty is well known and all that is needed is reassurance. It is characteristically unilateral. Other causes include Klinefelter's syndrome (XXY trisomy); drugs like cimetidine, digitalis, spironolactone; leprosy; liver failure; and teratoma of the testis. It can rarely also occur due to ectopic hormonal production in bronchial carcinoma, and in adrenal and pituitary lesions.

## 159. THEME: COMPLICATIONS OF BREAST CARCINOMA

OPTIONS

A. Cerebral metastases
B. Hypercalcaemia
C. Spinal cord compression
D. Lymphoedema
E. Virchow's node
F. Pathological fracture
G. Deep vein thrombosis
H. Ankle sprain

*For each of the scenarios described below, select the most appropriate complication of breast carcinoma from the list of options above. Each option may be used once, more than once, or not at all.*

1. A 55-year-old female known to have breast cancer presents with headache, nausea and vomiting. She is noted to have papilloedema.

2. A 50-year-old lady presents with a progressively increasing generalized swelling of the right upper limb. Past history includes a breast surgery for carcinoma on the right side.

3. A 40-year-old lady under treatment for breast cancer presents with thirst, polyuria and constipation.

4. A 50-year-old lady is known to have advanced breast cancer. She presents to you with persisting back pain and sudden onset bladder dysfunction.

5. A 55-year-old lady known to have advanced breast carcinoma presents with pain and inability to bear weight on the right leg following a small trip down a step at home. On examination the right lower limb is shortened and externally rotated.

## 159. ANSWERS

1. **A - Cerebral metastases**

Features may include headache which is often worse in the morning, nausea, vomiting, papilloedema, fits and focal neurological signs.

2. **D - Lymphoedema**

This is a troublesome complication of breast cancer treatment. It is less often seen now because radical axillary dissection and radiotherapy are rarely combined. It can occur months or years after treatment. It is however important to exclude a recurrent tumour. An oedematous limb is susceptible to bacterial infections following quite minor trauma, and these require vigorous antibiotic treatment. Lymphangiosarcoma is a rare complication of lymphoedema.

3. **B - Hypercalcaemia**

This is an oncological emergency encountered most commonly in myeloma. Causes in general include lytic bone metastasis, production of osteoclast activating factor or ectopic PTHrp release by the tumour. Features include lethargy, anorexia, nausea, polydipsia, polyuria, constipation, dehydration, confusion and weakness. Serum calcium will be > 3 mmol/L. Management involves rehydration. IV pamidronate may be needed.

4. **C - Spinal cord compression**

The history is classical. Features could also include lower limb weakness, sensory loss and bowel dysfunction. Urgent imaging will be needed followed by referral to the neurosurgeons.

5. **F - Pathological fracture**

Features suggesting a fractured neck of femur with a small trip suggest a pathological fracture since this lady is known to have advanced breast cancer.

## 160. THEME: EAR ACHE IN PAEDIATRICS

OPTIONS

A. Acute suppurative otitis media
B. Acute mastoiditis
C. Otitis externa
D. Herpes zoster
E. Furuncle
F. Tonsillitis
G. Adenoiditis
H. Acquired cholesteatoma

*For each of the clinical scenarios described below, select the most appropriate diagnosis from the list of options above. Each option may be used once, more than once, or not at all.*

1. An 8-year-old child presents with a rapid onset right sided ear ache following an episode of upper respiratory tract infection. He describes it as very painful. Parents have also noticed some subjective hearing loss. Examination reveals a red and bulging tympanic membrane.

2. A 12-year-old lad presents with persistent left ear problems for many years. He has had chronic ear discharge with decreased hearing on the affected side. Examination reveals a perforated tympanic membrane with a small whitish mass protruding through it.

3. A 7-year-old girl presents with severe pain in the left ear. Examination reveals left facial palsy with visible vesicles in the left ear canal.

4. A 5-year-old kid presents with severe otalgia. He saw his GP last week when he was treated for acute suppurative otitis media with antibiotics. Examination reveals swelling and tenderness behind the ears.

## 160. ANSWERS

1. **A - Acute suppurative otitis media**

The presence of a red and bulging tympanic membrane suggests suppurative otitis media. In chronic suppurative otitis media, a perforation will be evident.

2. **H - Acquired cholesteatoma**

Clues include chronic ear problems, perforation in the tympanic membrane and a visible cholesteatoma through the perforation.

3. **D - Herpes zoster**

This is likely to be Ramsay Hunt syndrome.

4. **B - Acute mastoiditis**

The disease seems to have progressed to cause mastoiditis.

## 161. THEME: ORAL SIGNS AND SYSTEMIC DISEASE

OPTIONS

A. Blue gum lines
B. Angular stomatitis
C. Macroglossia
D. Melanosis of the lips
E. Hairy leukoplakia
F. Gingival hyperplasia

*For each of the clinical scenarios described below, select the most appropriate oral sign from the list of options above. Each option may be used once, more than once, or not at all.*

1. Lead poisoning

2. Acromegaly

3. AIDS

4. Iron deficiency anaemia

## 161. ANSWERS

1. **A - Blue gum lines**

Ingestion is by far the most important exposure route. Lead may be in the air if dust is created by grinding or similar procedures, or if fumes are created by welding torches.

2. **C - Macroglossia**

Acromegaly results in gradual enlargement of body tissues including the bones of the face, jaw, hands, feet, and skull. It is caused by abnormal production of growth hormone after normal growth of the skeleton and other organs is complete. Excessive production of growth hormone in children causes gigantism rather than acromegaly.The cause of the increased hormone secretion is usually a benign tumour of the pituitary gland.

3. **E - Hairy leukoplakia**

Other important oral signs in AIDS include oral candidiasis and Kaposi's sarcoma.

4. **B - Angular stomatitis**

## 162. THEME: TERMINOLOGY IN ENT DISORDERS

OPTIONS

A. Dysphagia
B. Odynophagia
C. Laryngitis
D. Hoarseness
E. Stridor
F. Tonsillitis
G. Laryngomalacia
H. Pharyngitis

*For each of the descriptions below, select the most appropriate terminology from the list of options above. Each option may be used once, more than once, or not at all.*

1. This word describes pain on swallowing.

2. This describes the sound made when the laryngeal airway is narrowed.

3. Persons who abuse their voice commonly present with this symptom.

## 162. ANSWERS

1. **B - Odynophagia**

Dysphagia is actually difficulty in swallowing.

2. **E - Stridor**

This is caused by air flowing through a narrowed laryngeal or tracheal airway and is often louder on inspiration than expiration. Wheeze arises in the bronchioles and is usually expiratory. Stertor is caused by vibration of tissues above the larynx, and snoring by tissues in the oro- and nasopharynx.

3. **D - Hoarseness**

Vocal abuse causes trauma to the vocal cords and consequent swelling or nodule formation, thus resulting in hoarseness. These are called variously as singer's nodule, or screamer's nodule in young children.

## 163. THEME: DIAGNOSIS OF THROAT DISORDERS

OPTIONS

A. Post cricoid web
B. Epstein-Barr virus
C. Pharyngeal pouch
D. Infectious mononucleosis
E. Reinke's oedema
F. Laryngitis
G. Adenoid hypertrophy

*For each of the descriptions below, select the most appropriate diagnosis from the list of options above. Each option may be used once, more than once, or not at all.*

1. This disease may cause emergency tonsillectomy to protect the airway.

2. This problem may result in aspiration pneumonia.

## 163. ANSWERS

1. **D - Infectious mononucleosis**

Epstein-Barr virus causes infectious mononucleosis (glandular fever).

2. **C - Pharyngeal pouch**

Occasionally these may present with recurrent chest infections due to aspiration from regurgitation into the larynx.

## 164. THEME: DISEASES INVOLVING THE HEAD AND NECK

OPTIONS

A. Squamous cell carcinoma
B. Adenocarcinoma
C. Wegener's granulomatosis
D. Pleomorphic adenoma
E. Warthin's tumour
F. Leukoplakia

*For each of the descriptions below, select the most appropriate diagnosis from the list of options above. Each option may be used once, more than once, or not at all.*

1. This disease presents with crusting and bleeding from the nose. It can involve the kidneys and lungs also.

2. This is the commonest tumour found in the parotid gland.

3. This is the commonest malignant tumour of the maxillary sinus.

## 164. ANSWERS

1. **C - Wegener's granulomatosis**

This is a life threatening condition because of the necrotising glomerulonephritis that also occurs, leading to renal failure. An important clue is the presence of cANCA (antineutrophil cytoplasmic antibody).

2. **D - Pleomorphic adenoma**

The pleomorphic adenoma occurs at any age and has an equal sex incidence. It accounts for at least 75% of parotid tumours and more than 50% of submandibular tumours. Clinically, the tumour has the texture of cartilage and has an irregular and bosselated surface. Very rarely after a number of years the tumour may undergo malignant change and for this reason all patients presenting with pleomorphic adenoma should be advised to undergo surgical removal of the tumour.

3. **A - Squamous cell carcinoma**

Squamous cell carcinomas make up the vast majority of head and neck cancers. Adenocarcinoma is sometimes found in the ethmoid sinuses but usually occurs in people who work with hard woods, such as carpenters and cabinet makers.

## 165. THEME: VISUAL FIELD DEFECTS

OPTIONS

A. Contralateral upper homonymous quadrantanopia
B. Inferior homonymous quadrantanopia
C. Cortical blindness
D. Monocular blindness
E. Tunnel vision
F. Central scotoma
G. Bitemporal field defects
H. Non-peripheral homonymous hemianopic scotomas with macular sparing

*For each of the conditions described below, select the most appropriate visual field defect from the list of options mentioned above. Each option may be used once, more than once, or not at all.*

1. Pituitary tumour

2. Temporal lobe tumours

3. Parietal lobe tumour

4. Posterior cerebral artery ischaemia

5. Central retinal artery occlusion

## 165. ANSWERS

1. **G - Bitemporal field defects**

Fibres from the nasal retina of both eyes cross in the optic chiasma to join uncrossed temporal retinal fibres. Pituitary tumour may disrupt the chiasma affecting the fibres from the nasal retinas and hence the defect.

2. **A - Contralateral upper homonymous quadrantanopia**

Superior parts of the visual field fall inferiorly on the retina, temporal fields on the nasal retina and vice versa.

3. **B - Inferior homonymous quadrantanopia**

Yeah, you guessed rightly. Even though the word contralateral is missing, this is still the correct response.

4. **H - Non-peripheral homonymous hemianopic scotomas with macular sparing**

Posterior cerebral artery ischaemia causes posterior visual cortex lesion and hence the characteristic defect. Remember, it is the anterior visual cortex that deals with peripheral vision.

5. **D - Monocular blindness**

There is dramatic visual loss within seconds of occlusion. The retina appears white, with a cherry red spot at the macula. Occlusion is often thromboembolic. It is important to rule out temporal arteritis.

## 166. THEME: TRANSIENT VISUAL LOSS

OPTIONS

A. Aspirin
B. Warfarin
C. Clopidogrel
D. Heparin
E. No treatment
F. Antistatin

*For each of the scenarios described below, select the most appropriate treatment option from the list of options mentioned above. Each option may be used once, more than once, or not at all.*

1. A 60-year-old male presents with an episode of transient loss of vision in the left eye. General and systemic examination is normal.

2. A 60-year-old male presents with an episode of transient loss of vision in the left eye. General and systemic examination is normal apart from an irregularly irregular pulse.

## 166. ANSWERS

1. **A - Aspirin**

2. **B - Warfarin**

In the first case the most appropriate option is aspirin to prevent stroke. Since the second scenario suggests an atrial fibrillation, warfarin is indicated here.

## 167. THEME: DIAGNOSIS OF STRIDOR

OPTIONS

A. Croup
B. Acute epiglottitis
C. Ingestion of FB
D. Vocal cord palsy
E. Angioneurotic oedema
F. Foreign body inhalation
G. Diphtheria
H. Retropharyngeal abscess
I. Laryngomalacia

*For each of the scenarios mentioned below, select the most appropriate cause for stridor from the list of options mentioned above. Each option may be used once, more than once or not at all.*

1. A 16-year-old girl presents with facial oedema, dyspnoea and stridor. She is apyrexial. Past history is negative.

2. A week-old baby is brought in by concerned parents with noisy breathing. They describe loud noises brought on by certain positions in sleep.

3. A 21-month baby is brought in by concerned parents with intermittent loud breathing noises and barking cough for a day's duration. The baby has had an upper respiratory tract infection for the past week which has worsened in recent days. Examination reveals an inspiratory stridor. The baby is irritable but generally well.

4. A 5-year-old girl develops a choking episode while playing in the school. She recovers, but over the next day becomes unwell and develops stridor. She is noted to have marked intercostal recession.

## 167. ANSWERS

1. **E - Angioneurotic oedema**

The aetiology is unknown. It most commonly affects young girls and women. The main feature distinguishing this condition from an anaphylactic shock is the absence of a precipitation allergen.

2. **I - Laryngomalacia**

This may sometimes appear hours after birth. Floppy aryepiglottic folds and glottis increase the tendency of the larynx to collapse in inspiration in affected infants. Stridor may be characteristically seen in certain positions, during sleep or when upset. Majority need no treatment.

3. **A - Croup**

This is laryngotracheobronchitis and is most commonly viral in origin. It is usually self limiting and treatable at home with humidification +/- antibiotics. Severe cases may need admission to hospital. They tend to worsen in the night and hence it is preferable to admit kids even with mild illness, if they are seen in A&E in the evenings.

4. **F - Foreign body inhalation**

The history is classical.

## 168. THEME: VERTIGO

OPTIONS

A. Meniere's disease
B. Benign positional (postural) vertigo
C. Drug induced
D. Acoustic neuroma
E. Multiple sclerosis
F. Vestibular neuronitis

*For each of the scenarios mentioned below, select the most appropriate cause for vertigo from the list of options mentioned above. Each option may be used once, more than once or not at all.*

1. A 24-year-old male is seen with complaints of sudden onset vertigo, vomiting and prostration, which are exacerbated by head movements. He has been suffering with a cold for the past few days.

2. A 50-year-old lady is referred to you for an episode of severe vertigo that lasted a day accompanied with nausea and vomiting. She has also noticed a hearing loss in her left ear and feels that it has become progressively worse. Examination confirmed a left sided sensorineural hearing loss.

3. A teenager is recovering from a recent road traffic accident and 'minor' head injury that was diagnosed in A&E. She has recently noticed attacks of sudden onset vertigo lasting a minute brought on by head turning. Hallpike test is positive.

## 168. ANSWERS

1. **F - Vestibular neuronitis**

The history is classical. This condition usually follows a febrile illness in adults and is most probably viral. Treat with cyclizine. It is difficult to distinguish from viral labyrinthitis (note however that labyrinthitis is not part of the options).

2. **A - Meniere's disease**

The history is classical. Presence of uni or bilateral tinnitus may be an additional clue. There is progressive sensorineural deafness. Treatment for acute vertigo is symptomatic. Surgery may be needed later on.

3. **B - Benign positional (postural) vertigo**

This is again common after a head injury. Other causes include post viral illness, spontaneous degeneration of labyrinth, chronic middle ear infections. Hallpike test is positive. This is usually a self limiting condition. If persistent, physiotherapy referral for vestibular exercises may be needed.

## 169. THEME: EPISTAXIS

OPTIONS

A. Allergic sinusitis
B. Cocaine use
C. Haemophilia
D. Foreign body
E. Idiopathic thrombocytopenic purpura
F. Maxillary carcinoma
G. Non accidental injury
H. Cannabis use
I. Orf

*For each of the scenarios mentioned below, select the most appropriate cause for epistaxis from the list of options mentioned above. Each option may be used once, more than once or not at all.*

1. A 27-year-old male presents with a history of chronic sinusitis and epistaxis over the past few years. Rhinoscopy reveals nasal crusting and a septal defect. The patient appears unkempt. There is marked gingivitis and tooth decay.
2. A 6-year-old kid presents with epistaxis. Parents are concerned that he bruised with trivial trauma. Examination reveals a splenomegaly.
3. A 3-year-old kid presents with right sided epistaxis. His mom has noticed discharge from his right nostril for a few months. Examination reveals inflamed mucous membrane with the presence of bloody discharge.
4. A 50-year-old cabinet maker presents with an episode of epistaxis in the morning. On examination right maxillary prominence is noted. Rhinoscopy demonstrates the presence of a fleshy mass obstructing the right nasal cavity. He has an associated unilateral diplopia on the right side.
5. A 50-year-old sheep farmer presents with right sided epistaxis. Rhinoscopy confirms the presence of a polyp in the anterior aspect of his nasal septum. He does not have any past medical history.

## 169. ANSWERS

1. **B - Cocaine use**

2. **E - Idiopathic thrombocytopenic purpura (ITP)**

3. **D - Foreign body**

4. **F - Maxillary carcinoma**

5. **I - Orf**

Epistaxis is the commonest ENT emergency by far. However, in 80% the cause remains unknown. Trauma from nose picking and fractures is a common cause. The first scenario clearly describes a cocaine abuser. Nasal crusting, septal defect, unkempt patient, gingivitis and tooth decay all point towards the same. Another clue might be the presence of whistling noises coming from the nose during inspiration. The presence of epistaxis with easy bruising along with a splenomegaly points to ITP as the cause in scenario 2. The 3rd scenario is again classical. Foreign bodies are commonest in kids aged 2–3 years. The 4th scenario is again typical. The patient's occupation and findings all point to maxillary carcinoma. Though squamous cell carcinoma is the most common histology in head and neck cancers, for occupations involving hard wood (e.g., carpenters, cabinet makers), an adenocarcinoma is the commonest finding. In scenario 5, the most important clue is the occupation of sheep farming. That alone clinches the diagnosis.

## 170. THEME: DIAGNOSIS OF HOARSENESS OF VOICE

OPTIONS

A. Acute viral/bacterial laryngitis
B. Chronic laryngitis
C. Singer's nodules
D. Laryngeal papilloma
E. Gastro-oesophageal reflux disease
F. Recurrent laryngeal nerve palsy
G. Carcinoma of the larynx
H. Laryngeal trauma

*For each of the scenarios described below, select the most appropriate diagnosis from the list of options mentioned above. Each option may be used once, more than once, or not at all.*

1. A 5-year-old boy presents with a progressive hoarseness for the past couple of months. Examination of the vocal cords reveals multiple small pedunculated lesions on the vocal cords that are pinkish white in colour.

2. A 30-year-old male computer programmer reports hoarseness, which is most marked early in the morning. This resolves progressively as the day proceeds. He is a non smoker. Indirect laryngoscopy reveals slightly oedematous red cords.

3. A 35-year-old street hawker attends A&E after losing his voice since morning. He smokes about 10 cigarettes per day. Examination reveals oedema of the vocal cords with a small submucosal haematoma.

4. A 22-year-old amateur singer attends ENT clinic for a recent hoarseness in voice. Examination confirms several small nodules on both vocal cords at the junction of the anterior third and posterior two-thirds of the vocal cords.

5. A 70-year-old gentleman undergoes surgery for a pharyngeal pouch under a general anesthetic. Postoperatively the patient develops hoarseness of voice.

## 170. ANSWERS

1. **D - Laryngeal papilloma**

These are viral and are commonly seen between the ages of 2 and 5. They must be removed with care, as they can easily be spread to the whole of the larynx and trachea. Laser therapy is the treatment of choice. They are said to disappear at puberty.

2. **E - Gastro-oesophageal reflux disease**

The finding on indirect laryngoscopy along with the history of diurnal hoarseness suggests this diagnosis.

3. **H - Laryngeal trauma**

This man is a street hawker. The pathology is due to violent banging of the vocal cords.

4. **C - Singer's nodules**

The history and examination findings are again classical. The site of common occurrence of these nodules as mentioned in the question is the site for the most contact injury during speech. Nodules are often bilateral. Speech therapy can help in the early stages. The nodules can be removed surgically.

5. **F - Recurrent laryngeal nerve palsy**

With partial paralysis cords are fixed in the midline, while in complete paralysis they are fixed mid way (para-median position). Proposed reasons for this include the Semon's law and the Wagner–Grossman theory. Causes of paralysis include cancers (larynx most commonly, thyroid, oesophagus, hypopharynx, bronchus or any malignant node), iatrogenic (after thyroid surgery, oesophageal surgery, or pharyngeal pouch surgery). Unilateral cord palsies can be compensated for by movement of the contralateral cord, but may require formal medialization in the form of fat injections or a thyroplasty.

## 171. THEME: BACTERIAL SURGICAL INFECTIONS

OPTIONS

A. Clostridium difficile
B. Clostridium welchii/perfringens
C. Staphylococcus aureus
D. Escherichia coli
E. Pseudomonas aeruginosa
F. Klebsiella
G. MRSA
H. Bacteroides fragilis
I. Streptococcus pneumoniae

*For each of the patients described below, select the most likely causative organism from the list of options above. Each option may be used once, more than once, or not at all.*

1. A 79-year-old nursing home resident is seen in A&E for dehydration due to offensive greenish diarrhoea for 4 days. He had been to A&E last week with a UTI which was treated with cephradine.

2. A 40-year-old gentleman undergoes a Lichtenstein tension free mesh hernioplasty on the right. 5 days after surgery he visits his GP practice nurse with a discharge from the wound.

3. A 32-year-old traveler from the Mediterranean presents acutely unwell to hospital. He is pyrexial at 40°C and exhibits all the features of a septicaemia shock. His past history included a major organ resection for a blood disorder.

4. A patient undergoes an emergency resection for a perforated diverticular abscess. Postoperatively day 4 the patient develops fever. A blue–green discharge is noted on the wound swabs.

## 171. ANSWERS

1. **A - Clostridium difficile**

The use of cephalosporins promotes the proliferation of gut Clostridium difficile, which causes pseudomembranous colitis. The exotoxin produced results in damage to gut epithelial cell membrane. The C.difficile toxin can be identified rapidly. The patient should be barrier nursed for at least 48 hours until after the diarrhoea has settled.

2. **C - Staphylococcus aureus**

This is the commonest cause of wound infection. It classically causes suppuration, particularly skin abscesses. It may also cause cellulitis.

3. **I - Streptococcus pneumoniae**

The implication in the question is most probably on thalassaemia and splenectomy in the past. These patients are at increased risk of sepsis from encapsulated bacteria (which are mainly phagocytosed by the spleen) like Streptococcus pneumoniae, Neisseria meningitidis, Haemophilus influenzae and Babesia microti.

4. **E - Pseudomonas aeruginosa**

The blue-green discharge is characteristic. After bowel surgery most infections are caused by aerobic Gram-negative bacilli (AGNB) acting in synergy with Bacteroides. This is particularly true after appendicitis, diverticulitis and peritonitis. However, the blue-green discharge in this question is the most important clue. AGNB include E coli, Klebsiella and Proteus.

## 172. THEME: BACTERIAL SURGICAL INFECTIONS

OPTIONS

A. Clostridium difficile
B. Clostridium welchii/perfringens
C. Staphylococcus aureus
D. Escherichia coli
E. Pseudomonas aeruginosa
F. Pasteurella multocida
G. MRSA
H. Bacteroides fragilis
I. Streptococcus pneumoniae
J. Clostridium tetani

*For each of the patients described below, select the most likely causative organism from the list of options above. Each option may be used once, more than once, or not at all.*

1. A 75-year-old pensioner is out gardening when he stabs his foot in the garden with an unknown object. He presents to casualty in 3 days time with fever, malaise and severe pain in the leg. Examination reveals the presence of crepitus in the muscles of the leg.

2. A 22-year-old animal lover is bit by her cat on the index finger. There is cellulitis around the bite marks predominantly in the region of the 1st metacarpophalangeal joint.

3. A 75-year-old male becomes confused and drowsy less than 48 hours after a TURP for BPH. His urine is cloudy and offensive.

4. A 45-year-old lady with rheumatoid arthritis presents with an acutely hot, painful and swollen knee. Aspiration suggests frank pus. Microbiology suggests Gram-positive cocci.

## 172. ANSWERS

1. **B - Clostridium welchii/perfringens**

This is again a relatively straightforward question. The infection in question is caused by gas forming organisms. However, C. tetani can be excluded with confidence because of the short incubation period and the absence of muscle spasms.

2. **F - Pasteurella multocida**

This is a Gram-negative parvobacterium found in the majority of animal bites. Another favourite with the examiners includes Eikenella corrodens. Treatment needs to be broad spectrum and could include augmentin or an oral cephalosporin with metronidazole.

3. **D - Escherichia coli**

This is another classical Question. This is a Gram-negative facultative anaerobic bacillus. Fewer than $10^3$ organisms/mL of urine are not considered significant.

4. **C - Staphylococcus aureus**

## 173. THEME: ANAEROBES AND SURGERY

OPTIONS

A. Clostridium tetani
B. Clostridium botulinum
C. Clostridium difficile
D. Fusobacterium necrophorum
E. Porphyromonas gingivalis
F. Bacteroides fragilis

*For each of the patients described below, select the most likely causative organism from the list of options above. Each option may be used once, more than once, or not at all.*

1. Causes severe periodontal disease

2. Occurs following contaminat on with soil. Incubation period ranges from 3 weeks to 3 months. Produces an exotoxin and causes hyperreflexic spasm.

3. Associated with necrobacillosis—a severe tonsillitis with septicaemia and metastatic abscesses.

4. Causes antibiotic associated diarrhoea and pseudomembranous colitis.

## 173. ANSWERS

1. **E - Porphyromonas gingivalis**

2. **A - Clostridium tetani**

3. **D - Fusobacterium necrophorum**

4. **C - Clostridium difficile**
Treatment is needed with metronidazole or vancomycin.

## 174. THEME: LOIN PAIN

OPTIONS

A. Pyelonephritis
B. Renal stone
C. Pancreatitis
D. Pelvi-ureteric obstruction
E. Pelvic abscess
F. Renal adenocarcinoma
G. Ureteric colic
H. Urinary bladder carcinoma

*For each of the patients described below, select the most likely diagnosis from the list of options above. Each option may be used once, more than once, or not at all.*

1. A middle aged man presents with loin pain, haematuria and loin mass.

2. A teenager presents with agonising colicky right loin pain radiating to his groin. He is found tossing around on the examination couch.

3. A 25-year-old lady presents with a sensation of dragging heaviness in his left loin, which is made worse by binge drinking.

4. A 25-year-old man is referred to the urology clinic with intermittent attacks of right loin pain for which he has been repeatedly seen in A&E. The A&E staff have noticed a vague swelling in the loin on each occasion which 'disappears' after the patient passes urine.

5. A 22-year-old girl with multiple surgeries as a child for bilateral vesico-ureteric reflux presents with left loin pain, dysuria and fever.

## 174. ANSWERS

1. **F - Renal adenocarcinoma**

Haematuria is the commonest mode of presentation of a renal carcinoma. Three other common modes of presentation include general debility (as in this case), pain in the loin or a mass. Rarer presentations include ureteric colic (clot colic), bone pain, pathological fractures, pyrexia of unknown origin, hypertension and features of erythrocythaemia. Presentation with a varicocele is a favourite with many examiners.

2. **G - Ureteric colic**

Ureteric colic is agonising pain from loin to groin. Typically it starts suddenly. Strangury may occasionally occur if the stone is in the intramural ureter.

3. **D - Pelvi-ureteric obstruction**

4. **D - Pelvi-ureteric obstruction**

Unilateral hydronephrosis is twice more common in females and the right side is more commonly affected. Most common causes include an idiopathic pelviureteric junction obstruction or calculus. Presenting features may include an insidious onset with dragging pain, which is typically aggravated by excessive fluid intake, attacks of acute renal colic or a presentation with Dietl's crisis. Dietl's crisis is intermittent hydronephrosis characterized by a swelling in the loin, after an attack of acute renal pain, which disappears with the passage of urine.

5. **A - Pyelonephritis**

History of reflux with systemic features and loin pain suggests pyelonephritis.

## 175. THEME: RENAL CONDITIONS

OPTIONS

A. Renal calculi
B. Acute tubular necrosis
C. Horseshoe kidneys
D. Acute renal failure
E. Pyonephrosis
F. Polycystic kidneys
G. Renal tuberculosis
H. Renal tubular injury

*For each of the patients described below, select the most likely diagnosis from the list of options above. Each option may be used once, more than once, or not at all.*

1. A 35-year-old man presents to the emergency department with sudden onset agonising pain in the right lumbar region for 6 hours duration. The pain is colicky. Urine dipstick reveals the presence of blood.

2. An 87-year-old male presents with vomiting, anorexia and dehydration for 4 days. He has a large stag horn calculus in the right pelvis with a papery thin cortex for many years. He also suffers from recurrent renal colic on the left side. His urea is 31 and creatinine is 365.

3. A 24-year-old lady presents with an irregular abdominal mass, loin pain, haematuria and hypertension.

4. A 24-year-old male is admitted with a crush injury following a RTA. Overnight he develops compartment syndrome in his left leg. An emergency fasciotomy reveals the presence of ischaemic muscles. He develops myoglobinuria and develops a renal complication.

5. A 66-year-old immigrant from Asia presents with anaemia, fever and a vague cystic swelling in his left loin. A plain X-ray KUB demonstrates the presence of a calculus. An ultrasound shows dilatation of the renal pelvis and calyces.

## 175. ANSWERS

1. **A - Renal Calculi**
Pain is the leading symptom in 75% of people with urinary stone disease. Fixed renal pain may be worse on movement. Other symptoms at presentation can include haematuria and pyuria. The patient is restless and turns and tosses around in bed (unlike in acute appendicitis or peritonitis when the patient lies still). Urine dipstick usually shows red blood cells. White blood cells may be seen if there is associated infection.

2. **D - Acute renal failure**
This patient already has a nonfunctional kidney on one side. A renal calculus presumably has led to obstruction on the other side. This is a post renal cause of acute renal failure.

3. **F - Polycystic kidneys**
This is a hereditary condition and transmitted by either parent as an autosomal dominant trait. It does not usually manifest itself clinically before the age of 30 years. The kidneys are enlarged with the cysts giving the appearance of a collection of bubbles below the renal capsule. Clinical features may include an irregular mass, loin pain, haematuria and infection. Important clues may be the presence of hypertension (75% of patients) and uraemia.

4. **B - Acute tubular necrosis**
Crush syndromes and compartment syndromes are a cause of ischaemia; also fluid loss, disseminated intravascular coagulation, and myoglobin release can cause acute tubular necrosis. Dialysis may be needed.

5. **E - Pyonephrosis**
The features on investigation with the classic triad of anaemia, fever and a swelling in the loin suggest the diagnosis. An important clue in renal tuberculosis may be the presence of 'sterile' pyuria.

## 176. THEME: DISORDERS OF THE URINARY SYSTEM

OPTIONS

A. Pyonephrosis
B. Acute tubular necrosis
C. Horseshoe kidneys
D. Acute renal failure
E. Renal carcinoma
F. Bladder calculus
G. Renal tuberculosis
H. Carcinoma of the bladder

*For each of the patients described below, select the most likely diagnosis from the list of options above. Each option may be used once, more than once, or not at all.*

1. A 12-year-old African immigrant is referred with frequency, strangury and occasional interruption of the urinary stream.

2. A 35-year-old African immigrant is referred with anorexia, weight loss, frequency of micturition and dysuria. Urine investigations suggest a sterile pyuria.

3. A 75-year-old chronic smoker presents with a 6-week history of painless haematuria.

4. A 60-year-old chronic smoker presents with a 6-week history of a discomfort in the left loin. He also gives a history of haematuria. A mass is palpable in the left lumbar region which is both ballotable and bimanually palpable.

### 176. ANSWERS

1. **F - Bladder calculus**

Primary vesical calculus is commoner in poorer societies due to a poor diet. It is hence rare in the western world. Typical features have been mentioned in the question. Pain (strangury) usually occurs at the end of micturition and is referred to the tip of the penis or the labia majora. In very young boys, screaming and pulling at the penis with the hand at the end of micturition may be an important clue.

2. **G - Renal tuberculosis**

Presence of frequency, dysuria, renal pain with 'constitutional symptoms' like weight loss and evening rise of temperature should arouse suspicion especially in immigrant population. Sterile pyuria is an important give away here. Bacteriological examination—at least three full specimens of early morning urine should be sent for microscopy and culture before specific chemotherapy is started.

3. **H - Carcinoma of the bladder**

Over 90% of these are transitional cell in origin. Important aetiologies include smoking, working in dye and rubber industry, long term catheterization and schistosomiasis infestation of the bladder. Painless haematuria is the most common symptom and should be considered as a carcinoma arising from the bladder unless proven otherwise. Constant pain in the pelvis usually indicates extravesical spread. Investigations include urine examination including culture and cystoscopy. Transurethral resection of bladder tumour (TURBT) followed by a course of radiotherapy is useful in treating most tumours. Intravesical chemotherapy and immunotherapy (using BCG) have an important role in management.

4. **E - Renal carcinoma**

## 177. THEME: TREATMENT OF UROLOGICAL MALIGNANCIES

OPTIONS

A. Transurethral resection of bladder tumour
B. Chemotherapy
C. Intravesical BCG
D. Nephrectomy with preservation of perinephric fat
E. Nephroureterectomy
F. Radical cystectomy
G. Nephrectomy with removal of perinephric fat

*For each of the patients below, select the most appropriate treatment from the above list. Each option may be used once, more than once, or not at all.*

1. A 60-year-old male presents with a 6-week history of a discomfort in the left loin. He also gives a history of haematuria. A mass is palpable in the left lumbar region which is both ballotable and bimanually palpable. CT scan confirms a lesion confined to the left kidney without evidence of hilar lymphadenopathy or renal vein involvement.

2. A 60-year-old chronic smoker presents with painless haematuria. An intravenous urography shows a filling defect in the bladder. Rest of the examination is normal.

3. A 60-year-old male presents with a 6-week history of haematuria with a discomfort in the left loin. Investigations confirm an irregular filling defect in the left renal pelvis. Urine cytology suggests a transitional cell tumour.

## 177. ANSWERS

### 1. G - Nephrectomy with removal of perinephric fat

The transabdominal approach is widely preferred. The vascular pedicle should be ligated before the kidney is mobilized to prevent dissemination. If the renal vein or the inferior vena cava is invaded the surgeon must obtain control of the cava above and below as a first priority. Adenocarcinoma of the kidney does not respond well to radiotherapy or chemotherapy.

### 2. A - Transurethral resection of bladder tumour

This is recommended in a patient with bladder tumour. It also helps to serve as a biopsy to stage the muscle invasion. A single dose of mitomycin C instilled into the bladder prior to catheter removal decreases the risks of recurrence in patients with pTa, PT1 grade 1 and 2 disease.

### 3. E - Nephroureterectomy

Papillary transitional tumours of the renal pelvis tend to invade the renal parenchyma. Quite characteristically they are multifocal. Seeding down the lumen of the urinary tract may give rise to multiple ureteric tumours. This may also arise from a field change which renders the whole urothelium liable to metaplasia. The correct treatment would consist of the above procedure with removal of the entire ureter with a cuff of bladder wall.

## 178. THEME: UROLOGICAL CALCULI

OPTIONS

A. Ureteroscopic removal
B. Percutaneous nephrolithotomy (PCNL)
C. Conservative management
D. Percutaneous nephrostomy (PCN)
E. Nephrectomy
F. Extracorporeal shock wave lithotripsy
G. Open surgery

*For each of the patients below, select the most appropriate treatment from the above list. Each option may be used once, more than once, or not at all.*

1. A 24-year-old male presenting with right loin pain is diagnosed as having a 4-mm unimpacted right renal pelvic calculi.

2. A 24-year-old male presenting with agonising right loin to groin pain is diagnosed as having a 4-mm right ureteric calculus. He is pyrexial and extremely tender in the right loin. An ultrasound confirms a dilated pelvi-calyceal system.

3. A 24-year-old male presents with right loin pain and is diagnosed as having a 1.5-cm stone in the upper calyceal region of the right kidney. An intravenous urogram confirms normal renal function bilaterally without any evidence of obstruction.

4. A middle aged male presents with intermittent attacks of right loin pain. Investigations confirm a stag horn calculus in the right kidney. Renal function tests and split renal function test using a DMSA scan are normal.

5. A 24-year-old male presents with repeated attack of right loin to groin agonizing pain. Intravenous urography confirms a 3-mm stone calculus in the right lower ureter causing mild hydronephrosis and hydroureter.

## 178. ANSWERS

1. **C - Conservative management**

Calculi smaller than 5 mm will most likely pass spontaneously unless impacted.

2. **D - Percutaneous nephrostomy (PCN)**

Though the calculus is small, it has caused obstruction due to impaction and possibly secondary infection suggested by the systemic features. This needs an urgent PCN.

3. **F - Extracorporeal shock wave lithotripsy (ESWL)**

Stones up to 2 cm in diameter lying within the kidney with the exception of the lower pole calyx are best treated with ESWL. Stones more than 1 cm in size in the lower pole calyx are best treated with PCNL due to poor clearance rates.

4. **B - Percutaneous nephrolithotomy (PCNL)**

Complex stag horn calculi are best treated by a combination of PCNL for removal of the central part of the stone with ESWL being employed later for removal of the peripheral fragments.

5. **A - Ureteroscopic removal**

Features suggest that the stone is impacted. Indications for surgical removal of a ureteric calculus include a stone that doesn't move over a period of time, an enlarging stone, a stone causing complete obstruction of the kidney, evidence of infection, a stone which is deemed too large to pass and obstruction involving a 'precious' kidney (e.g., solitary kidney).

## 179. THEME: TREATMENT OF UROLOGICAL CONDITIONS

OPTIONS

A. Open prostatectomy
B. Radiotherapy
C. External beam radiotherapy
D. Medical management
E. Catheterization
F. TURP
G. Radical cystectomy with adjuvant radiotherapy

*For each of the patients below, select the most appropriate treatment from the above list. Each option may be used once, more than once, or not at all.*

1. An 80-year-old male presents with back pain due to metastatic prostate cancer. He has been on hormone therapy for 2 years.

2. A 55-year-old male is diagnosed with high grade muscle invasive transitional cell carcinoma of the bladder.

3. A 70-year-old male presents with frequency and nocturia. Investigations reveal a maximal flow rate of 12 mL/sec and a post-void residual volume of 90 mL. The prostate is clinically enlarged.

4. A 65-year-old male presents with acute retention of urine for 12 hours duration. He gives a history of progressively worsening frequency, nocturia, straining and a poor stream for a year. Digital rectal examination reveals a moderately enlarged smooth prostate.

5. A 65-year-old male presents with acute retention of urine for 8 hours duration. His residual volume was 1200 mL. Digital rectal examination suggested a huge benign prostate which was confirmed as 140 mL on transrectal ultrasound.

6. A 68-year-old male presents with anorexia, vague abdominal pain and frequency. Examination revealed a suprapubic swelling. This was confirmed as a full bladder on ultrasound (volume 1400 mL). His urea is 24 and creatinine 365.

## 179. ANSWERS

1. **C - External beam radiotherapy**

Hormone therapy should be continued.

2. **G - Radical cystectomy with adjuvant radiotherapy**

Best modality is controversial. Views are divided over whether radical cystectomy, radical radiotherapy or combinations of the two provide the best results. Many authors use a combination as in this answer.

3. **D - Medical management**

Indications for surgical treatment include severe symptoms of 'prostatism', acute retention, chronic retention with renal impairment and complications of bladder outflow obstruction and haemorrhage.

Two classes of drugs have been used in the medical management and include $\alpha$-adrenergic blocking drugs and the 5 $\alpha$-reductase inhibitors. $\alpha$-blockers work more quickly, but the other group has fewer side effects. They result in a 20% improvement in symptom scores.

4. **F - TURP**

Refer above for indications for surgical treatment.

5. **A - Open prostatectomy**

Open prostatectomy is recommended for large prostates (approximately more than 80–100 g). This is because the morbidity is lower with an open surgery in these patients. This is due to a reduced operating time. Also complications from excessive fluid absorption at TURP are avoided. A retropubic prostatectomy is commonly preferred.

6. **E - Catheterization**

For patients presenting with chronic retention of urine with uraemia, an urgent catheterization is mandatory to allow renal function to recover and stabilize. If renal function is good, a catheterization is not indicated. But the patient must be booked for a prostatectomy on the next available list.

## 180. THEME: CHEMISTRY OF RENAL CALCULI

OPTIONS

A. Calcium oxalate
B. Triple phosphate
C. Cystine
D. Uric acid
E. Pure oxalate
F. Pure lysine

*For each of the patients below, select the most appropriate answer from the list above. Each option may be used once, more than once, or not at all.*

1. These calculi are round or oval, smooth and yellow-brown in colour. They commonly occur in patients with gout. They are also known to occur in patients with ileostomies or with bladder outflow obstruction.

2. These calculi are irregular in shape and covered with sharp projections. The stone is usually dark brown or black because of the incorporation of blood pigment on it.

3. A 54-year-old lady known to have recurrent urinary tract infections presents with a renal colic. An X-ray reveals a large staghorn calculus filling the pelvi-calyceal system on the right side.

4. A young male presents to you in A&E with recurrent renal colic. He informs you that he has a familial tendency for calculi.

## 180. ANSWERS

1. **D - Uric acid**

The history of gout in this question alone clinches the diagnosis. These patients have acidic urine and the management involves reducing oral purine intake, alkalinizing the urine and taking allopurinol.

2. **A - Calcium oxalate**

These stones are hard and absorb X-rays well. They are hence easy to see radiologically.

3. **B - Triple phosphate**

The stone tends to grow in alkaline urine especially when Proteus organisms are present, which split urea to ammonium. Even very large stag horn calculi may be clinically silent for years.

4. **C - Cystine**

The incidence of these calculi is 1%. They appear in the urinary tract of patients with a congenital error of metabolism which leads to cystinuria. This is due to an autosomal recessive disease affecting transmembrane cystine transport in gut and kidney.

## 181. THEME: IMPOTENCE

OPTIONS

A. Physiological
B. Psychological
C. Spironolactone
D. Aspirin
E. Prolactinoma
F. Klinefelter's syndrome
G. Addison's disease
H. Haemochromatosis

*For each of the patients described below, select the most appropriate diagnosis from the above list. Each option may be used once, more than once, or not at all.*

1. A 55-year-old male presents with a 3-month history of impotence. He is aware of normal morning erections and has a normal sex drive. However, he has been unable to achieve and maintain a proper erection since acquiring a new partner 3 months ago. His sexual relations with his ex-wife whom he divorced 4 months ago were normal. Blood tests are normal.

2. A 50-year-old male presents with a 2-year history of deteriorating impotence and reduced libido. He has been troubled with arthritis in the recent past. He is also known to have hypertension and diabetes. He takes quite a few medications for the same. Though his testosterone levels in the blood are low, his FSH and LH levels are normal.

3. A 65-year-old male is on spironolactone and aspirin. He presents with impotence. His blood tests are all normal.

4. An 18-year-old lad presents with impotence and reduced libido. He is unaware of any morning erections. Examination reveals a tall thin individual with a small penis and absence of well developed secondary sexual characteristics. Testosterone is low; FSH and LH are high, while prolactin is normal.

## 181. ANSWERS

1. **B - Psychological**

This is the commonest cause of impotence. The history of normal morning erections, normal sex drive, inability to maintain an erection with a new partner and normal relations with the old partner till recently are important clues.

2. **H - Haemochromatosis**

The inappropriately normal FSH and LH in the presence of low testosterone indicates hypogonadotrophic hypogonadism. This in association with diabetes, hypertension and arthritis indicates haemochromatosis, which is an autosomal recessive disorder associated with excess iron deposition.

3. **C - Spironolactone**

Lot of medications can cause impotence. Important medications include: antidepressants including amitriptyline, chlorpromazine, diazepam, doxepin, fluoxetine, imipramine, lorazepam; antihistamines like hydroxyzine; antihypertensives like atenolol, enalapril, verapamil, spironolactone; chemotherapeutic agents and anti Parkinson medications.

4. **F - Klinefelter's syndrome**

A tall and thin individual, small penile size, absence of pubertal changes and blood picture suggestive of primary gonadal failure suggest Klinefelter's syndrome. This is characterized by an XXY trisomy.

## 182. THEME: DIAGNOSIS OF URINARY INCONTINENCE

OPTIONS

A. Acute retention of urine
B. Chronic retention with overflow
C. Urethral diverticulum
D. Detrusor inactivity
E. Stress incontinence
F. Fistula formation
G. Urethral stricture
H. Urge incontinence

*For each of the following patients presenting with urinary incontinence, select the most appropriate diagnosis from the list of options above. Each option may be used once, more than once, or not at all.*

1. A 50-year-old lady presents with a complaint of worsening urinary incontinence over the past few months. She reports loss of a small volume of urine when coughing or during physical exertion. Her gynaecological history stands as gravida 5, para 4 and all have been normal vaginal deliveries. There is an objective loss of urine on coughing.

2. A 55-year-old lady has been distressed with incontinence recently. She has wetted herself at a couple of social occasions recently and she is really concerned about this. She tells you that when 'she get the feeling to go, she has to go'.

3. A 50-year-old lady is seen in your follow up clinic after a radical hysterectomy and radiotherapy for cervical cancer. She complains of continuous trickling of urine onto her underpants which she has to keep changing continuously. Urinalysis and urodynamic investigations are normal.

## 182. ANSWERS

1. **E - Stress incontinence**

This is commoner in parous women. The history of multiple pregnancies with vaginal deliveries, with the history of incontinence while straining, coughing, sneezing are important clues which clinches the diagnosis. It is important to exclude a UTI and glycosuria. Mild stress incontinence improves with pelvic floor exercises or physiotherapy. Surgery may be needed for severe stress symptoms and includes urethroplasty, transabdominal colposuspension.

2. **H - Urge incontinence**

This is classical of urge incontinence. It is an 'urge' to open your bladder. The bladder is 'unstable' with high detrusor muscle activity. Unlike stress incontinence it may be present in nulliparous females also. Usually no organic cause is found. Though detrusor instability usually presents with urge incontinence, in about 25% it presents as stress symptoms.

3. **F - Fistula formation**

History of radical surgery followed by continuous incontinence should alert you to this possibility. Vesicovaginal, and less commonly urethrovaginal fistulae, is possible. Most patients would need surgical repair. If surgical repair is not possible, help is needed from a continence adviser.

## 183. THEME: TREATMENT OF URINARY INCONTINENCE

OPTIONS

A. Antibiotics
B. Pelvic floor exercises
C. Imipramine
D. Alarms with vibrations
E. Intermittent self catheterization
F. Bladder neck surgery

*For each scenario described below, select the most appropriate management option from the list of options above. Each option may be used once, more than once, or not at all.*

1. A 50-year-old lady presents with a complaint of worsening urinary incontinence over the past few months. She reports loss of a small volume of urine when coughing or during physical exertion. Her gynaecological history stands as gravida 5, para 4 and all have been normal vaginal deliveries. There is an objective loss of urine on coughing.

2. A 14-year-old boy has long term urinary incontinence from meningomyelocele.

3. An 8-year-old boy presents with secondary enuresis.

## 183. ANSWERS

1. **B - Pelvic floor exercises**

This is commoner in parous women. The history of multiple pregnancies with vaginal deliveries, with the history of incontinence while straining, coughing, sneezing are important clues which clinch the diagnosis. It is important to exclude a UTI and glycosuria. Mild stress incontinence improves with pelvic floor exercises or physiotherapy. Surgery may be needed for severe stress symptoms and includes urethroplasty, transabdominal colposuspension.

2. **E - Intermittent self catheterization**

3. **D - Alarms with vibrations**

Secondary enuresis implies wetness after >6 months' dryness. Bedwetting occurs on most nights in 15% of 5-year-olds. Avoiding blame, fluid restriction before going to bed and time usually helps. A system of rewards (e.g., star chart) and alarms may be tried. If needed imipramine or desmopressin can be used short term.

## 184. THEME: CARDIAC ABNORMALITIES

OPTIONS

A. Aortic stenosis
B. Aortic regurgitation
C. Mitral stenosis
D. Mitral regurgitation
E. Mitral valve prolapse
F. Tricuspid regurgitation
G. Atrial septal defect
H. Ventricular septal defect
I. Patent ductus arteriosus
J. Coarctation of aorta

*For each of the patients described below, select the most appropriate diagnosis from the above list. Each option may be used once, more than once, or not at all.*

1. A 78-year-old elderly male patient is admitted for an elective laparoscopic cholecystectomy. His blood pressure is 112/94 mm Hg. He has a harsh systolic murmur at the 2nd right intercostal space.

2. A 40-year-old lady attends pre-assessment clinic for an elective laparoscopic cholecystectomy. She has had dyspnoea and exercise syncope for some time now. Auscultation reveals an ejection systolic murmur radiating to the carotids. The pulse is slow rising in character.

3. A 25-year-old tall thin chap with long limbs and fingers is seen in the dental clinic for crowding of teeth. He is noted to have a high arched palate. He is noted to have a mid systolic click with a murmur at the apex.

4. A 70-year-old lady is seen in the pre assessment clinic for a left total knee replacement. Both cheeks appear ruddy. A low rumbling mid diastolic murmur is heard.

## 184. ANSWERS

1. **A - Aortic stenosis**

The presence of a harsh systolic murmur as mentioned along with a narrow pulse pressure suggests aortic stenosis. This would require further assessment with an echo. Senile stenosis is a result of thickening and calcification of the valve cusps but with no commissural fusion (unlike the appearances in rheumatic stenosis).

2. **A - Aortic stenosis**

Typical features are described again. Patients may also have angina. The apex beat may be displaced. In this age group, pathology is usually extensive calcification in a congenitally bicuspid valve. In younger patients, stenosis is almost always congenital.

3. **E - Mitral valve prolapse**

Features typically describe a young patient with Marfan's syndrome. It is a connective tissue disorder and three systems are predominantly involved: eyes, heart and skeleton including jaws. Well known features include subluxation or dislocation of lens, myopia, detachment of retina, high arched palate, crowding of teeth, tall thin build with arm span greater than height and heart lesions. Heart lesions include mitral valve prolapse, dilatation mainly of the ascending aorta, aneurysm and dissection of aorta.

4. **C - Mitral stenosis**

A serious complication of mitral stenosis is the development of atrial fibrillation. Infective endocarditis is a further hazard. The pulmonary component of the second heart sound may be loud depending on the severity of the pulmonary hypertension.

## 185. THEME: CARDIAC ABNORMALITIES

OPTIONS

A. Tetralogy of Fallot
B. Transposition of the great vessels
C. Total anomalous pulmonary venous drainage
D. Ventricular septal defect
E. Atrial septal defect
F. Coarctation of aorta
G. Mitral valve prolapse
H. Eisenmenger's syndrome
I. Patent ductus arteriosus
J. Aortic regurgitation
K. Atrial septal defect, atrioventricular septal and atrioventricular canal defects

*For each of the descriptions below, select the most appropriate match from the above list. Each option may be used once, more than once, or not at all.*

1. Eisenmenger's syndrome

2. Ankylosing spondylitis

3. This is a condition in which there is a VSD with an overriding aorta, pulmonary artery stenosis and right ventricular hypertrophy.

4. This occurs following the reversal of the left-to-right shunt. Cyanosis and dyspnoea are the most common clinical features.

5. This is a condition wherein the aorta arises from the right ventricle and the pulmonary artery from the left ventricle.

6. Turner's syndrome

7. Down's syndrome

## 185. ANSWERS

1. **D - Ventricular septal defect**

2. **J - Aortic regurgitation**

Ankylosing spondylitis like other seronegative arthropathies is associated more commonly with aortic regurgitation than mitral regurgitation.

3. **A - Tetralogy of Fallot**

Cyanosis is the most obvious clinical feature. Lethargy and tiredness are common presenting symptoms. There is usually polycythaemia and chest radiograph reveals a boot shaped heart with poorly developed lung vasculature. The diagnosis is confirmed by echocardiography and cardiac catheterisation.

4. **H - Eisenmenger's syndrome**

5. **B - Transposition of the great vessels**

The most obvious presentation is severe cyanosis in the neonatal period. Cardiac catheterisation and echocardiography confirm the diagnosis and delineate the anatomy.

6. **F - Coarctation of aorta**

7. **K - Atrial septal defect, atrioventricular septal and atrioventricular canal defects**

Remember this is an EMQ (EMI). Option E in isolation is also true, but in the presence of option K, it is not the most appropriate answer.

## 186. THEME: COMPLICATIONS OF THORACIC SURGERY

OPTIONS

A. Chylothorax
B. Haemothorax
C. Pneumothorax
D. Haemo-pneumothorax
E. Mediastinitis
F. Pleural effusion
G. Diaphragmatic paresis
H. Empyema

*For each of the patients described below, select the most appropriate diagnosis from the above list. Each option may be used once, more than once, or not at all.*

1. A 60-year-old male develops a swinging fever 4 days after a CABG. A chest X-ray shows a widening of the mediastinum, with a fluid level seen in the posterior mediastinum.

2. A 60-year-old immigrant male undergoes resection of his right lower lobe for lung abscess. Postoperatively he develops respiratory distress. He is found to have swinging pyrexia. A chest X-ray shows an effusion on the right side. CT scan confirms the presence of loculations.

3. A 65-year-old male undergoes a CABG using the left internal mammary artery as a graft. A routine postoperative X-ray shows a raised left hemi-diaphragm.

## 186. ANSWERS

1. **E - Mediastinitis**

This is most frequently seen after cardiac surgery. It is also well recognized after trauma or oesophageal rupture/perforation. The patient requires a thoracotomy, mediastinal drainage and broad spectrum antibiotics.

2. **H - Empyema**

Early empyema as in this case will need pleural drainage, with underwater seal and adequate dosage of appropriate antibiotics. Complete drainage and re-expansion of the lung should be achieved before the drains are removed.

3. **G - Diaphragmatic paresis**

This is due to damage to the left phrenic nerve. This nerve can also be involved directly by intrathoracic malignancy.

## 187. THEME: EMPYEMA

OPTIONS

A. Radiology guided aspiration
B. Intercostal drainage
C. Needle thoracocentesis
D. Thoracoplasty
E. Pleurodesis
F. Thoracotomy
G. Thoracoplasty

*For each of the patients described below, select the most appropriate intervention from the above list. Each option may be used once, more than once, or not at all.*

1. A 66-year-old insulin dependent diabetic obese lady undergoes laparoscopic cholecystectomy which had to be converted to open due to adhesions. Postoperatively she develops fever and tachycardia. Investigation confirms a parpneumotic effusion on the right side without loculations. Aspiration suggests frank pus.

2. A 60-year-old immigrant male undergoes resection of his right lower lobe for lung abscess. Postoperatively he develops respiratory distress. He is found to have swinging pyrexia. A chest X-ray shows an effusion on the right side. CT scan confirms the presence of pus without evidence of loculations.

3. A 60-year-old immigrant male undergoes resection of his right lower lobe for bronchiectasis. He continues to remain unwell. A chest X-ray few months after surgery confirms the presence of pus with evidence of multiple loculations which has failed to resolve despite repeated aspiration and antibiotics.

4. A middle aged lady is troubled with recurrent pleural effusion secondary to rheumatoid arthritis.

## 187. ANSWERS

1. **A - Radiology guided aspiration**
Since this is a small non loculated parpneumotic effusion, this is the treatment of choice.

2. **B - Intercostal drainage**
Early empyema as in this case will need pleural drainage, with under-water seal and adequate dosage of appropriate antibiotics. Complete drainage and re-expansion of the lung should be achieved before the drains are removed.

3. **F - Thoracotomy**
Thoracotomy is indicated for chronic empyema, or when initial measures fail to resolve an acute episode. This patient has developed chronic empyema. Because of the underlying fibrosis constricting the lung parenchyma, aspiration of pus alone will not lead to expansion of the lung. A formal thoracotomy is performed and the thickened parietal pleura and the fibrin peel overlying the lung are painstakingly removed, piecemeal if necessary.

4. **E - Pleurodesis**
This is obliteration of the pleural space and is achieved using tetracycline, bleomycin and talcum powder. Surgical pleurodesis is best avoided.

## 188. THEME: STAGING LUNG CANCER

OPTIONS

A. T1N0M0
B. T3N2M0
C. TXN0M0
D. T3N3M1

*For each of the scenarios below, select the most appropriate stage from the above list. Each option may be used once, more than once, or not at all.*

1. A chronic smoker presents with weight loss, anorexia, cough and haemoptysis. Sputum cytology shows carcinomatous cells. However, a chest X-ray is normal.

2. A 2-cm nodule picked up incidentally on 'routine' screening before a laparoscopic surgery in a chronic smoker.

3. A smoker presents with weight loss, cough and chest pain. He has a large bronchial cancer with widespread metastasis.

## 188. ANSWERS

1. **C - TXN0M0**

A rough estimate of classification is needed for the purpose of the exam. However, the purpose of the exam is not to confuse you. If you look carefully at the options, you should be able to find the answer, e.g., this is the only option showing TX which stands for presence of malignant cells and bronchial secretions in the absence of visualization by radiography or bronchoscopy.

2. **A - T1N0M0**

This is again straightforward. Primary tumour less than 3 cm is T1. We assume nodes and metastasis as N0, M0 since no history is given.

3. **D - T3N3M1**

Apply the same principle again. This is the only option with M1.

Please refer to any standard textbook for the complete TNM staging.

## 189. THEME: CARDIOTHORACIC EMERGENCIES

OPTIONS

A. Primary pneumothorax
B. Right tension pneumothorax
C. Aortic dissection
D. Right flail chest
E. Secondary pneumothorax
F. Empyema
G. Pleural effusion
H. Haemothorax

*For each of the scenarios below, select the most appropriate diagnosis from the above list. Each option may be used once, more than once, or not at all.*

1. A 26-year marathon runner collapses during a training session. He is rushed to A&E. On arrival, he is cyanosed and hypotensive. His trachea is deviated to the left and he has diminished breath sounds in his right hemithorax.

2. A 50-year-old lady with a long history of hypertension is admitted with severe chest pain and collapse. ECG is normal. A chest X-ray shows a widened mediastinum with a small left pleural effusion.

3. A 70-year-old diabetic is admitted with increasing breathlessness, fever, rigors and feeling unwell. She has been on antibiotics for a week's duration for a chest infection. On examination, she has diminished air entry in the right base. Her chest X-ray shows an opaque right lung base with obliteration of the costophrenic angle.

4. A 75-year-old male known to have chronic obstructive airways disease (COAD) presents to A&E with a sudden increase in breathlessness. He is afebrile. He has a hyperresonant left hemithorax with reduced breath sounds. There is no tracheal deviation.

## 189. ANSWERS

1. **B - Right tension pneumothorax**
This is a dire emergency. In addition to respiratory difficulty, the mediastinal shift may cause significant embarrassment of venous return and hence cardiac output. Initial treatment is to achieve a needle thoracocentesis. This will return the pneumothorax to a non tension state and allow insertion of a chest drain in a more stable patient.

2. **C - Aortic dissection**
Clues include a history of hypertension, history of severe chest pain and collapse coupled with a normal ECG. The chest radiology clinches the diagnosis. A contrast CT scan is needed to confirm the dissection further.

3. **F - Empyema**
This patient has typical features. An aspiration can be attempted to clinch the diagnosis.

4. **E - Secondary pneumothorax**
This usually develops in an older patient with underlying lung disease. History and findings as mentioned in the question are classical.

## 190. THEME: LUNG CANCER COMPLICATIONS

OPTIONS

A. Bony metastasis
B. Cerebellar ataxia
C. Ectopic ACTH secretion
D. Ectopic ADH secretion
E. Ectopic parathyroid hormone secretion
F. Horner's syndrome
G. Lambert-Eaton syndrome
H. Pancoast's syndrome
I. SVC obstruction

*For each of the scenarios for lung cancer described below, select the most appropriate complication of lung cancer from the above list. Each option may be used once, more than once, or not at all.*

1. A 55-year-old smoker recently diagnosed with lung carcinoma presents with sudden onset dyspnoea, facial and upper limb swelling, plethora, cyanosis and venous engorgement.
2. A 50-year-old smoker presents with chronic cough, haemoptysis, anorexia and weight loss for a month's duration. He has had severe pain in his left shoulder radiating down his left arm. There is some weakness in the intrinsic muscles of the left hand.
3. A 50-year-old smoker presents with chronic cough, haemoptysis, anorexia and weight loss for a month's duration. Examination reveals a smaller pupil on the left side.
4. A 78-year-old lady known to have advanced lung cancer is brought to A&E in a state of confusion and agitation. On examination, she is drowsy with a blood pressure reading of 170/86 mm Hg. Her biochemistry stands as: Sodium 118 mmol/litre, Potassium 3.1 mmol/litre, normal urea and creatinine and plasma osmolality-255 mOsm/kg.
5. A 70-year-old gentleman known to have small cell lung cancer complains of occasional double vision and of problems in chewing. Examination confirms weakness of girdle muscles and an oculomotor nerve palsy on the right with ptosis. However the weakness improves after repeated demonstration to medical students.

## 190. ANSWERS

1. **I - SVC obstruction**

History is suggestive of SVC obstruction. It is commonly from lung carcinoma or lymphoma. Features include dyspnoea, orthopnoea, facial and upper limb swelling, cough, plethora, cyanosis and venous engorgement. Dexamethasone is given first. Subsequently, urgent radiotherapy is needed for non small cell lung cancer, while chemotherapy is needed for lymphoma and small cell lung cancer.

2. **H - Pancoast's syndrome**

3. **F - Horner's syndrome**

Both the patients in scenario 2 and 3 most likely have pancoast's tumour which is an apically placed squamous cell carcinoma of the lung. It can invade directly into local structures. Invasion of brachial plexus as in scenario 2 leads to pancoast's syndrome. Involvement of sympathetic fibres leads to Horner's syndrome which is characterised by ptosis, miosis and enophthalmosis.

4. **D - Ectopic ADH secretion**

This is associated with small cell carcinoma of the lung. Inappropriate levels lead to hypervolaemic hyponatraemia. Severe hyponatraemia below 110 mmol/litre can lead to convulsions and coma.

5. **G - Lambert-Eaton syndrome**

This is seen with small cell carcinoma of the lung. There is impaired release of acetylcholine at the neuromuscular junction caused by autoantibodies directed to native calcium channels. The picture is similar to myasthenia gravis except that symptoms improve with repeated movements.

## 191. THEME: PATHOLOGY OF BREAST CARCINOMA

OPTIONS

A. Ductal carcinoma in-situ (DCIS)
B. Lobular carcinoma in-situ
C. Infiltrating ductal carcinoma (NOS)
D. Tubular carcinoma
E. Medullary carcinoma
F. Mucinous carcinoma
G. Signet ring carcinoma
H. Invasive lobular carcinoma
I. Invasive cribriform carcinoma

*For each of the characteristics described below, choose the single most appropriate diagnosis from the list of options above. Each option may be used once, more than once or not at all.*

1. Characterized by a proliferation of malignant breast epithelial cells confined to the duct system and does not invade the basement membrane.

2. Diagnosis by exclusion but it accounts for 65% of all invasive mammary cancers.

3. Most obvious histological characteristic is a prominent lymphocytic infiltration.

4. Microscopy reveals characteristic stromal invasion with a sieve-like pattern.

5. It is important because of its tendency to bilaterality and the fact that its clinical diagnosis may be difficult because of diffuse infiltrative nature, which frequently produces distortion of the breast rather than a lump.

## 191. ANSWERS

1. **A - Ductal carcinoma in-situ (DCIS)**
DCIS accounts for 5% of all cases of breast cancer in unscreened population. With a screening programme the incidence increases to 15 –20% because it is associated with mammographically visible microcalcification. The treatment is controversial. When it is extensive in the breast, mastectomy is usually recommended. For smaller tumours, wide excision with or without radiotherapy may be required.

2. **C - Infiltrating ductal carcinoma (NOS)**
No specific gross or microscopic features allow recognition of this type of cancer. It has a relatively poor prognosis. It is usually classified as intermediate or high grade. However, other features such as tumour size and axillary node involvement are of more prognostic importance than histological features alone.

3. **E - Medullary carcinoma**
It accounts for about 6% of all invasive mammary cancers. Macroscopically they tend to be soft, well circumscribed and have a uniform consistency. They have a smooth contour. They are less frequently associated with lymph node metastases and are therefore associated with better prognosis.

4. **I - Invasive cribriform carcinoma**
Classically presents with a firm mass and microscopy reveals characteristic stromal invasion with a cribriform pattern (sieve-like). It tends to be well-differentiated and has a good prognosis.

5. **H - Invasive lobular carcinoma**
It accounts for about 10% of all cases of breast carcinoma. There are five main subtypes – classic, solid, alveolar, mixed, pleomorphic. The most common type, classical lobular carcinoma, is characterized by the 'Indian filing' of invading malignant cells, often in a 'targetoid pattern'. Its prognosis is similar to invasive ductal cancer. The other types of lobular carcinoma, especially the pleomorphic variant, have a worse prognosis.

## 192. THEME: INVESTIGATION OF BREAST DISEASE

OPTIONS

A. Trucut core biopsy
B. Fine-needle aspiration cytology
C. Ultrasound examination
D. Reassurance
E. Mammography
F. Wide excision
G. Computed tomography (CT) scan
H. Magnetic resonance imaging (MRI)
I. Lymphangiography
J. Stereotype cone biopsy

*For each of the patients described below, choose the single most useful investigation from the list of options above. Each option may be used once, more than once or not at all.*

1. A 30-year-old woman comes to the clinic for screening of her breasts. She is asymptomatic and there is no positive family history.

2. A 35-year-old woman presents with a mass in the upper quadrant of her right breast. A smooth, firm, mobile, round mass is found on examination.

3. A 50-year-old woman comes to the clinic with a complaint of hard mass in her right breast. Examination reveals skin tethering. Mammography and ultrasound are inconclusive.

4. A 38-year-old woman presents with itching of her left nipple. On examination, no ulceration is seen, but a scaly lesion is observed around the nipple.

5. A 20-year-old woman feels that her breasts become lumpy and heavy during the time of her periods. She also feels anxious and irritable.

## 192. ANSWERS

1. **D - Reassurance**

As the woman is asymptomatic and there is no family history, there is no need for screening. All women in UK are screened for breast cancer by a three-yearly mammography starting at the age of 50 years till 64 years.

2. **C - Ultrasound examination**

This is suggestive of breast cyst or fibroadenoma. In young women under the age of 45 years, mammography is not very helpful because of the density of the breast tissue. Ultrasonography helps to distinguish cyst from fibroadenoma. A cyst can be aspirated. If suspicious, a fine needle aspiration cytology (FNAC) can be done.

3. **A - Trucut core biopsy**

Trucut core biopsy will provide definite evidence of carcinoma. It can be done as an outpatient procedure under local anaesthesia. Advantage is that it provides histological rather than cytological specimen. Hence *in situ* can be differentiated from invasive disease and ductal distinguished from lobular carcinoma. Grading and identification of oestrogen receptor is also possible.

4. **C - Ultrasound examination**

As there is no obvious ulceration or lump palpable, the woman can be reassured that there is nothing sinister. But an ultrasonography may be useful to rule out underlying impalpable lesions.

5. **D - Reassurance**

Features suggest cyclical mastalgia. Once reassured, patients tend to cope well with the symptoms. If the symptoms are persistent, drug therapy may be started with evening primrose oil. Other treatment options include danazol, bromocriptine and tamoxifen.

## 193. THEME: INVESTIGATION OF BREAST DISEASE

OPTIONS

A. Trucut core biopsy
B. Fine-needle aspiration cytology
C. Ultrasound examination
D. Reassurance
E. Mammography
F. Wide excision
G. Computed tomography (CT) scan
H. Magnetic resonance imaging (MRI)
I. Lymphangiography
J. Stereotype cone biopsy

*For each of the patients described below, choose the single most useful investigation from the list of options above. Each option may be used once, more than once or not at all.*

1. A 28-year-old woman presents with a mass in the upper lateral quadrant of her right breast. On examination a 2 cm firm, mobile mass is found. She has a morbid fear of needles.

2. A 24-year-old woman presents with a diffuse nodular breast swelling which seems to increase in size during her periods. There is no axillary involvement, and the swelling disappears after her menses.

3. A 59-year-old woman presents with a mass in the lower inner quadrant of her left breast. The skin is pulled in and there is no axillary involvement.

4. A 45-year-old woman underwent a mammography, which showed diffuse calcifications. She wants to know for certain that she has no malignancy.

5. A 50-year-old woman underwent a wide local excision for left breast carcinoma 3 years ago. She presents with hard mass in her left breast just below the previous scar. Mammography and ultrasound appear to be inconclusive.

## 193. ANSWERS

1. **C - Ultrasound examination**

This could be a breast cyst or fibroadenoma. Ultrasonography will help to differentiate between the two. If there are not much symptoms the lesion can be left alone with no further treatment.

2. **D – Reassurance**

This is suggestive of lumpy breasts because of aberrations of normal development and involution. A firm reassurance is all that is usually required. The patient may be reviewed after six weeks at a different point in the menstrual cycle and often the clinical signs will have resolved by that time. Pain chart may be useful. Evening primrose oil is also helpful to control pain. Other options are danazol, bromocriptine and tamoxifen.

3. **A – Trucut core biopsy**

This is suggestive of breast carcinoma. Though mammography and ultrasonography are usually performed initially, a trucut core biopsy will provide definite evidence of carcinoma and help in planning further management.

4. **J – Stereotype cone biopsy**

Stereotype cone biopsy is useful in such cases where there may be no palpable abnormality but mammography is suspicious. Biopsy can be taken from the suspicious area under mammography guidance.

5. **H – Magnetic resonance imaging (MRI)**

This is suggestive of possible recurrence of carcinoma. MRI is very useful in such cases in differentiating scar from recurrent carcinoma.

## 194. THEME: BENIGN BREAST DISEASE

OPTIONS

A. Absence of breast tissue
B. Accessory breast tissue
C. Cystosarcoma phyllodes
D. Idiopathic benign breast hypertrophy
E. Lipoma
F. Lobular mastitis
G. Mondor's disease
H. Peri-ductal mastitis
I. Sclerosing adenosis
J. Breast cyst

*The following scenario describes presentation of a woman with breast pathology. From the list above, choose the single most appropriate diagnosis. Each item may be used once, more than once, or not at all.*

1. A 50-year-old woman presents with a sudden appearance of painful lump in her right breast. On examination there is a 3 cm lump in the upper outer quadrant of her right breast that is smooth and tense on palpation. Overlying skin is free and the lump is mobile. There is no axillary lymphadenopathy.

2. A 55-year-old woman complains of a 2-day history of pain in her right breast. The pain is described as localised to the lateral aspect of the breast and of sudden onset. She has no significant risk factors for breast cancer; however, she is extremely anxious. On examination she has a tender, subcutaneous, linear cord in the right breast. The overlying skin is acutely inflamed and becomes puckered on raising the right arm. Mammography and breast ultrasound are unremarkable.

3. A 40-year-old woman presents with a rapidly growing painless lump in her right breast. On examination overlying skin appears reddened but free from the lump. The lump is mobile over the underlying structures. Axillary lymph nodes are not enlarged. FNAC reveals much hypercellularity, atypia and numerous mitoses.

## 194. ANSWERS

### 1. J - Breast cyst

Cysts are classically seen in perimenopausal women. They are usually single on presentation and appear suddenly. Their most characteristic feature is their smooth, tense nature on palpation. The diagnosis is straightforward as aspiration confirms the diagnosis. Mammography and ultrasonography may aid the diagnosis. Simple aspiration usually suffices. Main indications for surgical excision of the cyst are if the aspirate is bloodstained or if there is recurrence of the cyst.

### 2. G – Mondor's disease

In a patient complaining of sudden breast pain, the finding of a tender subcutaneous cord, attached to the skin, is pathognomonic of Mondor's disease. This rare condition is characterised by a sclerosing thrombophlebitis of the subcutaneous veins of the anterior chest wall, which gives rise to the clinical findings. Imaging studies tend to be unremarkable. The condition is benign and self-limiting although a fibrous subcutaneous band may remain. Treatment is symptomatic with non-steroidal anti-inflammatory drugs.

### 3. C - Cystosarcoma phyllodes

Phyllodes tumours occur in premenopausal women. They can grow rapidly to a large size and may involve much of the breast. The overlying skin may become reddened and in advanced cases can become frankly ulcerated. Histology reveals both epithelial and fibrous stromal elements, with the stroma showing hypercellularity, much atypia and numerous mitoses. The treatment ranges from simple enucleation in younger women to wider excision in older women.

## 195. THEME: PROGRESSION OF BREAST CANCER

OPTIONS

A. Asthma
B. Axillary recurrence
C. Bone-marrow infiltration
D. Bony metastases
E. Cerebral metastases
F. Left ventricular failure
G. Hypercalcaemia
H. Liver metastases
I. Local recurrence
J. Lymphangitis carcinomatosis
K. Peritoneal recurrence
L. Pleural effusion
M. Spinal cord compression

*For each of the patients described below, choose the single most likely diagnosis from the list of options above. Each option may be used once, more than once or not at all.*

1. A 60-year-old woman who underwent mastectomy for a breast tumour 6 years ago now complains of increasing breathlessness. On examination, she is noted to have decreased movement of the left hemithorax, which is dull to percussion and has absent breath sounds.

2. A 55-year-old woman is admitted to the Accident and Emergency department after having fallen in the street. She is complaining of pain in the right hip, and the right lower limb is lying in external rotation. She had breast-conserving surgery, radiotherapy and chemotherapy for breast cancer 8 years ago.

3. A 43-year-old woman who was treated 2 years ago for a grade 3 breast cancer presents with increasing confusion, headache and vomiting. On examination, she is drowsy but has no focal neurological signs. She has blurring of the optic disc margins.

4. A 40-year-old woman who was treated a year ago for a breast cancer presents with 2-day history of increasing confusion. She is drowsy and disoriented. Her daughter says she had been complaining of severe thirst during the last week.

5. A 50-year-old woman who was treated for breast cancer 2 years ago is unable to walk. She complains of increasing weakness in her left leg for the last 7 days. She has been constipated and unable to pass urine for the last 24 hours.

## 195. ANSWERS

### 1. L – Pleural effusion

Features are suggestive of pleural effusion which is because of spread of cancer to the pleural cavity and the lungs. Combination chemotherapy must be started if possible with the addition of steroids for symptomatic relief. Endocrine treatment is more appropriate for older patients with poor performance status.

### 2. D – Bony metastases

This is suggestive of pathological fracture as it resulted from a trivial fall. Given the past history, most likely cause is bone metastases. Pathological fractures require appropriate orthopaedic evaluation and surgical fixation where necessary. Bisphosphonates can reduce the symptoms of bone metastases. A short course of radiotherapy will also relieve the symptoms. Systemic therapy is indicated at the same time.

### 3. E – Cerebral metastases

Features suggest raised intracranial tension. As there is no focal neurological sign, the cause appears to be cerebral metastasis from the breast cancer. The treatment relies on radiation therapy and steroids. Systemic therapy has not been widely used as most agents fail to cross the blood-brain barrier.

### 4. G – Hypercalcaemia

Features are suggestive of hypercalcaemia from widespread bone metastasis, which may itself be asymptomatic. It may eventually progress to coma with renal failure. Initial treatment includes rehydration and forced diuresis and administration of steroids to enhance calcium excretion in the urine. Resistant cases may be treated with mithramycin.

### 5. M – Spinal cord compression

Features are suggestive of spinal cord compression because of metastases to the epidural space. Their treatment relies on radiation therapy. Surgery may be useful in these patients in the early stage.

## 196. THEME: DIAGNOSIS OF BREAST DISEASE

OPTIONS

A. Breast abscess
B. Fibroadenoma
C. Breast carcinoma
D. Duct ectasia/periductal mastitis
E. Benign mammary dysplasia
F. Paget's disease of the nipple
G. Cyst
H. Extraductal papilloma

*For each of the patients described below, choose the single most likely diagnosis from the list of options above. Each option may be used once, more than once or not at all.*

1. A 45-year-old woman presents with a lump in her left breast with axillary involvement. There is no supraclavicular lymphadenopathy.

2. A young mother who is breast-feeding her baby presents with complaints of pain in her right breast. On examination, the breast is found to be red, hot and tender on the outer side.

3. A 19-year-old girl presents with a breast lump which is mobile and disappears after menstruation.

4. A 50-year-old woman complains of a blood-stained discharge from the side of the nipple. There is no underlying lump present. She is a chronic smoker.

5. A 48-year-old woman presents with persistent crusty scaly nipple.

## 196. ANSWERS

1. **C – Breast carcinoma**

Features are suggestive of breast carcinoma. Diagnosis is by mammography and biopsy. Once diagnosed, further investigations for staging will be required.

2. **A – Breast abscess**

Features are suggestive of a breast abscess. Lactational breast abscess are caused by Staphylococcus aureus. If it is seen before frank abscess formation, antibiotic treatment alone is often successful. Aspiration should be done to be sure that no pus is present. A second-line penicillin or cephalosporin is useful. If pus is found, drainage is necessary. If formal drainage is done, further antibiotic therapy is no longer required.

3. **E – Benign mammary dysplasia**

Features suggest cyclical nodularity. The diffuse nodular swellings usually resolve by the next menstrual cycle. As long as malignancy is excluded, patients can simply be reassured.

4. **D – Duct ectasia/periductal mastitis**

Features suggest duct ectasia. If lump is present, appropriate management of the lump is instituted. If these symptoms persist, then exploration is indicated. If a conservative approach is chosen, the patient should be reviewed after 3 months.

5. **F - Paget's disease of the nipple**

Features suggest Paget's disease. It usually represents an underlying intraductal carcinoma that may be quite extensive in the breast and may be invasive. The differential diagnosis is with eczema, which is usually bilateral and associated with disease elsewhere. Traditional treatment included mastectomy with lower axillary clearance. However, in the elderly, wide local excision of the nipple and underlying ducts may suffice.

## 197. THEME: FIRST LINE MANAGEMENT OF BREAST CANCER

OPTIONS

A. Primary radiotherapy
B. Lumpectomy
C. Wide local excision + radiotherapy with axillary sampling
D. Primary hormonal treatment
E. Total mastectomy
F. Modified radical mastectomy
G. Primary chemotherapy

*For each of the patients described below, choose the single most likely first line management from the list of options above. Each option may be used once, more than once or not at all.*

1. A 40-year-old woman presents to the breast clinic with a 5-cm lump in outer upper quadrant of right breast. Axillary nodes are palpable. Trucut biopsy shows invasive ductal carcinoma. There is no evidence of distant metastases.

2. An 85-year-old woman presents with a firm 2-cm lump in the lower inner quadrant of the left breast. The lump is mobile and axillary nodes are not palpable. FNAC shows C5 with oestrogen receptor positive.

3. A 45-year-old woman presents with a firm 3-cm lump in the lower outer quadrant of right breast. There is no skin tethering. Axillary nodes are not palpable. FNAC shows C5. Mammography does not show multicentricity.

4. A 55-year-old woman is noted to have widespread microcalcification throughout the breast on screening mammography. FNAC shows C2. Stereotactic core biopsies show DCIS but no invasive cancer.

5. A 40-year-old woman presents with a firm 3-cm lump in the outer upper quadrant of right breast. The lump is mobile with no lymph nodes palpable in the axilla. Her mother died from breast cancer. Mammography and ultrasonography are suggestive of fibroadenoma. FNAC is C2.

## 197. ANSWERS

1. **G - Primary chemotherapy**

Features suggest locally advanced cancer (Stage III). Induction chemotherapy is recommended in such cases. This has to be followed by surgery. Neoadjuvant chemotherapy improves the survival in excess of 50% at 5 years.

2. **D - Primary hormonal treatment**

Tumours in the elderly are slow growing, are associated with a high oestrogen receptor status and have a good prognosis. Treatment with the anti-oestrogen tamoxifen has therefore been advocated. This may be followed by lumpectomy. Tamoxifen alone may be used in the very frail patients.

3. **C - Wide local excision + radiotherapy with axillary sampling**

The indications of breast conservation treatment are tumour size less than 4 cm, no fixation to underlying muscle or overlying skin and no evidence of multicentricity on mammography. Centrally located tumours and poor tumour differentiation are a relative contraindication to breast conservation. Patient choice is important. If a patient prefers total mastectomy then her wishes should be adhered to.

4. **E - Total mastectomy**

The treatment of DCIS is controversial. When it is widespread and extensive in the breast, mastectomy is usually recommended. As the risk of axillary metastases in screen-detected carcinoma is very less, there is no place for surgical clearance of the axilla in its management.

5. **B - Lumpectomy**

In women under the age of 25 years, routine removal is unnecessary. Here the age and family history are the indications for removal of the fibroadenoma. Removal of fibroadenoma is recommended by some authorities after the age of 25 years.

## 198. THEME: HEAD AND NECK LUMPS

OPTIONS

A. Medial ectopic thyroid gland
B. Thyroglossal cyst
C. Meningocele
D. Cystic hygroma
E. Ranula
F. Branchial cyst
G. Inclusion dermoid

*For each of the patients described below, choose the single most likely diagnosis from the list of options above. Each option may be used once, more than once or not at all.*

1. A newly born baby is brought with swelling in the right posterior triangle. On examination, it transmits light and is partially compressible.

2. A 20-year-old female presents with a soft cystic swelling in the neck along the anterior border of sternomastoid. It is not painful or tender.

3. A child presents with a midline swelling in the head which feels putty-like and does not transmit light.

4. A 12-year-old boy presents with a swelling in the neck which is slightly to the right of midline. It moves up on protrusion of tongue.

5. An infant is brought with a posterior midline skin-covered swelling which is transilluminant.

## 198. ANSWERS

1. **D – Cystic hygroma**

Cystic hygroma usually manifests in the neonate or in early infancy. Often the posterior triangle of the neck is mainly involved. As a result of intercommunication of its many compartments, the swelling is soft and partially compressible. It visibly increases in size when the child coughs or cries. It is brilliantly translucent. The cheek, axilla, groin and mediastinum are other sites for a cystic hygroma. The lesion may become infected, when it becomes inflamed and painful. Definitive treatment is excision of the entire cyst at an early stage.

2. **F - Branchial cyst**

A branchial cyst develops from the vestigial remnants of the second branchial cleft. It usually appears in the upper neck in early or middle adulthood and is found at the junction of the upper and middle third of the sternomastoid muscle. It is a fluctuant swelling which may transilluminate sometimes. Occasionally it may be difficult to differentiate from a tuberculous abscess. Ultrasound and fine needle aspiration both aid the diagnosis. Treatment is by complete excision.

3. **G – Inclusion dermoid**

It occurs due to dermal cells being buried along the line of closure of embryonic clefts and sinuses by skin fusion. The cyst contains paste-like desquamated material. The usual sites are the midline of the body, above the outer canthus and behind the ear. Because of the contents it is not transilluminant. Treatment is by complete excision.

4. **B – Thyroglossal cyst**

It represents a persistence of the thyroglossal track. It may be found anywhere in or adjacent to the midline from the tongue base to the thyroid isthmus. It characteristically moves up on protrusion of the tongue. Treatment is by excision of the whole thyroglossal tract which includes removal of the body of the hyoid bone and suprahyoid tract till the foramen caecum. This is known as Sistrunk's operation.

5. **C – Meningocele**

Features are suggestive of meningocele. Management includes ruling out myelomeningocele and concomitant hydrocephalus. If there is hydrocephalus a concomitant ventriculoperitoneal shunt is generally preferred.

## 199. THEME: GOITRE

OPTIONS

A. Anaplastic carcinoma
B. Multinodular goitre
C. Plummer's syndrome
D. Graves disease
E. Pendred's syndrome
F. Colloid goitre
G. Physiological goitre
H. Thyroiditis

*For each of the patients described below, choose the single most likely diagnosis from the list of options above. Each option may be used once, more than once or not at all.*

1. A 60-year-old woman has suffered from slight enlargement of thyroid since many years. Recently it has enlarged rapidly in size and her voice has become hoarse.

2. A 25-year-old woman presents with recent swelling in the neck and weight loss. She looks very anxious and her palms are very moist.

3. A deaf and dumb brother and sister both presented with a smooth enlargement of the thyroid gland.

4. A 35-year-old woman presents with pain in the neck, fever, malaise and enlargement of thyroid gland. Her serum $T_4$ levels are normal.

5. A 23-year-old woman presents with slight enlargement of thyroid gland. She is 5-month pregnant. She is otherwise asymptomatic.

## 199. ANSWERS

1. **A - Anaplastic carcinoma**

Features suggest carcinoma of the thyroid. Hoarseness of voice is a very characteristic sign. It has got a high prevalence in the endemic goitrous areas. Treatment is by total thyroidectomy followed by external radiotherapy. But an attempt at curative resection is only justified if there is no infiltration through the thyroid capsule and no evidence of metastases.

2. **D - Graves disease**

Features suggest Graves disease. Typical symptom is weight loss despite increased appetite. Tiredness, emotional lability and heat intolerance are other characteristic features. Treatment would be with antithyroid drugs. Surgery is indicated in large goitres. Radioiodine is reserved for patients over 45 years of age.

3. **E - Pendred's syndrome**

Features suggest Pendred's syndrome. It is goitre associated with congenital deafness. This is due to a deficiency of peroxidase, the enzyme responsible for organification of trapped iodine.

4. **H – Thyroiditis**

Features are suggestive of subacute thyroiditis. This is due to a virus infection. Clinical features are of painful enlargement of the thyroid with fever and malaise. There is raised ESR and the serum $T_4$ levels may be high or normal. The condition is self-limiting. If diagnosis is in doubt, it may be confirmed by FNAC, radioactive iodine uptake and by a rapid symptomatic response to prednisone. Specific treatment for an acute case with severe pain is to give prednisone for 7 days and then reduce the dose gradually.

5. **G - Physiological goitre**

Simple euthyroid goitre can develop at times of increased demand like puberty and pregnancy. No treatment is required as it tends to be self-limiting.

## 200. THEME: MANAGEMENT OF GOITRE

OPTIONS

A. Antithyroid drugs
B. Surgery
C. Radioiodine
D. Reassurance
E. Thyroxine
F. Prednisolone

*For each of the patients described below, choose the single most useful management from the list of options above. Each option may be used once, more than once or not at all.*

1. A 30-year-old woman presents with mild diffuse enlargement of the thyroid gland. She has recently lost 2 stones despite a good appetite. Her serum $T_4$ levels are found to be very high.

2. A 50-year-old woman presents with a long-standing history of goitre. She has recently developed palpitations. On examination she has a moderately large multinodular goitre.

3. A 35-year-old woman presents with a small swelling in the neck slightly on the right side of the midline. It moves up on deglutition. She says that she has developed intolerance to hot weather. Her serum TSH levels are found to be very low.

4. A 40-year-old woman who was operated for a toxic goitre 2 years ago presents with slight swelling in the neck. Her serum $T_4$ levels are very high. She does not want to have any further children.

5. A 45-year-old woman presents with fever, malaise and painful enlargement of the thyroid gland. Her serum $T_4$ levels are slightly elevated.

## 200. ANSWERS

1. **A - Antithyroid drugs**

Features suggest Graves disease. Typical symptom is weight loss despite increased appetite. Tiredness, emotional lability and heat intolerance are other characteristic features. Treatment would be with antithyroid drugs. Surgery is indicated in large goitres. Radioiodine is reserved for patients over 45 years of age.

2. **B - Surgery**

Features are suggestive of toxic multinodular goitre. It does not respond as well or as rapidly to radioiodine or antithyroid drugs as does a diffuse toxic goitre. The goitre itself is often large and uncomfortable. Hence the treatment of choice is surgery.

3. **B - Surgery**

Features suggest a toxic nodule of the thyroid. Resection is easy and without morbidity. Radioiodine is a good option over the age of 45. Now radioiodine is being increasingly used in younger patients, particularly when they have completed their families.

4. **C - Radioiodine**

Features are suggestive of recurrent thyrotoxicosis after surgery. In general, radioiodine is preferred treatment. Antithyroid drugs may be used in younger women intending to have children. Further surgery is not recommended.

5. **F - Prednisolone**

Features are suggestive of subacute thyroiditis. This is due to a virus infection. Clinical features are of painful enlargement of the thyroid with fever and malaise. There is raised ESR and the serum $T_4$ levels may be high or normal. The condition is self-limiting. If diagnosis is in doubt, it may be confirmed by FNAC, radioactive iodine uptake and by a rapid symptomatic response to prednisolone. Specific treatment for an acute case with severe pain is to give prednisolone for 7 days and then reduce the dose gradually.

## 201. THEME: THYROID DISEASE

OPTIONS

A. Subtotal thyroidectomy
B. Hemithyroidectomy
C. Total thyroidectomy
D. Radioiodine treatment
E. Enucleation
F. Radiotherapy/chemotherapy

*For each of the patients described below, choose the single most useful management from the list of options above. Each option may be used once, more than once or not at all.*

1. A 30-year-old woman with Graves disease who is thyrotoxic. Medical treatment has failed to control her symptoms and is hoping to start a family in the next few years.

2. A 55-year-old woman presents with a painless swelling in her thyroid. Investigations have revealed it to be a lymphoma.

3. A 50-year-old man presented with a lump in the right lobe of the thyroid. Fine needle aspiration has revealed it to be follicular in nature.

## 201. ANSWERS

### 1. A - Subtotal thyroidectomy

Graves disease is initially treated medically with drugs such as carbimazole or propylthiouracil. Subtotal thyroidectomy carries the risk of nerve damage and damage to the parathyroid glands. Furthermore patient may become hypo- or hyperthyroid after surgery.

### 2. F - Radiotherapy/chemotherapy

Lymphoma stages Ia and IIa are treated with radiotherapy and stages IIa–IVb with chemotherapy.

### 3. B - Hemithyroidectomy

FNAC will not differentiate between follicular adenoma and follicular carcinoma. Hence, thyroid lobectomy is required. With minimally invasive lesions, total lobectomy and suppression of TSH with thyroxine are all that is required. If, however, overt capsular or vascular invasion is seen, reoperation in the form of total thyroidectomy is strongly advised: total thyroidectomy should ideally be performed within 7–10 days.

## 202. THEME: MANAGEMENT OF THYROID LUMPS

OPTIONS

A. Observation
B. Radioactive iodine
C. Thyroxine suppressive therapy
D. Tracheostomy
E. Right hemithyroidectomy
F. Subtotal thyroidectomy
G. Right hemithyroidectomy, followed by radioactive iodine
H. Total thyroidectomy with lymph node clearance
I. Total thyroidectomy, followed by external-beam radiotherapy

*For each of the clinical scenarios described below, choose the option that best describes the initial management from the above list. Each option may be used once, more than once, or not at all.*

1. A 60-year-old man has a 5-cm right thyroid mass. He is clinically and biochemically euthyroid. Ultrasound-guided fine-needle aspiration cytology (FNAC) has confirmed papillary carcinoma.

2. A 33-year-old euthyroid woman has a 0.8-cm right thyroid mass. Ultrasound-guided FNAC has confirmed a follicular neoplasm.

3. A 33-year-old woman has a 0.8-cm right thyroid mass. Ultrasound-guided FNAC has confirmed a colloid nodule. She has no other complaints and is euthyroid.

4. A 40-year-old euthyroid woman has a multinodular goitre with retrosternal extension. She complains of mild long-standing stridor and difficulty swallowing. Ultrasound-guided FNAC of a prominent nodule has confirmed a colloid nodule.

## 202. ANSWERS

1. **H - Total thyroidectomy with lymph node clearance**
This is a high-risk patient. 15% of patients with papillary carcinoma fall in high-risk group (older patient, poorly differentiated tumours, local invasion, distant metastases and large primary lesions). Total thyroidectomy is reserved for such patients. This should always include clearance of nodes in the primary lymphatic drainage zone. When local invasion or distant spread not amenable to surgery occur, radioiodine may show uptake in approx. 20% of cases and then the option of therapeutic radioiodine can be considered.

2. **E - Right hemithyroidectomy**
This is a low-risk patient with a low-risk tumour. FNAC cannot reliably differentiate between benign and malignant follicular pathology. Hence thyroid lobectomy is required. With minimally invasive lesions, total lobectomy and suppression of TSH with thyroxine are all that is required. If, however, overt capsular or vascular invasion is seen, reoperation in the form of total thyroidectomy is strongly advised: total thyroidectomy should ideally be performed within 7–10 days.

3. **A - Observation**
This is a low-risk patient with FNAC indicative of benign pathology. Observation with repeat FNAC is the best treatment option.

4. **F - Subtotal thyroidectomy**
This patient requires thyroidectomy (total or subtotal) to relieve the pressure symptoms. As there is no suggestion of malignancy, radioactive iodine is not indicated. The stridor is mild and long standing; therefore, tracheotomy is unlikely to be necessary.

## 203. THEME: COMPLICATIONS OF THYROID SURGERY

OPTIONS

A. Recurrent laryngeal nerve palsy
B. External laryngeal nerve palsy
C. Hypocalcaemia
D. Hypercalcaemia
E. Hypothyroidism
F. Tracheomalacia
G. Wound haemorrhage
H. Keloid

*For each of the patients described below, choose the single most likely diagnosis from the list of options above. Each option may be used once, more than once or not at all.*

1. A 45-year-old woman who underwent subtotal thyroidectomy is found to have hoarse voice on the next postoperative day.

2. A 55-year-old woman underwent total thyroidectomy 1 year ago for thyroid carcinoma. At the follow-up clinic she gives history of weight gain and feeling lethargic.

3. A 50-year-old woman undergoes a lobectomy of the thyroid gland. 6 hours after the surgery she complains of severe pain in the neck and difficulty in breathing.

4. A 40-year-old woman underwent a total thyroidectomy. On the 2nd postoperative day she complains of tingling and numbness in the face and fingers.

5. A 60-year-old black woman who underwent subtotal thyroidectomy 5 years ago presents with an unsightly swelling over the scar of the surgery. She also complains of itching over the swelling.

## 203. ANSWERS

**1. A - Recurrent laryngeal nerve palsy**

Features suggest recurrent laryngeal nerve palsy. Hoarseness of voice usually becomes evident 2–3 days after surgery. This is most likely due to oedema and is relieved by local anaesthetic lozenges or humidified air. Persistence of symptoms may indicate neuropraxia. This is reversible and recovers over several weeks or months. Permanent nature of damage should not be accepted unless it lasts for more than 9 months.

**2. E - Hypothyroidism**

Hypothyroidism is inevitable after total thyroidectomy. Hypothyroidism with rising TSH concentrations should be allowed to develop over 6 weeks after total thyroidectomy for malignancy. A radioiodine scan will then identify possible distant metastases, which can be ablated. Thereafter, $T_3$ is administered in preference to $T_4$ as its shorter biological half-life allows repeat scans to be performed with minimal delay. Once isotope ablation of residual disease has been achieved, conversion to $T_4$ is appropriate.

**3. G - Wound haemorrhage**

It is typically reactionary and is a potential problem in the first 24 hours after surgery. It presents with significant pallor, respiratory difficulty, stridor and swelling of the wound. Any haematoma should be evacuated immediately and intubation or tracheostomy may be necessary.

**4. C - Hypocalcaemia**

Hypocalcaemia due to parathyroid efficiency will usually be evident within 1 week of operation and should be suspected if the patient appears unduly agitated or depressed, or hyperventilates. Circumoral tingling is the first and most sensitive indicator of a low serum calcium. Paraesthesia in the fingers and toes is seen when hypocalcaemia is profound. IV infusion of 10 mL of 10 per cent calcium gluconate is required. Vitamin D and 2–3 g oral calcium per day are given until a normocalcaemic state is achieved.

**5. H - Keloid**

The deposition of excessive collagen in the scar to form a keloid is an unpredictable complication. It is more prevalent in blacks. Reoperation is unlikely to confer any improvement but topical steroids and low-dose irradiation may help.

## 204. THEME: THYROID DISEASE

OPTIONS

A. Medullary thyroid carcinoma (MTC)
B. Anaplastic carcinoma
C. Follicular carcinoma
D. Lymphoma
E. Follicular adenoma
F. Papillary carcinoma

*For each patient described below, select the most likely single diagnosis from the list of options above. Each option may be used once, more than once or not at all.*

1. A 13-year-old girl presents to the surgical outpatient department with a neck swelling. Clinical examination shows a 2-cm solid lump in the left thyroid lobe, and two enlarged cervical lymph nodes lateral to the thyroid mass. Ultrasonography confirms the solid nature of the thyroid nodule. FNA biopsy of the thyroid nodule reveals malignant cells with vesicular appearance of nuclei.

2. A 60-year-old man presents to the surgical outpatient department with rapidly enlarged thyroid swelling and hoarseness. Clinical examination shows a 3-cm solid lump in the left thyroid lobe and two enlarged cervical lymph nodes lateral to the thyroid mass. Ultrasonography confirms the solid nature of the thyroid nodule. FNA biopsy of the thyroid nodule reveals malignant cells with vesicular appearance of nuclei.

## 204. ANSWERS

1. **F - Papillary carcinoma**

The presence of regional lymphadenopathy, the age of the patient and the characteristic vesicular appearance of the nuclei support the diagnosis of papillary carcinoma. The treatment consists of total thyroidectomy and removal of enlarged lymph nodes.

2. **B - Anaplastic carcinoma**

The presence of regional lymphadenopathy, the age of the patient and the characteristic vesicular appearance of the nuclei support the diagnosis of anaplastic carcinoma. The patient may benefit from total thyroidectomy followed by external radiotherapy, although tumour cells may be implanted in the surgical incision.

## 205. THEME: LUMPS IN THE NECK

OPTIONS

A. Chemodectoma
B. Branchial cyst
C. Hodgkin's lymphoma
D. Cystic hygroma
E. Thyroglossal cyst
F. Pharyngeal pouch
G. Dermoid cyst
H. Goitre
I. Collar stud abscess

*For each of the patients described below, choose the single most likely diagnosis from the list of options above. Each option may be used once, more than once or not at all.*

1. A 40-year-old woman from India presents with a swelling in the neck. She suffers from weight loss and decreased appetite. On examination, there is a 2-cm swelling in the anterior triangle, which is fluctuant. Overlying skin appears red-purple in colour. The temperature over the swelling is normal.

2. An 18-year-old man presents with a swelling in the neck since a month. On examination, there is a 2-cm lump in the right supraclavicular region which is firm rubbery, smooth and well-defined. No other abnormality is found on examination.

3. A 20-year-old man presents with a swelling in the neck. On examination, there is 1-cm swelling in the midline. It is nontender, smooth, firm and well-defined. It moves up when he pokes his tongue out.

4. A 45-year-old man presents with a slowly enlarging swelling in the neck. On examination, there is 4-cm size lump in the anterior triangle which is firm, rubbery and pulsatile. It is possible to move it from side-to-side but not up and down.

5. A 12-year-old girl presents with a midline neck swelling. On examination, there is 3-cm lump which is soft and fluctuant. It does not move with deglutition or protrusion of tongue. There is no cervical lymphadenopathy.

## 205. ANSWERS

1. **I - Collar stud abscess**
Tuberculosis (TB) is still a common cause of cervical lymphadenopathy. If treatment is not instituted, the caseated node may liquefy and form a cold abscess. The pus may erode the deep cervical fascia and may point beneath the superficial fascia. This is a collar stud abscess. The patient should be treated with appropriate chemotherapy. If an abscess fails to resolve despite appropriate chemotherapy, occasionally excision of the abscess and its surrounding fibrous capsule is necessary.

2. **C - Hodgkin's lymphoma**
Features are suggestive of Hodgkin's lymphoma. Firm, rubbery nodes are present. Excisional biopsy is required for diagnosis. Radiation therapy is used to treat localized disease with the addition of chemotherapy for systemic or diffuse disease.

3. **E - Thyroglossal cyst**
It represents a persistence of the thyroglossal track. It may be found anywhere in or adjacent to the midline from the tongue base to the thyroid isthmus. It characteristically moves up on protrusion of the tongue. Treatment is by excision of the whole thyroglossal tract which includes removal of the body of the hyoid bone and suprahyoid tract till the foramen caecum. This is known as Sistrunk's operation.

4. **A - Chemodectoma**
Features suggest a chemodectoma. The tumour arises from the chemoreceptor cells on the medial side of the carotid bulb and at this point the tumour is adherent to the carotid wall. It can sometimes be emptied by firm pressure, after which it will slowly refill in a pulsatile manner. A bruit may also be present. Diagnosis is by duplex study or if indicated, a carotid angiogram. Biopsy or FNAC is contraindicated. The need for surgical removal must be considered carefully as complications are potentially dangerous.

5. **G - Dermoid cyst**
Features suggest a dermoid cyst. It occurs due to dermal cells being buried along the line of closure of embryonic clefts and sinuses by skin fusion. The cyst contains paste-like desquamated material. The usual sites are the midline of the body, above the outer canthus and behind the ear. Because of the contents it is not transilluminant. Treatment is by complete excision.

## 206. THEME: NECK LUMPS

OPTIONS

A. Branchial cyst
B. Carotid body tumour
C. Cervical rib
D. Cystic hygroma
E. Parotid tumour
F. Pharyngeal pouch
G. Sternocleidomastoid tumour
H. Submandibular tumour
I. Thyroglossal cyst
J. Thyroid swellings
K. Tonsillitis

*The following scenarios describe various presentations of neck lumps. From the above list choose the most likely diagnosis. Each item may be chosen once, more than once, or not at all.*

1. A 30-year-old man presents with a lump in his neck. On examination, it is situated in the left carotid triangle, and appears to be deep to the upper third of the sternocleidomastoid muscle. It feels cystic on palpation. Aspiration reveals 10 mL of thick yellow fluid. He is otherwise fit and well.

2. An 80-year-old woman presents with a history of dysphagia, halitosis, regurgitation and recurrent chest infections. She is otherwise well.

3. A 4-month-old infant is brought to clinic with a unilateral swelling on the right side of the neck. The child is noted to posture her head awkwardly. She is otherwise well but her mother reports that she was born by a difficult forceps delivery for a breech presentation.

4. A 20-year-old woman presents with an asymptomatic painless lump in the midline below her chin. The lump is smooth, measures 1 cm, is non tender and moves on swallowing.

## 206. ANSWERS

1. **A – Branchial cyst.** A branchial cyst is a remnant of, usually, the second branchial cleft. It is lined by squamous epithelium and if infected, a small sinus may develop tracking to the skin at the anterior border of the sternocleidomastoid muscle. Presentation is often as in the scenario, with the cyst arising from the junction between the upper and middle thirds of the sternocleidomastoid muscle. Treatment is surgical excision with concomitant antibiotic treatment of any pre-existing infection. Care must be taken to excise the entire cyst to prevent recurrence but it is not necessary to trace and excise any tract to the pharynx. Patients must be made fully aware of and give full consent regarding the risks of damage to the accessory, vagus and hypoglossal nerves. Rarely a chronically infected cyst may become adherent to the internal jugular vein.

2. **F – Pharyngeal pouch.** Also known as Zenker's diverticulum, pharyngeal pouches often present in the elderly where they have had opportunity to develop without many symptoms. Patients eventually present as in this scenario with dysphagia and subsequent weight loss. Pulmonary overspill occurs and hoarseness and recurrent chest infections may be the only presenting feature. A low, anterior triangular mass may be felt and fluid within the pouch can sometimes be displaced on deeper palpation. Their aetiology is unknown but imaging studies have suggested a neuromuscular incoordination resulting in herniation of the mucosa through the muscular coat. The weakest point is Killian's dehiscence between the thyropharyngeal and cricopharyngeal muscles that constitute the inferior constrictor muscle. Management involves surgical excision using an open or endoscopic technique where appropriate.

3. **G – Sternocleidomastoid tumour.** These appear 1–2 months after birth and are usually accompanied by a history of a complicated or breech birth. The 'tumour' is unilateral and situated as described in this scenario. It is initially a haematoma with associated muscle degeneration. It is often tender at first and associated with a torticollis. Early treatment is imperative, to prevent permanent disability, with active stimulation and passive stimulation which can be achieved at home by the infant's parents. This normally reduces the 'tumour' over the first 4–6 months. Only those that are noted late or fail to respond to conservative treatment require surgery.

4. **I – Thyroglossal cyst.** In the embryo, the thyroid gland develops from the thyroglossal duct that originates at the foramen caecum at the base of the tongue. Occasionally the duct may remain patent and a structure known as a thyroglossal cyst can persist. These cysts are the commonest midline neck masses of infancy, and may be confused with epidermoid cysts, dermoid cysts and pyramidal lobe thyroid nodules. They are lined with squamous or ciliated pseudo stratified columnar epithelium. Occasionally they contain lymphoid or thyroid tissue, and any of its constituents may undergo malignant change. Management involves surgical excision of the cyst and the central portion of the hyoid bone in a procedure known as Sistrunk's operation, to ensure that the condition does not recur.

## 207. THEME: NECK LUMPS

OPTIONS

A. Laryngocele
B. Thyroglossal cyst
C. Branchial cyst
D. Desmoid cyst
E. Dermoid cyst
F. Lymphangioma
G. Chemodectoma

*For each of the patients below, chose the most appropriate diagnosis from those above. Each may be used once, more than once or not at all.*

1. A 55-year-old gentleman presented with a long-standing history of mild stridor and hoarseness that had suddenly worsened. On palpation a large soft swelling over the thyrohyoid membrane was felt; when pressure was applied, this swelling disappeared.

2. A 7-year-old girl presented with a painless cystic swelling anterior to the thyroid cartilage. The swelling was transilluminable, mobile in all directions and moved on protrusion of the tongue.

## 207. ANSWERS

**1. A – Laryngocele**

When the laryngeal saccule is expanded with air it is termed a laryngocele. These may spread superiorly and present in the false cord (internal laryngocele) or may pass through the thyrohyoid membrane and present as a lump in the neck.

**2. B - Thyroglossal cyst**

A thyroglossal cyst is a fluctuant midline swelling which moves on tongue protrusion. It develops in cell nests in the thyroid gland's migration path.

## 208. THEME: CERVICAL LYMPHADENOPATHY

OPTIONS

A. Idiopathic histiocytic necrotising lymphadenitis
B. Infectious mononucleosis
C. Lymphoreticular disease
D. Metastatic malignancy
E. Sarcoidosis
F. Scalp infection
G. Tonsillitis
H. Toxoplasmosis
I. Tuberculosis

*For each of the patients described below, choose the single most appropriate diagnosis from the list of options above. Each option may be used once, more than once or not at all.*

1. A 60-year-old man presents with an asymptomatic slowly growing painless lump in the neck. On examination he has a hard 2-cm mass lying laterally in the submandibular triangle of his neck, deep to the middle third of the right sternocleidomastoid muscle. The patient is noted to have a dysphonia.

2. A 14-year-old girl presents with recurrent sore throats and on examination she has a soft 2-cm mass lying laterally within the anterior triangle of the neck, just below the angle of the mandible.

3. A 30-year-old Caucasian presents with a 3-month history of night sweats, weight loss and a unilateral enlargement of his left tonsil. There is also a rubbery enlarged level III lymph node in the left posterior triangle.

## 208. ANSWERS

### 1. D – Metastatic malignancy

The characteristic position described is that of cervical lymph nodes that drain the oropharynx and larynx. The lymphatic system of the neck can be divided into levels 1–5. This man has palpable Level 3 nodes that also drain levels 1 and 2, which receive lymph from the scalp, face and lips. The most likely diagnosis here is a laryngeal carcinoma given the history of dysphonia.

### 2. G – Tonsillitis

This acute history and anatomical description of involved lymph nodes is typical of tonsillitis, remembering that the tonsil itself is a lymphoid structure. Other acute causes of cervical lymphadenopathy include pharyngitis/laryngitis and Epstein–Barr virus infection. Chronic causes include tuberculosis and sarcoidosis.

### 3. C – Lymphoreticular disease

This is fairly obvious given the history. The differential would be tuberculosis/human immunodeficiency virus in at-risk individuals.

## 209. THEME: THYROID NEOPLASMS

OPTIONS

A. Anaplastic carcinoma
B. Papillary carcinoma
C. Medullary thyroid carcinoma
D. Malignant lymphoma
E. Follicular carcinoma
F. Secondary thyroid carcinoma

*For each of the following described below, choose the single most likely diagnosis from the list of options above. Each option may be used once, more than once or not at all.*

1. Characteristic histology feature is 'Orphan Annie' type cells.
2. Associated with lack of iodine and more common in areas with a high incidence of endemic goitre.
3. Highly malignant tumour with early local infiltration and distant spread.
4. Most are radiosensitive.
5. Originates from parafollicular cells.

## 209. ANSWERS

1. **B- Papillary carcinoma**

These account for 80% of thyroid tumours in patients less than 40 years of age. Infiltration to cervical nodes is the usual mode of spread. Histologically, tumours are characterized by papillary pattern. The diagnosis is established by the characteristic 'orphan Annie' cells. Another characteristic is presence of psammoma bodies. Low-risk patients are treated by total lobectomy on the side of the tumour with isthmusectomy. Total thyroidectomy is reserved for the patients categorized as 'high-risk'.

2. **E - Follicular carcinoma**

It is associated with lack of iodine and is therefore probably induced by TSH. Spread is via blood stream mostly to lung, bones and brain. Treatment is by thyroid lobectomy with intraoperative frozen section. If capsular or vascular invasion is clearly present, total thyroidectomy should be performed.

3. **A - Anaplastic carcinoma**

Features suggest anaplastic carcinoma of the thyroid. It has got a high prevalence in the endemic goitrous areas. Treatment is by total thyroidectomy followed by external radiotherapy. But an attempt at curative resection is only justified if there is no infiltration through the thyroid capsule and no evidence of metastases.

4. **D - Malignant lymphoma**

This occurs mainly in elderly women and grows rapidly. It may arise in pre-existing Hashimoto's disease. Most are radiosensitive and regress after external-beam radiotherapy. Chemotherapy is reserved for patients with disseminated disease.

5. **C - Medullary thyroid carcinoma**

It arises from the parafollicular C cells. It may be associated with phaeochromocytoma and parathyroid adenomas – MEN type IIA. Rarely there may be medullary carcinoma with phaeochromocytoma with absence of parathyroid adenomas – MEN type IIB. Total thyroidectomy is the procedure of choice. The primary lymphatic drainage areas must also be resected. A coexisting phaeochromocytoma or parathyroid tumour needs to be excluded.

## 210. THEME: LARYNGEAL CANCER

OPTIONS

A. Total laryngectomy and neck dissection
B. Radiotherapy
C. Chemotherapy
D. Excision of vocal cord mucosa

*For each of the patients below, select the most likely single treatment from the options listed above. Each option may be used once, more than once or not at all.*

1. A 50-year-old man presents with a hoarse voice. Clinical examination and investigations reveal a small invasive carcinoma of the left vocal cord. The left vocal cord is paralysed and there is a 4-cm lymph node in the left anterior neck.

2. A 65-year-old man is found to have a $T_1$ carcinoma of the vocal cord. There is no involvement of the anterior commissure.

3. A 60-year-old woman is found to have a carcinoma in situ of the left vocal cord.

4. A 55-year-old woman is found to have a glottic carcinoma involving the anterior commissure.

5. A 70-year-old woman with a large supraglottic carcinoma.

## 210. ANSWERS

1. **A - Total laryngectomy and neck dissection**

The tumour stage is $T_3 N_{2a}$. Partial laryngectomy is inadequate; therefore total laryngectomy combined with neck dissection is the surgical treatment of choice. Radiotherapy may be given postoperatively. Chemotherapy is indicated for inoperable disease.

2. **B - Radiotherapy**

Radiotherapy is as effective as surgery in the treatment of T1 tumours. However, the resulting voice quality is better than after surgery.

3. **D - Excision of vocal cord mucosa**

Close monitoring is required.

4. **B - Radiotherapy**

In the UK most teams would opt for radiotherapy and close follow up with total laryngectomy as an option for failure after radiotherapy.

5. **A - Total laryngectomy and neck dissection**

Nodal metastases are found in 55% of supraglottic tumours. Therefore radical neck dissection is often required for large supraglottic tumours.

## 211. THEME: SOFT TISSUE TUMOURS

OPTIONS

A. Lipoma
B. Neurofibroma
C. Malignant fibrous hystiocytoma
D. Ganglion
E. Haemangioma
F. Leiomyoma
G. Dermatofibrosarcoma
H. Rhabdomyosarcoma
I. Kaposi's sarcoma

*For each of the conditions described below, choose the single most likely diagnosis from the list of options above. Each option may be used once, more than once or not at all.*

1. They are fibrous wall cysts most commonly seen on the dorsal surface of the wrist.

2. Although they are benign and do not metastasize but tend to recur after excision.

3. They arise from the smooth muscle of gastrointestinal tract.

4. They are more commonly seen in patients suffering from AIDS.

5. Although classified as soft tissue sarcoma, it may arise from bone and a variety of other tissues.

## 211. ANSWERS

### 1. D - Ganglion

They result from an excrescence of synovial tissue and are filled with synovial fluid. Simple excision is usually curative. They are easily confused with giant cell tumour of the tendon sheath, which are also seen most commonly in the wrist and are also treated by simple excision.

### 2. G - Dermatofibrosarcoma

Dermatofibrosarcoma protuberans arises in the skin or subcutaneous tissue. These tumours do not metastasize but they behave locally as though malignant. It is important to achieve control at the time of first resection with at least 2 cm margin to minimize the risk of further recurrence.

### 3. F - Leiomyoma

They are benign tumours arising from smooth muscles of the uterus and gastrointestinal tract. Leiomyoblastomas are similar to leiomyoma but tend to grow larger. Both are treated by simple excision.

### 4. I - Kaposi's sarcoma

It is clinically characterised as multiple pigmented sarcoma nodules, usually beginning on the legs as red nodules and spreading slowly. It may also occur on chest, arms, head and neck. It frequently involves mucosa of mouth and anus. Treatment depends on the extent of the disease and symptoms, i.e., weight loss, fever or ongoing infection. Minimal tumour without symptoms may be treated with interferon. More extensive tumour or presence of symptoms requires chemotherapy.

### 5. C - Malignant fibrous histiocytoma

It implies high-grade sarcoma that lacks specific features of differentiation. Treatment depends upon size and grade of the tumour. For large size or high grade tumours surgery is combined with radiotherapy.

## 212. THEME: MANAGEMENT OF SKIN AND SOFT TISSUE LESIONS

OPTIONS

A. Simple excision
B. Reassurance – wait and watch
C. Radiotherapy
D. Cryotherapy
E. Chemotherapy
F. Wide local excision
G. Radical excision

*For each of the patients described below, choose the single most useful management from the list of options above. Each option may be used once, more than once or not at all.*

1. A 40-year-old presents with 3-cm lump over his arm. It is painless. On examination, it is soft, mobile, lobulated, and slip sign is positive.

2. A 45-year-old presents with a 4-cm lump on his abdomen. He is otherwise well with no complaints related to the lump. On examination, there is 4-cm lump present over a previous midline scar of laparotomy which was done as emergency procedure. It is not reducible and there is no impulse on coughing. The lump is not very mobile and overlying skin is tethered.

3. A 38-year-old man presents with a rapidly enlarging swelling on his right calf. On examination, there is a 5-cm lump present which appears to be arising from the muscle. Core needle biopsy reveals grade II rhabdomyosarcoma.

4. A 2-month-old boy is brought because the parents have noticed a strawberry like swelling over his arm. They say it appeared in the first month and is increasing in size. On examination, the sign of emptying is demonstrable.

5. A 34-year-old man presents with a 1-cm swelling over the dorsum of his right finger distal phalanx. On examination, it is red, moderately firm pedunculated nodule. The surface shows some crusts.

## 212. ANSWERS

1. **A - Simple excision**

Features are suggestive of lipoma. Treatment is by simple excision.

2. **F - Wide local excision**

Features suggest desmoid tumour. They arise from the muscular wall of the abdomen and often in association with abdominal incisions. Wide resection is the preferred treatment. If resected to clear margins they seldom recur.

3. **G - Radical excision**

Treatment of soft tissue sarcomas depends on grading and size of tumour. For grade II or III with tumour size more than 2 cm, treatment of choice is radical resection. If this is not possible, preoperative radiation may be given followed by resection with 5 mm margin of normal tissue.

4. **B - Reassurance – wait and watch**

Features are suggestive of haemangioma. From the age of 3 months to 1 year the haemangioma grows with the child and then it ceases to grow. Eventually the colour fades and flattening occurs and by the age of 9 years 90% demonstrate complete involution.

5. **A - Simple excision**

Features are suggestive of pyogenic granuloma. It is common acquired, reactive, proliferative vascular lesion of the skin and mucous membranes, arising after minor trauma. The lesion looks like a haemangioma. It is most commonly seen on the face, fingers and toes. Treatment is by excision.

## 213. THEME: MALIGNANT MELANOMA

OPTIONS

A. Acral lentiginous melanoma
B. Amelanotic melanoma
C. Lentigo maligna melanoma
D. Nodular melanoma
E. Superficial spreading melanoma

*For each of the scenarios given below, select the correct type of cutaneous malignant melanoma from the above list. Each option may be used once, more than once, or not at all.*

1. Occurs within a Hutchinson's melanotic freckle.
2. Has a predilection for sites with thick epidermis such as the sole of the feet.
3. Commonest type of cutaneous malignant melanoma.

## 213. ANSWERS

1. **C – Lentigo maligna melanoma**

These account for 10–15% of cutaneous melanomas. They typically occur on the sun-exposed areas of the head and neck and hands. Clinically, they are large, flat, tan lesions with areas of dark brown or black colouration that look like a stain on the skin. They are characterized by a prolonged radial growth phase. They do not have the same propensity to metastasise as melanomas of other growth patterns.

2. **A – Acral lentiginous melanoma**

These characteristically occur on the palms or soles or beneath the nail beds. They make up 2–8% of melanomas in Caucasian people as opposed to 40–60% of melanomas in people of black or Asian descent.

3. **E – Superficial spreading melanoma**

These are the most common variety of melanoma, seen in about 70% of cases. The lesion usually arises within a pre-existing nevus. There is often a history of a slowly evolving change in the precursor lesion over several years. The initial growth is above the basement membrane.

## 214. THEME: SALIVARY GLAND DISEASE

OPTIONS

A. Acute suppurative sialadenitis
B. HIV-associated sialadenitis
C. Mikulicz's syndrome
D. Sarcoidosis
E. Sialolithiasis
F. Sialosis
G. Sjögren's syndrome
H. Viral parotitis
I. Xerostomia

*From the list above, select the most likely diagnosis for the following patients who all present with disease affecting the salivary glands. The items may be used once, more than once, or not at all.*

1. A 50-year-old man presents with severe, sudden onset submandibular pain. He has experienced similar pain previously precipitated by eating, but never as severe as this. Past history includes hypertension. On examination, he is afebrile and there is a diffuse submandibular swelling that is only minimally tender on bimanual palpation.

2. A 30-year-old woman presents with enlargement of her parotid gland. She reports intermittent painless swelling over the last few months. Past medical history includes hypothyroidism and chronic back pain, for which she takes thyroxine 100 g and co-proxamol, respectively. On examination, there is soft enlargement of the parotid gland.

3. A 50-year-old woman presents with a recent history of a dry mouth. She reports irritation of her eyes, although denies arthralgia. There is no relevant past medical or drug history. Clinical examination of the salivary glands is unremarkable. Full blood count is normal; erythrocyte sedimentation rate and C-reactive protein are both grossly elevated.

## 214. ANSWERS

1. **E – Sialolithiasis.** Calculi can occur in the submandibular or parotid glands, although the former is most commonly affected. Predisposing factors include chronic sialadenitis, reduced salivary flow rates, dehydration and duct obstruction. Calculi are associated with diabetes mellitus, hypertension and chronic liver disease. A stone within a gland may be asymptomatic, whereas a stone in the duct is likely to cause painful swelling that is precipitated by eating. Acute suppurative sialadenitis may supervene, and this is characterised by fever and severe pain that may give rise to spasm of the adjacent muscles of mastication, leading to 'trismus'; such a patient may be toxic. Twenty per cent of submandibular and 66% of parotid calculi are radiolucent, and so sialography is indicated to demonstrate filling defects. Stones may be removed surgically by lithotomy (distal stones) or excision of the duct with the gland (proximal stones).

2. **F – Sialosis.** Sialosis refers to recurrent swelling of the salivary glands in the absence of neoplasia or inflammation. The swelling is typically painless and bilateral. An important distinguishing feature from other causes of parotidomegaly is the fact that the gland, although enlarged, remains soft and not indurated. Sialosis occurs in association with endocrine disorders (myxoedema, Cushing's disease, diabetes mellitus etc.), metabolic disturbances (nutritional disorders, vitamin deficiencies etc.), and certain drugs (e.g., dextropropoxyphene [co-proxamol], oral contraceptives, anti-psychotics, clonidine etc.).

3. **G – Sjögren's syndrome.** The salivary glands may be damaged by autoimmune disease. Sjögren's syndrome is characterised by the presence of two of the following triad: keratoconjunctivitis sicca (dry eyes); xerostomia (dry mouth); and rheumatoid arthritis or other connective tissue disorder (e.g., scleroderma, systemic lupus erythematosis, polyarteritis nodosa etc.). The clinical scenario presented describes a patient with primary Sjögren's syndrome, which consists of xerostomia and xerophthalmia, with no connective tissue component. By contrast, secondary Sjögren's syndrome refers to the presence of all three features. The main differential in 'at risk' groups is that of human immunodeficiency virus-associated sialadenitis, which is clinically indistinguishable. This diagnosis should be considered, especially in female patients because Sjögren's has a 10:1 female predominance. Mikulicz's syndrome is also an autoimmune syndrome that describes enlargement of the salivary glands, xerostomia and enlargement of the lacrimal glands that cause a bulge below the outer end of the eyelids, and a narrowing in the palpebral fissures.

## 215. THEME: SUTURE MATERIAL

OPTIONS

A. '0'Vicryl
B. 3'0' PDS
C. 6'0' PDS
D. 6'0' Prolene
E. 2'0' Prolene
F. 2'0' Silk
G. 1 PDS
H. Stainless steel wire
I. 4'0' Vicryl

*For each of the following situations, select the most appropriate suture material for the procedure from the above list. Each option may be used once, more than once, or not at all.*

1. Bowel anastomosis.
2. Mid-line abdominal wound closure.
3. Sternotomy wound.
4. Distal end of femoro-popliteal bypass.
5. Securing a prosthetic mesh for incisional hernia repair.
6. Urethroplasty.

## 215. ANSWERS

1. **B – 3 '0' PDS**

Numerous suture materials can be used for bowel anastomosis. The most popular materials are the absorbable ones: PDS (polydioxanone) and Vicryl (polyglactin 910). The size of the suture would vary from 2'0' to 4'0'. Stapling techniques have become commonplace with the advantage of speed and a wider functional side-to-side anastomosis. There is no evidence that anastomotic leak rates are any higher between suturing and stapling.

2. **G – 1 PDS**

The abdominal wall can be closed through a variety of techniques: layered closure or mass closure. The latter is quicker and currently the most popular technique in the UK. The suture material may be absorbable or non-absorbable, loop or non-loop. However, it must be strong and heavy (usually a 1 PDS or 1 Nylon).

3. **H – Stainless steel wire**

Sternotomy wounds in adults are closed with stainless steel wires. However, sternotomy wounds in paediatric patients are closed with a heavy PDS suture.

4. **D – 6 '0' Prolene**

Arterial anastomoses are fashioned with prolene (polypropylene), an non-absorbable material. For small calibre anastomoses fine material must be used, otherwise narrowing would occur.

5. **E – 2 '0' Prolene**

Prosthetic mesh techniques have become the accepted means for repairing incisional hernias. The aim is for the mesh to be secured in position and not migrate; therefore, a non-absorbable suture such as 2 '0' prolene is most appropriate.

6. **I – 4'0' Vicryl**

Absorbable suture has to be used for repair of urethra or bladder. Nonabsorble suture may lead to encrustation and stone formation. For urethra 3'0' or 4'0' Vicryl is used.

## 216. THEME: SURGICAL COMPLICATIONS

OPTIONS

A. IV broad-spectrum antibiotics
B. Correction of ketoacidosis
C. Immediate laparotomy
D. Laparoscopic evaluation
E. Enteral nutrition
F. Observation
G. Correction of hyperglycaemia

*From the list above, select the most likely initial management for the following patients. The items may be used once, more than once, or not at all.*

1. After an abdominal penetrating injury a 25-year-old man undergoes resection of the distal ileum and ascending colon, which were severely damaged. End-to-end ileo-transverse anastomosis is done. On postoperative day four the patient, who is afebrile and without abdominal symptoms, begins to drain small bowel content through the lower end of the incision.

2. A 60-year-old woman is admitted to the emergency department with evidence of spreading peritonitis. Her temperature is 40 degree C with a pulse rate of 120/minute and blood pressure of 96/60. Her blood sugar is 960mg%. Urine specific gravity is 1.030, and marked glucosuria and ketonuria are present.

## 216. ANSWERS

1. **F - Observation**
This patient has no fever and no general abdominal findings. Hence, this is a controlled fistula. Without sepsis, antibiotics are not indicated. TPN is at least as effective as enteral nutrition in these patients. This fistula can be managed conservatively with the expectation that it will close spontaneously. Fluid replacement should be pursued vigorously in order to maintain appropriate renal function. The patient's oral intake should be limited initially but there is no need for a nasogastric tube unless mechanical obstruction is present.

2. **B - Correction of ketoacidosis**
This patient is critically ill and she is not an appropriate candidate for any diagnostic study such as CT scan, laparoscopy, or laparotomy until her ketoacidosis is addressed. The hyperglycaemia is less critical and will improve while the ketoacidosis is treated with IV hydration and crystalline insulin. The patient also needs IV antibiotics once steps to correct the ketoacidosis are underway.

## 217. THEME: SALIVARY GLAND TUMOURS

OPTIONS

A. Warthin's tumour
B. Low-grade mucoepidermoid carcinoma
C. Pleomorphic adenoma
D. Carcinoma

*From the list above, select the most likely diagnosis for the following patients who all present with disease affecting the salivary glands. The items may be used once, more than once, or not at all.*

1. A 30-year-old woman presents with a 2-cm mass below her right earlobe. She has been aware of the mass for 4 years. Examination reveals a firm, non-tender, movable mass with intact facial nerve function. Cervical lymph nodes are not palpable.

2. A 60-year-old man presents with a slowly growing painless swelling over the angle of jaw. On examination a 3-cm soft and well-defined mass is found in the right parotid.

3. A 65-year-old man presents with a rapidly growing mass over the right angle of his jaw. Examination reveals a hard, irregular mass with facial nerve palsy on the right side.

## 217. ANSWERS

1. **C - Pleomorphic adenoma**

Benign mixed tumours (pleomorphic adenomas) are the most common tumours of the salivary glands. The peak incidence occurs between 30 and 40 years of age. The tumour is slow-growing, firm, smooth and movable and it most frequently appears in the tail of the parotid gland. Recurrence of the tumour is the result of incomplete removal. Facial nerve weakness in a patient who has a parotid tumour almost always indicates the presence of a malignant lesion.

2. **A - Warthin's tumour**

This is a benign cystic tumour which contains epithelial lymphoid element. It occurs in middle and old age, more common in males. There is slow growing painless swelling over the angle of jaw. Characteristically it is soft and well defined. Treatment is by surgical excision. Recurrence is rare.

3. **D - Carcinoma**

Usually affects parotid and may arise in a pleomorphic adenoma. The gland becomes hard, irregular and painful. Facial nerve palsy may develop. Treatment is by radical parotidectomy with sacrifice of the facial nerve. Block dissection of the neck may be required. Radiotherapy is of limited value. The prognosis is poor.

## 218. THEME: BENIGN LESIONS OF SKIN

OPTIONS

A. Pedunculated papillomas (skin tags)
B. Keloid
C. Keratoacanthoma
D. Sebaceous cysts
E. Seborrhoeic keratosis
F. Fibrous histiocytoma
G. Hidradenitis suppurativa
H. Pyogenic granuloma
I. Furuncle

*From the list above, select the most likely diagnosis for the following conditions. The items may be used once, more than once, or not at all.*

1. Small polypoid lesions occur in adults, most frequently on the trunk, neck, axilla and groin.

2. Found in elderly patients, and often multiple, well-demarcated raised lesions with varying degrees of pigmentation.

3. Nodular lesion with a central crater containing a keratin 'plug'.

4. Dark red nodule of exuberant granulation tissue and polymorphs. There is rapid initial growth often at the site of trauma.

5. Chronic indolent disease of skin and subcutaneous tissue in apocrine gland-bearing areas, e.g., axilla, groin. The involved area is indurated, fibrotic and inflamed with sinuses draining pus.

## 218. ANSWERS

1. **A - Pedunculated papillomas (skin tags)**
They may catch on clothes and bleed, and are often cosmetically unacceptable. They are removed by excision under local anaesthetic.

2. **E - Seborrhoeic keratosis**
It may be difficult to differentiate from malignant melanoma if deeply pigmented. Treatment is to leave alone or treat by surgical excision or curettage.

3. **C - Keratoacanthoma**
They progress rapidly in 2 weeks to 2 months. Probably of viral aetiology, they often show spontaneous regression. Treatment is by excision biopsy unless the lesion is obviously regressing.

4. **H - Pyogenic granuloma**
Occasionally surface may ulcerate and then must be distinguished from amelanotic melanoma. Treatment is by excision.

5. **G - Hidradenitis suppurativa**
Staphylococcus aureus is the usual organism grown but occasionally coliforms may be cultured. Differential diagnosis includes furunculosis, carbuncle, and cellulitis. Biopsy confirms the diagnosis. Treatment is initially with antibiotics. Abscesses are incised and drained. Advanced cases may need wide excision and grafting.

## 219. THEME: PREMALIGNANT LESIONS OF SKIN

OPTIONS

A. Squamous cell carcinoma
B. Basal cell carcinoma
C. Kaposi's sarcoma
D. Metastatic carcinoma
E. Bowen's disease
F. Solar keratoses
G. Malignant melanoma
H. Neurofibrosarcoma

*For each of following skin lesions described, select an appropriate diagnosis from the list of options above. Each option may be used once or more than once or not at all.*

1. A well-defined erythematous plaque with occasional crusting. It may be associated with internal malignancy.

2. Rough scaly epidermal lesions on sites of exposure to the sun.

3. These may grow rapidly. It metastasizes via lymphatics and rarely via the bloodstream.

4. Raised purplish nodules, initially single, but gradually multiple nodules appear. Commonly seen in patients with AIDS.

5. Seen on areas exposed to sunlight. Locally invasive and rarely metastasise.

## 219. ANSWERS

1. **E - Bowen's disease**
This is an intra-epidermal squamous cell carcinoma. Diagnosis is confirmed by biopsy. Treatment is by curettage, excision, grafting or topical 5-fluorouracil.

2. **F - Solar keratoses**
10–20% of these undergo malignant change. Treatment is by excision. Topical 5-fluorouracil has been used in patients with malignant lesions.

3. **A - Squamous cell carcinoma**
It starts as a lump which ulcerates with bleeding and discharge. Treatment is wide local excision or radiotherapy. Block dissection of regional lymph nodes is required if these are affected.

4. **C - Kaposi's sarcoma**
The nodules may ulcerate. The solitary nodule should be excised. Local radiotherapy or cytotoxic therapy is useful for multiple lesions.

5. **B - Basal cell carcinoma**
The commonest area affected is the face above a line drawn from the angle of the mouth to the lobule of the ear. It starts as a nodule which ulcerates. Treatment includes surgical excision or radiotherapy.

## 220. THEME: PERI-ANAL PAIN

OPTIONS

A. Rectal prolapse
B. Thrombosed haemorrhoids
C. Fissure in-ano
D. Peri-anal haematoma
E. Anorectal abscess
F. Fistula-in-ano
G. Pruritus ani
H. Anal warts

*For each of following patients with anal pain, select an appropriate diagnosis from the list of options above. Each option may be used once or more than once or not at all.*

1. A 30-year-old man presents with acute peri-anal pain. It is worse on sitting, walking and defaecation. A tense, smooth, tender blue lump is seen at the anal verge on examination.

2. A 35-year-old woman presents with constant, throbbing, peri-anal pain worse on sitting. There is an indurated tender mass peri-anally. A boggy mass is felt on digital examination.

3. A 16-year-old woman presents with acute anal pain, severe on defaecation. She also complains about occasional blood on the toilet paper. Examination reveals an acute sphincter spasm.

4. A 25-year-old man presents to the Accident and Emergency department with acute anal pain. Examination reveals an oedematous, congested purplish mass at the anal margin.

## 220. ANSWERS

**1. D - Peri-anal haematoma**

Symptoms may subside spontaneously after 2–3 days during which time analgesia is given. If in acute phase, incision under LA should be carried out.

**2. E - Anorectal abscess**

The patient may have fever. A boggy mass may be felt on digital examination. Treatment is prompt surgical drainage to prevent fistula formation. There is no role for antibiotics except in diabetics and the immunocompromised and then only as an adjunct to surgery.

**3. C - Fissure in-ano**

Part the buttocks and the fissure may be apparent. A per rectal examination is impossible. Occasionally a 'sentinel pile' may be seen. Management could be conservative if symptoms are mild – LA gel or suppository. This is best applied some half an hour before defaecation. Correct constipation with a stool softening laxative and high-fibre diet. Acutely painful fissures should be treated as a surgical emergency. A sphincter stretch or a lateral subcutaneous internal sphincterotomy may be carried out to relieve spasm and to allow the fissure to heal.

**4. B - Thrombosed haemorrhoids**

These may be treated by bed rest, analgesia and ice packs.

## 221. THEME: COMPLICATIONS OF GALL STONES

OPTIONS

A. Chronic cholecystitis
B. Acute cholecystitis
C. Biliary colic
D. Mucocele
E. Empyema
F. Obstructive jaundice
G. Carcinoma
H. Cholangitis
I. Gallstone ileus

*Select the most appropriate diagnosis from the list above for each of the patients described below. Each option may be used once or more than once or not at all.*

1. A 40-year-old woman presents with acute abdominal pain in the epigastrium and the right upper quadrant. The patient rolls in agony and has had two episodes of vomiting. On examination she is tachycardic and sweating. There is rigidity in the upper abdomen.

2. A 45-year-old woman presents with acute pain in the right upper quadrant. On examination she has fever of 38.5°C, tachycardia and hypotension with a BP of 90/70 mm Hg. A tender mass is felt in the right upper quadrant.

## 221. ANSWERS

1. **C - Biliary colic**

This is a symptom rather than a complication of gallstones. The pain is not confined to the right upper quadrant. Severe spasms of colic occur against the background of continuous severe pain. Beware making a diagnosis of peritonitis – in peritonitis the patient does not roll around but remains still. An attack may last 2–4 hours.

2. **E - Empyema**

Diagnosis is by total white cell count and ultrasound examination. Treatment is with intravenous fluids, NG suction, antibiotics - cefuroxime and metronidazole. A cholecystectomy is needed. Occasionally there is so much inflammation that it is impossible to safely carry out cholecystectomy acutely. Drainage of the gallbladder with formation of cholecystotomy may be appropriate in these circumstances. Cholecystectomy may be undertaken at a later date.

## 222. THEME: CONSENT FOR SURGERY

OPTIONS

A. No need for consent, surgery can proceed
B. Surgery cannot proceed
C. Obtain consent from patient
D. Obtain consent from partner
E. Apply to make the child a ward of court

*For each of the scenarios below, select the most appropriate option for consent from the list of options mentioned above. Each option may be used once, more than once, or not at all.*

1. A 65-year-old male known to have a large abdominal aortic aneurysm refuses any form of surgery or radiological intervention though he is fully aware of the risk of aneurysm rupturing. He even refuses surgery should the aneurysm rupture. A day after refusing intervention again in a follow up clinic, he presents with massive abdominal distention, shock and confusion. Even in his confused state he continues to refuse surgery. His grand daughter however insists on surgery saying that her grandfather has always been afraid of needles and that he couldn't make an intelligent choice in his confused state.

2. A 65-year-old male Mr. X is involved in a road traffic accident. He is brought in with a GCS of 8/15 and CT scan shows a large extradural haematoma. His wife and daughter, however, refuse surgery. They tell you that Mr. X has always been afraid of hospitals and operations and that he had refused a hernia surgery 15 years ago. There is however no written directive.

3. An 8-year-old boy is brought in by anxious parents with abdominal pain for a week's duration. He is noted to have generalized peritonitis and CT scan confirms a perforated appendix. Parents however refuse surgery because their older son died after a surgery for similar reasons in the past.

## 222. ANSWERS

1. **B - Surgery cannot proceed**

The patient has clearly expressed his desire in the past. So, unfortunately, his surgery cannot proceed. Nobody, including the patient's wife or mother (forget the granddaughter), can consent or request a surgery on the patient's behalf against the patient's wishes.

2. **A - No need for consent, surgery can proceed**

While it is always a good idea to involve the family in these decisions, nobody in the family can legally consent or refuse a surgery. There is no advance directive to indicate that the patient would have refused such a life saving surgery. So, surgery can proceed.

3. **E - Apply to make the child a ward of the court**

The two options available are: (1) Respect the decision of the parents, or (2) Make the child a ward of the court and proceed with appropriate surgical management. Most surgeons would choose option 2 in the UK.

## 223. THEME: PHARMACOLOGY

OPTIONS

A. Morphine
B. Lignocaine
C. Tramadol
D. Paracetamol

*For each mechanism of action listed below, select the most appropriate drug from the list of options above. Each option may be used once, more than once, or not at all.*

1. Action is by a membrane stabilizing effect, impairing membrane permeability to sodium, so blocking impulse propagation.

2. They produce effects on neurons by acting on receptors located on neuronal cell membranes. Three major types of receptor are known- μ, δ and κ (mu, delta and kappa).

3. Binding of parent and M1 metabolite to mu-opioid receptors and weak inhibition of reuptake of norepinephrine and serotonin.

## 223. ANSWERS

1. **B - Lignocaine**

This is an important question for the examination. This mechanism of action is true for all local anaesthetics. The aim is to prevent or reduce nerve conduction of painful impulses to higher centres (via the thalamus), where the perception of pain occurs.

2. **A - Morphine**

Opioids produce effects on neurons by acting on receptors located on neuronal cell membranes. Three major types of opioid receptor, μ, δ and κ (mu, delta and kappa), were defined pharmacologically several years ago. Recently, the 3 opioid receptors have been cloned, and their molecular structures described. These receptors belong to the large family of receptors which possess 7 transmembrane-spanning domains of amino acids.

Pharmacological studies have shown that the naturally-occurring opioid peptide, β endorphin, interacts preferentially with μ receptors, the enkephalins with δ receptors and dynorphin with κ receptors. Morphine has considerably higher affinity for μ receptors than for other opioid receptors. The opioid antagonist, naloxone, inhibits all opioid receptors, but has highest affinity for μ receptors. All 3 receptors produce analgesia when an opioid binds to them. However, activation of κ receptors does not produce as much physical dependence as activation of μ receptors.

3. **C - Tramadol**

Opioid activity is due to both low affinity binding of the parent compound and higher affinity binding of the O-demethylated metabolite M1 to mu-opioid receptors.

It is a synthetic analogue of codeine and produces low dependence. In addition to a weak opioid effect, it enhances serotonergic and adrenergic pathways. It is of value in treating severe pain conditions. It is step II on the WHO analgesic ladder.

## 224. THEME: LOCAL ANAESTHETIC AGENTS

OPTIONS

A. Amethocaine
B. Cocaine
C. Bupivacaine
D. Prilocaine
E. Tetracaine

*For each of the descriptions below, select the most appropriate drug from the list of options above. Each option may be used once, more than once, or not at all.*

1. This drug is used in Bier's block.

2. Can be used topically as an alternative to EMLA®.

3. Commonly used for conjunctival anaesthesia.

4. This agent is used prior to nasal intubation or nasal surgery.

## 224. ANSWERS

1. **D - Prilocaine**
It has very low toxicity potential and hence is used in Bier's block.

2. **E - Tetracaine**
Though EMLA® is used most often before cannulation or blood collection in children, tetracaine is an alternative for topical application.

3. **A - Amethocaine**
This is an ester that rapidly diffuses into the conjunctiva.

4. **B - Cocaine**
It is highly toxic. It causes sympathetic stimulation and vasoconstriction. Hence it is used as a paste preparation before nasal intubation or nasal surgery.

## 225. THEME: MODE OF TUMOUR SPREAD

OPTIONS

A. Blood borne metastasis
B. Local invasion
C. Lymphatic spread
D. Transcoelomic metastasis

*For each of the scenarios mentioned below, select the option that most appropriately describes the mode of spread from the list of options above. Each option may be used once, more than once, or not at all.*

1. Renal cell carcinoma

2. Basal cell carcinoma of skin

3. Ovarian carcinoma

4. Papillary carcinoma of thyroid

5. Testicular tumours

## 225. ANSWERS

1. **A - Blood borne metastasis**
The tumour is prone to spread via the renal vein. Cannon ball metastases occur in the lungs. Highly vascular metastasis may pulsate.

2. **B - Local invasion**
They invade local structures and hence are called the 'rodent ulcers'.

3. **D - Transcoelomic metastasis**

4. **C - Lymphatic spread**
Papillary carcinoma of thyroid has a predominant lymphatic spread. In contrast, a follicular carcinoma has a predominantly haematogenous spread.

5. **C - Lymphatic spread**

## 226. THEME: JAUNDICE

OPTIONS

A. Hepatocellular jaundice
B. Post-hepatic jaundice
C. Pre-hepatic jaundice

*For each of the following scenarios, select the most likely type of jaundice from the list of options above. Each option may be used once, more than once, or not at all.*

1. Paracetamol induced jaundice

2. Physiological jaundice

3. Lymph nodes around porta hepatis

4. Primary biliary cirrhosis

5. Wilson's disease

## 226. ANSWERS

1. **A - Hepatocellular jaundice**

Common drugs include paracetamol overdose, antituberculosis drugs, statins, sodium valproate and halothane. They result predominantly from hepatocytes damage.

2. **C - Pre-hepatic jaundice**

Pre-hepatic jaundice is due to excess bilirubin production (haemolysis, decreased liver uptake or decreased conjugation). As unconjugated bilirubin is water insoluble, it does not enter the urine resulting in acholuric hyperbilirubinaemia. Causes include physiological, Gilbert's syndrome and Crigler-Najjar syndrome.

3. **B - Post-hepatic jaundice**

4. **B - Post-hepatic jaundice**

This is due to blockage of the common bile duct. Most causes are hence surgical and include biliary duct calculi, lymph nodes at porta hepatis, cholangiocarcinoma, primary biliary cirrhosis, biliary atresia and choledochal cyst. Drugs include antibiotics like flucloxacillin, co-amoxiclav and fusidic acid, oral contraceptives, anabolic steroids, chlorpromazine and sulfonylureas.

5. **A - Hepatocellular jaundice**

Common causes include viral hepatitis, alcoholic hepatitis, cirrhosis, liver abscess, Wilson's disease and alpha1-antitrypsin deficiency. Medications causing the same have already been mentioned above.

## 227. THEME: ORIGIN OF MEDIASTINAL MASSES

OPTIONS

A. Anterior mediastinum
B. Middle mediastinum
C. Posterior mediastinum
D. Superior mediastinum

*For each of the descriptions below, select the most appropriate location in the mediastinum from the list of options mentioned above. Each option may be used once, more than once, or not at all.*

1. Thymoma
2. Thyroid mass
3. Lymphoma
4. Neural tumours
5. Germ cell tumours

## 227. ANSWERS

1. **A - Anterior mediastinum**
This is the most common mediastinal tumour accounting for 25% of total. They generally occur after childhood. Other anterior mediastinal tumours include lymphoma and germ cell tumours.

2. **D - Superior mediastinum**
Other masses here include the parathyroids and lymphoma.

3. **A - Anterior mediastinum**
This is a common cause of a mediastinal mass lesion, particularly the anterior mediastinum leading to obstruction of the superior vena cava.

4. **C - Posterior mediastinum**
These may derive from the sympathetic nervous system or the peripheral nerves. They are most commonly discovered accidentally on routine chest radiography. Other tumours in this location include the mesenchymal tumours and cystic lesions.

5. **A - Anterior mediastinum**
They account for 13% of all mediastinal masses and cysts and are usually found in the anterior mediastinum. 75% are benign and cystic. Malignancy is suspected if elevated levels of alpha-fetoprotein, human chorionic gonadotrophin and carcinoembryonic antigen are detected.

Lesions involving the middle mediastinum include cystic lesions, lymphoma and mesenchymal tumours.

## 228. THEME: TERMINOLOGY IN TRANSPLANTATION

OPTIONS

A. Allograft
B. Isograft
C. Orthotopic graft
D. Heterotopic graft
E. Xenograft
F. Autograft

*For each of the descriptions below, select the most appropriate answer from the list of options mentioned above. Each option may be used once, more than once, or not at all.*

1. A transplant between identical twins.

2. A transplant placed in its normal anatomical site.

3. A graft performed between different species.

4. A tissue transplanted from one individual to another.

5. A transplant placed in a site different to that where the organ is normally located.

6. A transplant sited from one organ to another in the same individual.

## 228. ANSWERS

1. **B - Isograft**
It is also called the syngeneic graft.

2. **C - Orthotopic graft**
This is also called the syngeneic graft.

3. **E - Xenograft**

4. **A - Allograft**
This is synonymous with the old term homograft.

5. **D - Heterotopic graft**
An example of this is renal transplant which is placed in the iliac fossa usually.

6. **F - Autograft**
Skin grafting is an example of the same.

## 229. THEME: TYPES OF ALLOGRAFT REJECTION

OPTIONS

A. Hyperacute rejection
B. Acute rejection
C. Chronic rejection

*For each of the scenarios mentioned below, select the most appropriate option from the list of options mentioned above. Each option may be used once, more than once, or not at all.*

1. This rejection occurs within the first 6 months.

2. This rejection occurs immediately.

3. This is due to the presence in the recipient of preformed cytotoxic antibodies against HLA class I antigens expressed by the donor.

4. This rejection is mediated predominantly by T-lymphocytes.

5. This rejection is usually due to antibody and cell mediated effector mechanisms.

6. Pre-sensitisation is responsible for this.

## 229. ANSWERS

1. **B - Acute rejection**

2. **A - Hyperacute rejection**

3. **A - Hyperacute rejection**

These may arise from blood transfusion, a failed transplant or previous pregnancy. This type of rejection also occurs if an ABO blood group incompatible organ graft is performed.

4. **B - Acute rejection**

5. **C - Chronic rejection**

This occurs after 6 months. All types of transplant are susceptible to chronic rejection and it is the major cause of allograft failure. Chronic rejection causes functional deterioration in the graft resulting after months or years in graft failure.

6. **A - Hyperacute rejection**

## 230. THEME: SURGICAL MICROBIOLOGY

OPTIONS

A. Escherichia coli
B. Clostridium difficile
C. Borrelia vincentii
D. Streptococcus pneumoniae
E. Neisseria meningitides

*For each of the conditions enlisted below, select the most appropriate causative organism from the list of options mentioned above. Each option may be used once, more than once, or not at all.*

1. Vincent's angina

2. Ludwig's angina

## 230. ANSWERS

1. **C - Borrelia vincentii**
Vincent's angina is a pharyngeal infection with ulcerative gingivitis.

2. **D - Streptococcus pneumoniae**
Ludwig's angina is brawny swelling of the submandibular region combined with inflammatory oedema of the mouth. The infection encompasses both sides of the mylohyoid muscle causing oedema and inflammation such that the tongue may be displaced upwards and backwards giving rise to dysphagia. This can subsequently lead to obstruction of the airways.

## 231. THEME: RENAL IMAGING

OPTIONS

A. DMSA scan
B. DTPA scan
C. IVU
D. CT urogram
E. Ultrasound
F. X-ray KUB

*For each of the scenarios described below, select the most appropriate option from the list of options mentioned above. Each option may be used once, more than once, or not at all.*

1. A 35-year-old immigrant presents with repeated urinary tract infections. He is investigated further and this reveals a large stag horn calculus on the right side. The right kidney fails to excrete contrast on IVU. The kidney in question has a thin parenchyma with loss of cortico-medullary differentiation.

2. A 19-year-old girl presents with history that classically suggest a Dietl's crisis on the right. An IVU confirms a right PUJ (pelvi-ureteric junction) narrowing.

## 231. ANSWERS

1. **A - DMSA scan**

The split function of the kidneys needs to be found out. A DMSA scan is thus indicated.

2. **B - DTPA scan**

MAG-3 isotope is most commonly used.

Dietl's crisis is the presence of a swelling in the loin after an attack of acute renal pain. Some hours later, the pain and swelling subside, following the passage of large volume of urine. An important clue may be the relation to alcohol intake in a teenager.

## 232. THEME: CHEST TRAUMA

OPTIONS

A. Cardiac tamponade
B. Flail chest
C. Open pneumothorax
D. Tension pneumothorax
E. Haemothorax

*For each presentation listed below, select the most likely diagnosis from the options above. Each option may be used once, more than once, or not at all.*

1. A 24-year-old male is seen in A&E following a stab wound to his chest. Examination reveals a small wound to his left chest just beneath his nipple. He looks clinically well with good bilateral air entry. He deteriorates while in the ward and has tachycardia, hypotension and dyspnoea. He has a weak pulse and his JVP is raised.

2. A 24-year-old male is seen in A&E following a stab wound to his chest. Examination reveals a small wound to his left chest laterally. Examination reveals decreased breath sounds on the left with hyperresonant lung fields. His JVP is raised and his trachea is deviated to the right.

3. A 24-year-old male is seen in A&E following a stab wound to his chest. Examination reveals a small wound to his left chest. Examination reveals decreased breath sounds on the left with dullness on percussion in the left lower lung fields. His JVP is normal with a centrally situated trachea.

## 232. ANSWERS

### 1. A - Cardiac tamponade

Never underestimate a wound in the chest. This patient has most likely sustained a pericardial injury. In addition to trauma as in this case, other causes of pericardial tamponade include pericarditis, lung/breast cancer, myocardial infarction, bacterial infections and rarely radiation and myxoedema. Please remember the signs: falling BP, rising JVP, and muffled heart sounds- constituting the Beck's triad; JVP ↑ on inspiration (Kussmaul's sign); pulsus paradoxus (pulse fades on inspiration). Since the air entry is bilaterally equal, a pneumothorax can be excluded.

### 2. D - Tension pneumothorax

Features clearly point to this cause. Urgent needle decompression is mandatory. A chest X-ray obtained in a patient with tension pneumothorax actually demonstrates an error in judgement.

### 3. E - Haemothorax

Presence of a penetrating chest wound with decreased air entry on the left suggest either a haemo or a pneumothorax. However, the dullness on percussion clinches the diagnosis in favour of haemothorax.

## 233. THEME: TRAUMA IN UROLOGY

OPTIONS

A. Bladder
B. Kidney
C. Membranous urethra
D. Bulbar urethra
E. Testis
F. Prostate

*The following patients have all presented with urological trauma. Please select the most appropriate organ of injury from the list of options above. Each option may be used once, more than once or not at all.*

1. A 45-year-old gymnast sustains a blow to his perineum as a result of a fall astride the beam while at practice. He is in a lot of pain and has not passed urine since the accident a few hours ago. Examination reveals perineal haematoma and bleeding from the external meatus.

2. A 45-year-old male is involved in a road traffic accident. He sustains severe pelvic trauma with significant displacement of the pubic bones. Digital examination confirms a high riding prostate.

## 233. ANSWERS

1. **D - Bulbar urethra**

Rupture of the bulbar urethra is the most common urethral injury. The triad of signs of a ruptured bulbar urethra is retention of urine, perineal haematoma and bleeding from the external urinary meatus. Treat with analgesics for pain and a percutaneous suprapubic catheter insertion.

2. **C - Membranous urethra**

The most common causes of pelvic fracture are road traffic accidents, severe crush injuries and falls. The urethral injury can be managed in the short term by a suprapubic catheter. A major urethral injury should be suspected if there is significant displacement of the pubic bones. If the prostate is displaced, it may be impossible to reach or appear to be high on rectal examination.

## 234. THEME: MAJOR INJURY

OPTIONS

A. Major pelvic fracture
B. Severe diffuse axonal injury
C. Skull base fracture
D. Extradural haematoma
E. Secretions in mouth

*For the scenarios mentioned below, please select the most appropriate pathology from the list of options above. Each option may be used once, more than once or not at all.*

1. Hypercarbia

2. Inadequate cerebral perfusion

3. CSF rhinorrhoea and anosmia

4. Deep coma immediately after accident

## 234. ANSWERS

1. **E - Secretions in mouth**

This indicates upper airway obstruction. A blocked airway or inadequate ventilation is a potent cause of hypercarbia and hypoxia. This is an important cause of secondary brain damage. Hypercarbia causes brain oedema and a rise in intracranial pressure by causing cerebral vasodilatation.

2. **A - Major pelvic fracture**

Never underestimate the amount of blood loss in a major pelvic fracture. It is in the range of 2–3 liters. If this volume is not promptly replaced, the resulting cardiovascular shock can lead to inadequate cerebral perfusion, another significant cause of secondary brain damage.

3. **C - Skull base fracture**

They are relatively frequent fractures and are usually diagnosed on clinical grounds. Anterior fossa fractures present with subconjunctival haematomas, anosmia, epistaxis and CSF rhinorrhoea. Raccoon eyes indicate subgaleal haemorrhage and not necessarily base of skull fractures. Middle fossa fractures present with CSF otorrhoea or rhinorrhoea via the eustachian tube, haemotympanum, ossicular disruption, battle sign or 7/8 cranial nerve palsies.

4. **B - Severe diffuse axonal injury**

This occurs as a result of mechanical shearing following deceleration, causing disruption and tearing of axons, especially at the grey/white matter interface. Severity can vary from mild confusion to coma and even death.

## 235. THEME: BRAIN AND SPINAL TUMOURS

OPTIONS

A. Thoracic neurofibroma
B. Fronto-parietal meningioma
C. Frontal lobe tumour
D. Metastatic carcinoma
E. Pituitary tumour

*For each of the descriptions below, select the most appropriate diagnosis from the list of options above. Each option may be used once, more than once, or not at all.*

1. Progressive loss of temporal visual fields

2. Multiple lesions in the brain on CT scan

3. Focal motor seizures worsening over several months

4. Change of personality with impaired cognition

5. Increasingly stiff legs for the last few months

## 235. ANSWERS

1. **E - Pituitary tumour**

Pituitary tumours can compress the optic chiasm and cause progressive damage to the visual fields. Initially the central nerve fibres are damaged resulting in bitemporal hemianopia.

2. **D - Metastatic carcinoma**

3. **B - Fronto-parietal-meningioma**

These are slow growing and typically produce symptoms over a period of months or years.

4. **C - Frontal lobe tumour**

This is again a classical presentation.

5. **A - Thoracic neurofibroma**

A spinal tumour usually causes a progressive myelopathy below the spinal segmental level of origin. Features of an upper motor neurone lesion will be seen. Initially the tone and reflexes will be increased in the lower limbs and this will be expressed by the patient as an increasing stiffness in the legs.

## 236. THEME: CHEST AND THORACIC WALL INJURIES

OPTIONS

A. Diaphragmatic rupture
B. Flail chest
C. Myocardial contusion
D. Cardiac tamponade
E. Tension pneumothorax
F. Oesophageal perforation

*For each of the scenarios mentioned below, select the most appropriate diagnosis from the list of options above. Each option may be used once, more than once, or not at all.*

1. A 40-year-old male is involved in a RTA and is subsequently rushed into resus in A&E. Examination reveals bowel sounds in the left hemithorax.

2. A 40-year-old chronic alcoholic presents with severe chest pain following an episode of vomiting. Chest X-ray reveals gas in the mediastinum.

## 236. ANSWERS

1. **A - Diaphragmatic rupture**

Diaphragmatic rupture occurs in high speed blunt abdominal trauma against a closed glottis. Diaphragmatic rupture is more common on the left (the location of the liver on the right acts as a protective mechanism). An X-ray may reveal bowel gas in the lung fields as the colon and the stomach may herniate into the thorax. Quite a few of these injuries tend to be missed at initial presentation. Delayed presentation with diaphragmatic rupture is the subject of many a case report.

2. **F - Oesophageal perforation**

This patient is likely to have Boerhaave's syndrome. It is an important cause of the so called 'spontaneous' perforation. Always suspect perforation if pain follows vomiting. It is usually due to severe barotraumas when a person vomits against a closed glottis. The oesophagus bursts at its weakest point in the lower third. It is the most serious type of perforation because of the volume of infected material that is released under pressure. The finding on the X-ray is an important clue.

## 237. THEME: HEAD INJURY

OPTIONS

A. Extradural haematoma
B. Subdural haematoma
C. Basal skull fracture
D. Subgaleal haematoma
E. Depressed skull fracture
F. Compound skull fracture
G. Subarachnoid haemorrhage

*For each of the descriptions below, select the most appropriate option from the list of options above. Each option may be used once, more than once, or not at all.*

1. A 50-year-old male presents to A&E 4 days after a fall at home. He is a businessman by occupation and fell off a high step while doing a DIY (do it yourself) at home. He gives a history of hitting his head against the edge of the table. There is no history of loss of consciousness or bleeding. Examination reveals a left frontal haematoma with the presence of bilateral raccoon eyes.

2. A 74-year-old chronic alcoholic is brought to the emergency department with a right sided hemiparesis. He has had a few falls in recent days. His neighbours have noted fluctuating level of consciousness in recent days.

3. A 24-year-old male is brought in following a high speed RTA. ATLS has been instituted. He had a momentary loss of consciousness after the accident. His GC scale when brought into hospital is 15/15. However, while in A&E, he suddenly becomes confused and later unconscious. His GC scale drops to 8/15. His right pupil is dilated.

4. A 25-year-old male is brought in following a high speed RTA. ATLS has been instituted. His GC scale is 9/15 and a CT scan is planned on him. Examination reveals thin fluid mixed with blood coming out of the nostrils. The fluid does not clot.

## 237. ANSWERS

1. **D - Subgaleal haematoma**

The presence of left frontal haematoma with periorbital ecchymoses (raccoon eyes) is suggestive of subgaleal bleeding from frontal trauma. They gradually resolve over a couple of weeks.

2. **B - Subdural haematoma**

A history of alcoholism should ring a bell (as far as answering the question in the examination is concerned). Alcoholics, epileptics and patients on anticoagulants are particularly susceptible. Chronic subdural haematomas most commonly occur in infants and adults over 60 years of age. They present with progressive neurological deficit more than 2 weeks after the trauma.

3. **A - Extradural haematoma**

The history is classical. Fluctuating level of consciousness with the presence of a lucid interval should raise suspicion. An acute extradural haematoma is usually associated with trauma and seen in young adults. They occur usually as a result of squamous temporal bone fractures with laceration of the middle meningeal artery. Patients do well if delay to surgery is minimized.

4. **C - Basal skull fracture**

They are relatively frequent fractures and are usually diagnosed on clinical grounds. Anterior fossa fractures present with subconjunctival haematomas, anosmia, epistaxis and CSF rhinorrhoea. Raccoon eyes indicate subgaleal haemorrhage and not necessarily base of skull fractures. Middle fossa fractures present with CSF otorrhoea or rhinorrhoea via the eustachian tube, haemotympanum, ossicular disruption, battle sign or 7/8 cranial nerve palsies. Blood mixed CSF otorrhoea/rhinorrhoea classically does not clot.

## 238. THEME: LOWER ABDOMINAL PAIN

OPTIONS

A. Appendicitis
B. Perforated duodenal ulcer
C. Right ureteric colic
D. Mittelschmerz
E. Ectopic pregnancy
F. Urinary tract infection

*For each of the patients described below, select the most likely diagnosis from the list of options above. Each option may be used once, more than once, or not at all.*

1. A 20-year-old lady comes in with a 3-day history of lower abdominal pain. She is diffusely mildly tender in the hypogastrium and both iliac fossae. Urine dipstick shows ++ proteins, ++ blood. Pregnancy test is negative.

2. A 50-year-old lady presents with an 8-hour history of severe abdominal pain. Initially per umbilical but has then shifted to the right iliac fossa. Rovsing's sign is positive and she has rebound tenderness in the right iliac fossa.

3. A 70-years-old lady presents with a 6-hour history of severe abdominal pain. She has a past medical history of rheumatoid arthritis and is taking regular NSAIDs for the same. On examination, she is diffusely tender all over her abdomen.

4. A 30-years-old lady presents with sudden onset of right sided colicky loin to groin pain. On examination she is mildly tender in the right iliac fossa. There is no rebound tenderness. Pregnancy test is negative and urine dipstick is NAD.

5. A 25-years-old lady presents with a 8-hour history of severe right iliac fossa pain. Her last menstrual period is 2 weeks back. On examination, she is tender in the right iliac fossa. On questioning, she says that she feels hungry. Pregnancy test is negative.

## 238. ANSWERS

1. **F - Urinary tract infections.** UTIs are common in young females and often present as a diagnostic conundrum with appendicitis. However, the fact that there is diffuse tenderness all over lower abdomen makes a diagnosis of appendicitis less likely.

Clues: Urine dipstick is + for proteins and blood. Diffuse lower abdominal tenderness.

2. **A - Appendicitis.** Shifting pain from per umbilical to right iliac fossa region. Rebound tenderness and Rovsing's sign point towards the diagnosis.

Clues: Shifting pain, Rovsing's sign, rebound tenderness.

3. **B - Perforated duodenal ulcer.** As the fluid tracks down the right paracolic gutter, perforated DU can sometimes present with right lower abdominal pain. An erect chest X-ray will be diagnostic in this case.

Clues: Patient on long term NSAIDs, diffuse abdominal tenderness

4. **C - Right ureteric colic.** Right loin to groin pain with absence of rebound tenderness makes it more likely to be a ureteric colic.

Clues: Loin to groin pain, rebound tenderness

5. **D - Mittelschmerz.** This is lower abdominal pain caused by midcycle rupture of a follicular cyst with bleeding. Differentiation from appendicitis can sometimes be very difficult. However, systemic upset is rare. A diagnostic laparoscopy may be required sometimes.

Clues: Midcycle, young patient, patient feels hungry.

## 239. THEME: DIAGNOSIS OF ALTERED BOWEL HABIT

OPTIONS

A. Colorectal carcinoma
B. Inflammatory bowel disease
C. Sigmoid volvulus
D. Overflow diarrhoea
E. Irritable bowel syndrome
F. Amoebic dysentery
G. Diverticular abscess
H. Radiation colitis
I. Ischaemic colitis
J. Infective colitis
K. Collagenous colitis

*For each of the patients described below, select the most likely diagnosis from the list of options above. Each option may be used once, more than once, or not at all.*

1. An 80-year-old male with a long standing history of constipation presents with a history of constipation for a week followed by diarrhoea for a day's duration. Digital examination of rectum reveals hard impacted stools.

2. A 26-year-old young business executive presents to you with alternating diarrhoea and constipation for 3 months duration. She tells you that she has been passing small hard stools. She denies anorexia or weight loss.

3. A 61-year-old business executive presents to you with a 3-month history of altered bowel habit. He has had anorexia and admits to some weight loss over this period.

4. A 62-year-old business executive presents with tenesmus and early morning diarrhoea.

5. A 78-year-old lady with senile dementia is referred to you by the nursing home with high temperature and diarrhoea. She is tender in the left iliac fossa.

## 239. ANSWERS

1. **D - Overflow diarrhoea**

This is a classical presentation of faecal impaction with overflow diarrhoea. It is also important to rule out faecal impaction/constipation as a cause of retention of urine.

2. **E - Irritable bowel syndrome**

Age of the patient, stressful lifestyle and absence of anorexia and weight loss fetch the diagnosis.

3. **A - Colorectal carcinoma**

Altered bowel habits, anorexia and weight loss is a cancer unless proven otherwise. Expect at least one theme on this in the exam.

4. **A - Colorectal carcinoma**

Bleeding per rectum, tenesmus and early morning diarrhoea are classical features of rectal cancer.

5. **G - Diverticular abscess**

This is commoner in patients over 60 years of age. Complications of diverticulosis include diverticulitis, abscess, perforation, haemorrhage, strictures, intestinal obstruction and fistula formation. Sigmoid colon is involved in 90%. The association of this along with gallstones and hiatus hernia constitutes the Saint's triad. Surgery for perforated diverticulitis involves a Hartmann's procedure and is another favourite with the MRCS examiners (expect one question on it).

## 240. THEME: DIAGNOSIS OF ALTERED BOWEL HABIT

OPTIONS

A. Colorectal carcinoma
B. Ulcerative colitis
C. Sigmoid volvulus
D. Overflow diarrhoea
E. Irritable bowel syndrome
F. Amoebic dysentery
G. Diverticular abscess
H. Radiation colitis
I. Ischaemic colitis
J. Infective colitis
K. Collagenous colitis
L. Crohn's disease

*For each of the patients described below, select the most likely diagnosis from the list of options above. Each option may be used once, more than once, or not at all.*

1. A 26-year-old male presents with 2-month history of passing bloody diarrhoea mixed with mucus about 8 times per day with crampy lower abdominal pain. On examination he is pale and abdominal examination reveals lower abdominal tenderness. Sigmoidoscopy demonstrates active proctitis.

2. A 26-year-old is referred to your outpatient clinic by the GP with a 2-month history of diarrhoea and lower abdominal pain. Colonoscopy reveals patchy active inflammation involving predominantly the right sided colon.

3. A 62-year-old man is seen in A&E with a history of sudden onset abdominal pain, vomiting and bleeding per rectum. On examination, he is tender with guarding in the left iliac fossa. He is pyrexial (38.3°C), tachycardic (122/min) with an irregular pulse and hypotensive (blood pressure 78/40 mm Hg).

4. A 65-year-old renal transplant patient is referred to you with acute onset severe bloody diarrhoea. He looks clinically unwell.

5. A 55-year-old African immigrant known to have AIDS presents with acute onset severe bloody diarrhoea. He looks clinically unwell.

## 240. ANSWERS

1. **B - Ulcerative colitis**

The presence of classical features on history and investigation clinches the diagnosis in this case.

2. **L - Crohn's disease**

Though the information on the question is limited, the presence of patchy active inflammation should make one suspicious for Crohn's. Rectal sparing with skip lesions is classical.

3. **I - Ischaemic colitis**

This is again a classical presentation. The triad of acute abdominal pain, bleeding per rectum and shock in an elderly patient should clinch the diagnosis. The presence of an irregular pulse (implying an atrial fibrillation) is an important clue in this question. Urgent resuscitation followed by early laparotomy is indicated.

4. **J - Infective colitis**

5. **J - Infective colitis**

Infective colitis caused by cytomegalovirus infection in immunocompromised patients is well recognized. This diagnosis should always be considered first in patients on immunosuppression. Other responsible organisms include herpes virus and Cryptosporidium. Infections can result in severe bloody colitis, toxic megacolon or colonic perforation, which may be life threatening.

## 241. THEME: INVESTIGATIONS OF THE UPPER GI TRACT

OPTIONS

A. Abdominal ultrasound
B. CT scan of abdomen
C. MRI abdomen
D. Chest X-ray
E. Videofluoroscopic study
F. Barium meal
G. Endoscopic ultrasound (EU)
H. Endoscopy
I. ERCP
J. Laparoscopy
K. MRCP

*For each of the patients described below, select the most appropriate investigation from the list of options above. Each option may be used once, more than once, or not at all.*

1. A 70-year-old male presents with painless jaundice. He has a palpable gallbladder.

2. A 65-year-old male is referred to your consultants outpatient clinic with dysphagia. Subsequent endoscopy confirms a biopsy proven adenocarcinoma of the oesophagus. Your consultant plans to operate on him further. He asks you to arrange an investigation to stage the local invasion of the tumour and lymphadenopathy.

3. A 65-year-old man presents with dysphagia and an intermittent swelling in his neck. He has recently been treated by his GP for recurrent chest infections. He has also noticed gurgling sounds from the neck on swallowing.

4. A patient is referred to your Upper GI cancer unit from a peripheral district hospital with a diagnosis of CT and biopsy proven gastric adenocarcinoma. The mass appears to be locally advanced and your consultant wants to stage this further.

## 241. ANSWERS

1. **B - CT Scan of abdomen**

The history is suggestive of carcinoma of the head of the pancreas. The preferred test now for a tumour in the head of the pancreas is a contrast-enhanced spiral CT scan specific to the pancreas.

2. **G - Endoscopic ultrasound (EU)**

Accurate staging is a prerequisite in any cancer surgery. Ultrasonography of the liver and computerized tomography scanning of the chest and abdomen is mandatory before resection. However, a CT (and even a MRI) is inaccurate for staging the primary lesion and for staging lymph nodes. Endoscopic ultrasound (EU) is the best method for preoperative staging of oesophageal cancer. Bronchoscopy should be done in lesions of the upper or middle thirds where there is potential for tracheobronchial invasion. EU has an important role in staging rectal cancers as well.

3. **E - Videofluoroscopic study**

A thin emulsion of barium is given to the patient as part of this study. Alternatively, a barium swallow can be performed. In addition to barium outlining the pharyngeal pouch and upper oesophagus, the study gives good information about the pharyngeal contraction waves and the performance of the upper oesophageal sphincter. A chest X-ray is important to exclude aspiration pneumonitis.

4. **J - Laparoscopy**

Accurate estimation of local invasion and peritoneal metastasis can be achieved with laparoscopy thus avoiding a potentially negative laparotomy.

## 242. THEME: PATTERNS OF LYMPHATIC DRAINAGE

OPTIONS

A. Internal iliac lymph nodes
B. Superficial inguinal lymph nodes
C. Deep inguinal lymph nodes
D. Superficial epigastric
E. Para-aortic nodes
F. Inferior mesenteric lymph nodes

*For each of the scenario enlisted below, select the first portal of lymph node drainage from the list of options above. Each option may be used once, more than once, or not at all.*

1. Testicular carcinoma

2. Distal anal carcinoma

3. Scrotal skin

4. Cervical cancer

## 242. ANSWERS

1. **E - Para-aortic nodes**

2. **B - Superficial inguinal lymph nodes**

3. **B - Superficial inguinal lymph nodes**

4. **A - Internal iliac lymph nodes**

The proximal anal canal drains into the internal iliac nodes. Testicular cancer drains into the para-aortic nodes at the level of L2. Cervical cancer drains into internal and external iliac nodes.

## 243. THEME: MANAGEMENT OF THROMBOEMBOLISM

OPTIONS

A. Aspirin
B. Warfarin
C. Clopidogrel
D. Low molecular weight heparin
E. Intravenous heparin
F. Thrombolysis
G. Caval filter
H. Catheter embolectomy

*For each of the patients described below, select the most appropriate management option from the list of options above. Each option may be used once, more than once, or not at all.*

1. A 40-year-old lady undergoes hysterectomy. 4 days after surgery she develops marked oedema on the left side which is confirmed as an above knee deep vein thrombosis. A few days later she develops tachycardia, tachypnoea and hypotension.

2. A 50-year-old lady with cervical cancer and pelvic spread has had repeated pulmonary embolisms despite being on warfarin.

3. A 75-year-old lady undergoes a left total knee replacement. Post operatively she develops swelling and tenderness in her left calf. An ultrasound Doppler scan confirms the presence of DVT.

4. A 75-year-old lady with known protein C deficiency presents with an acutely swollen, cyanosed, painful right lower limb. A venous duplex confirms an extensive above knee DVT. Though she is started on heparin therapy, her symptoms fail to resolve.

## 243. ANSWERS

**1. H - Catheter embolectomy**

Pulmonary embolism causing a severe drop in cardiac output requires either an embolectomy or pulmonary artery thrombolysis. However thrombolysis is contraindicated in the postoperative period. Catheter embolectomy is performed on cardiac bypass.

**2. G - Caval filter**

Indications for caval filters include failure or complications from anti-coagulation, PE in the presence of severe right heart failure and pulmonary hypertension, extensive embolic occlusion of pulmonary circulation and during thrombolysis of a PE.

**3. B - Warfarin**

The question requests the most appropriate (and not the initial) management. Though a low molecular weight heparin is started initially, warfarin is the most appropriate management in this patient.

**4. F - Thrombolysis**

This woman has features to suggest phlegmasia caerula dolens (extension of thrombus to the venular and capillary level +/- acute arterial ischaemia). It occurs most frequently in hypercoagulable states. Failure to improve after a 24-hour trial with limb elevation and intravenous heparin necessitates thrombectomy or thrombolysis.

## 244. THEME: INVESTIGATION OF DIARRHOEA

OPTIONS

A. Sigmoidoscopy
B. Stool culture
C. Colonoscopy
D. C. difficile toxin titre
E. Thyroid function tests
F. HIV test
G. Serum gastrin estimation
H. Serum $B_{12}$ estimation
I. Barium enema
J. OGD

*For each of the patients described below, select the most appropriate investigation from the list of options above. Each option may be used once, more than once, or not at all.*

1. A 40-year-old lady presents with a history of heat intolerance, weight loss despite an increased appetite, tachycardia, tremors and diarrhoea.

2. A 40-year-old male has had a surgery on the neck in the past. He presents with abdominal pain and diarrhoea. Examination reveals numerous duodenal and gastric ulcers.

3. A 65-year-old has been on broad spectrum antibiotics for cellulitis involving his lower limb for 5 days. He starts with greenish foul smelling watery diarrhoea.

4. A 32-year-old intravenous drug abuser who lives off the street presents with weakness, lethargy, anorexia, weight loss and diarrhoea. He has had chronic diarrhoea for the past 2 months. On examination he looks pale and cachectic.

## 244. ANSWERS

1. **E - Thyroid function tests**

History is suggestive of thyrotoxicosis. Hypothyroidism in contrast causes constipation.

2. **G - Serum gastrin estimation**

This patient most likely has MEN 1. The surgery on the neck may indicate a surgery on the parathyroids. The suspicion is of Zollinger-Ellison syndrome and hence serum gastrin estimation should help clinch the diagnosis.

3. **D - C. difficile toxin titre**

4. **F - HIV test**

Chronic diarrhoea is defined as diarrhoea lasting more than 28 days. All the features in the patient's history strongly point to immunodeficiency/HIV and hence this is the most appropriate investigation here.

## 245. THEME: ABDOMINAL CONDITIONS

OPTIONS

A. Pernicious anaemia
B. Autoimmune hepatitis
C. Primary sclerosing cholangitis
D. Primary biliary cirrhosis
E. Ascending cholangitis
F. Acute cholecystitis
G. Hepatocellular failure
H. Hepatitis A

*For each of the scenarios described below, select the most appropriate diagnosis from the list of options above. Each option may be used once, more than once, or not at all.*

1. A 35-year-old lady presents with fever, malaise, amenorrhoea, anorexia and weight loss. She has been passing dark urine and pale stools. Examination suggests hepatomegaly. Liver function tests show a raised AST. Tests are positive for antismooth muscle antibodies (SMA).

2. A 45-year-old lady presents with recent onset jaundice. She has had lethargy and pruritus for many months which she has self treated with over-the-counter 'energy' pills and 'antihistamines'. Examination reveals jaundice, hepatomegaly and splenomegaly. Tests for antimitochondrial antibody (AMA) are positive.

3. A 50-year-old lady presents with tiredness, weakness, dyspnoea on mild exertion, a sore red tongue and diarrhoea. Test for anti intrinsic factor antibodies is positive.

4. A 50-year-old obese lady presents with fever, intermittent, colicky right upper quadrant abdominal pain and jaundice. Examination elicits tenderness in the epigastrium and right hypochondrium.

## 245. ANSWERS

1. **B - Autoimmune hepatitis**

This is an inflammatory liver disease of uncertain aetiology characterized by suppressor T- cell defects and the production of autoantibodies directed against hepatocytes surface antigens. Female sex, features of liver cell failure, raised AST, and presence of antibodies like SMA, ANA (anti nuclear antibodies), antiliver/kidney microsomal type 1 (LKM1) are important clues.

2. **D - Primary biliary cirrhosis**

Damage to the interlobular bile ducts by chronic granulomatous inflammation causes progressive cholestasis, cirrhosis and portal hypertension. 90% of patients are women with the peak age being between 40–60 years. The most important clue is the presence of the antimitochondrial antibody which is seen in 98% of patients. Other features on the blood tests include increased alkaline phosphatase with gamma GT with only mildly elevated AST/ALT.

3. **A - Pernicious anaemia**

Common features have been mentioned in the question. Other features include a low haemoglobin on the blood tests, MCV >110 fL, hyper segmented polymorphs, low serum $B_{12}$ and megaloblasts in the marrow. Important associations include thyroid disease, vitiligo, Addison's disease and carcinoma of stomach.

4. **E - Ascending cholangitis**

The three features mentioned comprise the Charcot's triad.

## 246. THEME: DIARRHOEA

OPTIONS

A. Irritable bowel disease
B. Infective diarrhoea
C. MRSA diarrhoea
D. Pseudomembranous colitis
E. Overflow diarrhoea
F. Amoebic dysentery
G. Gastroenteritis
H. Post vagotomy
I. Colorectal cancer

*For each of the scenarios described below, select the most appropriate diagnosis from the options listed above. Each option may be used once, more than once or not at all.*

1. A 70-year-old lady develops offensive smelling, greenish coloured loose stools following 5 days of treatment with a second generation cephalosporin.

2. A 70-year-old lady is admitted in hospital for a left total knee replacement. She has been treated with generous doses of codeine for postoperative knee pain to ensure early mobilization. She remains constipated for a week after surgery and then develops diarrhoea. Digital examination however reveals hard impacted stools.

3. A 75-year-old man presents to the surgical outpatients with a 2-month history of constipation. He has recently had irregular bowel habits and has experienced intermittent episodes of diarrhoea. He does not use any antibiotics and has no family history of colorectal cancer.

## 246. ANSWERS

**1. D - Pseudomembranous colitis**
Treatment is needed with metronidazole. In metronidazole-allergic patients, vancomycin is indicated.

**2. E - Overflow diarrhoea**
Old age, major surgery, impaired mobility and codeine can all add to cause constipation. This is classically spurious diarrhoea. If conservative measures fail, manual evacuation of stools under anesthesia may be needed.

**3. I - Colorectal cancer**
Past history or no past history, colorectal carcinoma should always be excluded with those symptoms. Many patients with colorectal carcinoma present with altered bowel habits and report loose stools or diarrhoea. This represents 'overflow' of proximal bowel content because of narrowing of the lumen in the affected segment of bowel.

## 247. THEME: COMPLICATIONS OF GALLSTONE DISEASE

OPTIONS

A. Acute cholecystitis
B. Acute pancreatitis
C. Ascending cholangitis
D. Sclerosing cholangitis
E. Biliary colic
F. Empyema of gallbladder
G. Mucocele of gallbladder
H. Gallbladder perforation
I. Gallstone ileus

*For each of the scenarios described below, select the most appropriate diagnosis from the options listed above. Each option may be used once, more than once or not at all.*

1. A 75-year-old lady presents with severe colicky central abdominal pain and vomiting. Examination reveals right upper quadrant tenderness and abdominal distention. Bowel sounds are hyper peristaltic and tinkling in nature. Supine abdominal film confirms the presence of multiple central fluid levels and an air-fluid level in the biliary tree.

2. A 48-year-old obese lady presents with a 4-day history of severe upper abdominal pain radiating to the back, and vomiting. Examination reveals marked tachycardia and generalized upper abdominal tenderness.

## 247. ANSWERS

### 1. I - Gallstone ileus

Clinical picture suggests small bowel obstruction. It occurs in the elderly and is due to erosion of a large gallstone through the gallbladder into the duodenum (choledochoduodenal fistula). Classically, there is impaction about 60 cm proximal to the ileocaecal valve. The stone may not always be visible (remember that 90% of gallstones are radiolucent). Presence of air or an air-fluid level in the biliary tree with intestinal obstruction clinches the diagnosis.

### 2. B - Acute pancreatitis

The history is classical of acute pancreatitis. Biliary calculi are the most important cause of pancreatitis in the western world.

## 248. THEME: PRESENTATIONS OF LYMPHOEDEMA

OPTIONS

A. Lymphoedema tarda
B. Lymphoedema praecox
C. Lymphoedema artefacta
D. Milroy's disease
E. Filariasis
F. Arteriovenous malformation
G. Secondary lymphoedema

*For each of the scenarios described below, select the most appropriate diagnosis from the options listed above. Each option may be used once, more than once or not at all.*

1. A 1-year-old boy is brought by anxious parents with bilateral lower limb swelling involving the whole leg which has been steadily increasing in size from the age of 2 months.

2. A 14-year-old girl presents with a swelling involving her left leg up to knee which has been present since menarche. Lymphangiography shows hypoplasia of the left lower limb lymphatics.

3. A 40-year-old obese lady presents with a swelling involving her left leg. There is no family history of lymphoedema.

4. A 50-year-old known to have rheumatoid arthritis presents with a progressively increasing swelling involving the entire limb.

## 248. ANSWERS

1. **D - Milroy's disease**

Congenital lymphoedema is more common in males, more likely to be bilateral and usually presents within a year of birth. Milroy's disease is the familial form that is present at birth or is noticed shortly afterwards. Congenital lymphoedema is associated with Pierre-Robin syndrome.

2. **B - Lymphoedema praecox**

This classically occurs before the age of 35 years, but peaks in incidence shortly after menarche. It usually is unilateral and extends only to the knee. Familial form is referred to as Meige's syndrome (different from the ovarian Meigs syndrome referred to in one theme).

3. **A - Lymphoedema tarda**

By definition, it happens after the age of 35 years. It is often associated with obesity. Lymphoedema presenting for the first time in later life should prompt a thorough search for underlying malignancy, particularly of the pelvic organs, prostate and external genitalia.

4. **G - Secondary lymphoedema**

Rheumatoid arthritis is a relatively rare but well documented cause of lymphoedema. It is due to chronic inflammation and lymph node fibrosis. It is important to remember that secondary lymphoedema is the commonest form of lymphoedema. The commonest cause worldwide is filariasis and should be suspected if the question mentions migrants/visitors from tropical countries, India and South America. In the developed countries malignancy is the commonest cause.

## 249. THEME: INVOLVEMENT OF NERVES

OPTIONS

A. Hypoglossal nerve
B. Trigeminal nerve
C. Facial nerve
D. Mandibular branch of the facial nerve
E. Great auricular nerve
F. Zygomatic branch of the facial nerve
G. Lingual nerve

*For each of the scenarios described below, select the most appropriate involvement from the options listed above. Each option may be used once, more than once or not at all.*

1. Chvostek's sign

2. Anaesthesia of the ear lobe after parotid surgery

3. Branch of the facial nerve at risk in submandibular gland surgery

## 249. ANSWERS

1. **C - Facial nerve**

Tapping over the branches of the facial nerve at the angle of the jaw will produce twitching at the corner of the mouth, the ala of the nose and the eyelids. This is a sign to demonstrate latent tetani.

2. **E - Great auricular nerve**

This can be troublesome especially in females who find it difficult to wear earrings. Recovery can take up to 18 months.

3. **D - Mandibular branch of the facial nerve**

Three cranial nerves are at risk during removal of the submandibular salivary gland—the mandibular branch of the facial nerve, the lingual nerve (a branch of the third division of the trigeminal nerve) and the hypoglossal nerve.

## 250. THEME: HAND

OPTIONS

A. Ganglion
B. Boutonniere's lesion
C. Heberden's node
D. Osler's node
E. Dermoid cyst
F. Ganglioneuroma
G. Bouchard's nodes
H. Swan neck deformity

*For each of the scenarios described below, select the most appropriate diagnosis from the options listed above. Each option may be used once, more than once or not at all.*

1. A 70-year-old male is seen in the pre-assessment clinic for bilateral total knee replacement. He has tri-compartmental osteoarthritis involving both knees. He complains of pain in his fingers. On examination you note nodes around the distal interphalangeal joint of both the right middle and ring fingers.

2. A 70-year-old male is seen in the pre-assessment clinic for bilateral total knee replacement. He has tri-compartmental osteoarthritis involving both knees. He has also had bilateral hip replacement for osteoarthritis. On examination you note nodes around the proximal interphalangeal joint of his right index finger.

3. A middle age lady with known rheumatoid arthritis for many years presents with a deformity involving her right middle finger. On examination you note that there is flexion at the proximal interphalangeal joint and extension at the distal interphalangeal joint.

4. A middle age lady with known rheumatoid arthritis for many years presents with a deformity involving her right middle finger. On examination you note that there is flexion at the metacarpophalangeal joints, extension at the proximal interphalangeal joint and flexion at the distal interphalangeal joint.

## 250. ANSWERS

1. **C - Heberden's nodes**

2. **G - Bouchard's nodes**

In osteoarthritis, nodes occurring at the proximal interphalangeal joint are called the Bouchard's nodes. Conversely those occurring at the distal interphalangeal joint are called Heberden's nodes.

3. **B - Boutonniere's lesion**

4. **H - Swan neck deformity**

These are classical deformities associated with rheumatoid arthritis. See a few clinical pictures in any of the standard textbooks and try and memorize the descriptions to help you answer these very important questions in the exam without getting confused.

## 251. THEME: INVESTIGATIONS FOR POSTOPERATIVE COMPLICATIONS

OPTIONS

A. No investigations
B. Blood tests
C. Upper GI endoscopy
D. ECG
E. Ventilation perfusion scan
F. Barium enema
G. Colonoscopy
H. Dye test
I. Cystoscopy
J. Chest X-ray

*For each of the scenarios described below, select the most appropriate investigation from the options listed above. Each option may be used once, more than once or not at all.*

1. A 55-year-old male who underwent a gastroenterostomy for benign gastric outlet obstruction 2 years ago presents with eructation of foul gas and diarrhoea after each meal.

2. A 65-year-old lady undergoes a left total knee replacement. 12 hours postoperatively she develops sudden onset chest pain with breathlessness.

3. A 65-year-old lady presents to A&E with a history of sudden onset chest pain and breathlessness 8 days after being discharged from hospital after a left total knee replacement.

4. A 55-year-old lady undergoes a radical hysterectomy for malignancy. She presents to hospital a fortnight later with a complaint of continuous soakage of undergarments with urine.

## 251. ANSWERS

1. **F - Barium enema**

This patient most likely has developed a gastrocolic fistula as a complication of surgery. The history is classical. A barium enema should help clinch the diagnosis.

2. **D - ECG**

12 hours postoperative is too early for a pulmonary embolism. It is likely to be an acute myocardial infarction.

3. **E - Ventilation perfusion scan**

This sounds more like pulmonary embolism. Though ECG is one of the options, a V/Q scan is the most appropriate option.

4. **H - Dye test**

This patient most likely has developed a vesicovaginal fistula from radical surgery. The most appropriate answer is the dye test. Intravenous indigo-carmine is injected and coloured urine visualized identifying the exact site of fistula.

## 252. THEME: TUMOUR MARKERS

OPTIONS

A. α Fetoprotein
B. β- hCG
C. Carcinoembryonic antigen (CEA)
D. Paraproteins
E. PSA
F. Alkaline phosphatase
G. CA-125
H. CA 19-9

*For each of the scenarios described below, select the most appropriate investigation from the options listed above. Each option may be used once, more than once or not at all.*

1. Hepatoma

2. Ovarian carcinoma

3. Prostate carcinoma

4. Colorectal carcinoma

5. Multiple myeloma

6. Pancreatic carcinoma

### 252. ANSWERS

1. **A - α Fetoprotein**

2. **G - CA-125**

3. **E - PSA**

4. **C - Carcinoembryonic antigen (CEA)**

5. **D - Paraproteins**

6. **H - CA 19-9**

This is an important question from the point of view of exams. Tumour markers are commonly used as a screening test for cancers or to follow up patients after treatment. An example of screening is the use of PSA (prostate specific antigen) in prostate cancers. Multiple myeloma is associated with the secretion of paraproteins, which may be seen on an electrophoretic strip. Light chain protein (Bence Jones) is secreted into the urine in myeloma. Hepatomas/Hepatocellular carcinomas secrete α fetoprotein. They are useful for follow up in recurrence. Apart from PSA, acid phosphatase can be used as a tumour marker for prostate cancer. However, it is much less specific and is now rarely used.

## 253. THEME: ARTERIAL BLOOD GAS ANALYSIS

OPTIONS

A. Metabolic acidosis
B. Metabolic alkalosis
C. Respiratory alkalosis
D. Respiratory acidosis

*For each of the scenarios mentioned below, select the most appropriate blood gas analysis from the list of options enlisted above. Each option may be used once, more than once, or not at all.*

1. A 74-year-old male known to have a pyloric outflow obstruction presents with nausea, vomiting, anorexia and weight loss. He has been throwing up everything he has had for the past 1 week. His blood gases in A&E read as: pH 7.52, $Pco_2$ 7.0 kPa, $Po_2$ 14 kPa and bicarbonates 44 mmol/L.

2. A 24-year-old student is brought to the A&E cyanotic and profoundly weak. His roommate has just returned from a semester in Africa. The patient had been observed admiring his roommate's authentic African blowgun and had scraped his finger on the tip of one of the poison darts (curare). Electrolytes and ABG results: Na 138, $Cl^-$ 100, $HCO_3^-$ 26, ABG/$Pco_2$/$Po_2$- 7.08/80 mm Hg /37 mm Hg.

3. A 23-year-old female presents to the Emergency Room complaining of chest tightness and light-headedness. Other symptoms include tingling and numbness in her fingertips and around her mouth. Her medications include alprazolam and birth control pills, but she recently ran out of both. Her electrolytes are: $Na^+$ 135, $Cl^-$ 113, and $HCO_3^-$ 22. ABG/$Pco_2$/$Po_2$: 7.54/22 mm Hg /115 mm Hg on room air.
4. A 65-year-old male is found collapsed on admission to A&E. Blood gases show: pH 7.05, $Pco_2$ 3.2 kPa, $Po_2$ 12 kPa and bicarbonates 8 mmol/L.

## 253. ANSWERS

### 1. B - Metabolic alkalosis

Develop a methodical system for interpreting blood gas analysis. The best and the easiest way to do it is to interpret pH → $Pco_2$ → Bicarbonates.

The pH indicates alkalosis. However, the $Pco_2$ is high (and thus does not correspond with an alkalosis picture). The bicarbonate is high and thus corresponds. Thus this is a metabolic alkalosis with respiratory compensation (that is why the $Pco_2$ is high). Important clue is the pyloric outflow obstruction. Metabolic alkalosis from excessive vomiting is a well known feature.

### 2. D - Respiratory acidosis

Respiratory processes predominantly affect the $Pco_2$, and this patient's $Pco_2$ is markedly abnormal at 80 mm Hg. A rise in the $Pco_2$ is consistent with a respiratory acidosis.

Though most hospitals use kPa as a measure of $Pco_2$ and $Po_2$, it is still important to remember the traditional mm Hg values.

It is also easy to find out that the changes are acute. Acute respiratory changes affect the pH by 0.08 for every mm Hg the $Pco_2$ changes. This patient's $Pco_2$ is 80 mm Hg, which is a change of 40 mm Hg from normal. 40/10 x 0.08 = 0.32, so you would expect the pH to change by 0.32 if this is an acute respiratory acidosis. Chronic respiratory changes affect the pH by 0.03 for every mm Hg the $Pco_2$ changes. If this patient had a chronic respiratory acidosis causing his $Pco_2$ to rise to 80, his pH would change by 0.12 (40 x 0.03), corresponding to a pH of 7.28. The pH in fact did change by 0.32 from normal of 7.4, leaving a pH of 7.08. Therefore the acidaemia is from acute respiratory acidosis.

### 3. C - Respiratory alkalosis

Use the same principles as outlined above. This patient has acute respiratory alkalosis.

### 4. A - Metabolic acidosis

Use the same principles again. The pH is low suggesting acidosis. The $Pco_2$ however does not correspond. The bicarbonate value does.

## 254. THEME: ULCERATION

OPTIONS

A. Marjolin's ulcer
B. Curling's ulcer
C. Cushing's ulcer
D. Pyoderma gangrenosum

*For each of the scenarios mentioned below, select the most appropriate ulceration from the list of options enlisted above. Each option may be used once, more than once, or not at all.*

1. Crohn's disease

2. Rheumatoid arthritis

3. Neurosurgery

4. Major burns

5. Squamous cell carcinoma in a chronic venous ulcer

## 254. ANSWERS

1. **D - Pyoderma gangrenosum**

2. **D - Pyoderma gangrenosum**

Pyoderma gangrenosum is an uncommon cause of skin ulceration. It may affect any part of the skin, but the lower legs are the most common site. It is thought to be an autoimmune disorder. Pyoderma gangrenosum often affects a person with an underlying internal disease such as:

- Inflammatory bowel diseases (ulcerative colitis and Crohn's disease)
- Rheumatoid arthritis
- Myeloid blood dyscrasias
- Chronic active hepatitis
- Wegener's granulomatosis
- Miscellaneous less common associations

Pyoderma gangrenosum usually starts quite suddenly, often at the site of a minor injury. It may start as a small pustule, red bump or blood-blister. The skin then breaks down resulting in an ulcer. The ulcer can deepen and widen rapidly. Characteristically, the edge of the ulcer is purple and undermined as it enlarges. It is usually very painful. Several ulcers may develop at the same time.

Untreated, the ulcers may continue to enlarge, persist unchanged or may slowly heal. Treatment is usually successful in arresting the process, but complete healing may take months.

3. **C - Cushing's ulcer**

This is also known as von Rokitansky-Cushing syndrome. This is an acute ulceration of the stomach, proximal duodenum, or oesophagus, frequently leading to haemorrhage or perforation, associated with intracranial injury or increase in intracranial pressure, associated with gastric acid hypersecretion. Eponym is used to indicate the gastrointestinal haemorrhagic complication arising after head injury or neurosurgery.

4. **B - Curling's ulcer**

5. **A - Marjolin's ulcer**

## 255. THEME: CHOICE OF COLORECTAL SURGERY

OPTIONS

A. Abdomino-perineal resection
B. Anterior resection
C. Hartmann's procedure
D. Left hemicolectomy
E. Panproctocolectomy
F. Subtotal colectomy
G. Transverse loop colostomy

*For each of the scenarios mentioned below, select the most appropriate choice of surgery from the list of options enlisted above. Each option may be used once, more than once, or not at all.*

1. A 25-year-old male known to have ulcerative colitis presents to A&E with abdominal pain, distention, vomiting, and bleeding per rectum. X-ray shows a colonic diameter of 5.5 cm. He does not respond to conservative management. His white cell count stands at 27.5 x $10^9$/L. His colonic diameter on abdominal X-ray increases to 7 cm.

2. A 60-year-old male is brought into A&E with abdominal pain, distention and constipation. Examination reveals generalized peritonitis. At laparotomy a 6-cm perforated mass is found in the sigmoid colon. There is gross faecal contamination of the peritoneal cavity.

## 255. ANSWERS

1. **F - Subtotal colectomy**

This patient has features to suggest fulminating colitis and toxic dilatation (megacolon). Dilatation should be suspected in patients with active colitis who develop severe abdominal pain. It is an indication that inflammation has gone through all the muscle layers of the colon. The diagnosis is confirmed by the presence on a plain abdominal radiograph of the colon with a diameter more than 6 cm. Plain abdominal radiographs should be obtained daily in patients with severe colitis and a progressive increase in diameter despite medical therapy is an indication for surgery. This patient needs a subtotal colectomy with ileostomy. The rectum is not increased as this would increase the length of surgery and increase morbidity.

2. **C - Hartmann's procedure**

This patient has a perforated sigmoid carcinoma which needs resection. However, a primary anastomosis is not advisable in the presence of gross faecal contamination. This is another favourite question with the examiners.

## 256. THEME: DIAGNOSIS OF FRACTURES

OPTIONS

A. Anterior shoulder dislocation
B. Posterior shoulder dislocation
C. Colles fracture
D. Scaphoid fracture
E. Smith's fracture
F. Monteggia fracture dislocation
G. Galeazzi fracture dislocation
H. Mallet finger
I. Femoral neck fracture
J. Calcaneum fractures

*For each of the patients described below, select the most appropriate diagnosis from the above list. Each option may be used once, more than once, or not at all.*

1. A 75-year-old lady residing alone falls out of her bed and injures her left hip. On examination her leg is shortened and externally rotated. The hip is tender on palpation and she is unable to weight bear.

2. A 40-year-old man falls from the roof of his house and lands on his feet. He presents to A&E with painful and swollen heels. His soles are bruised and he is unable to weight bear.

3. A 15-year-old girl fell off a tree and injured her left forearm. She is tender over the distal aspect of her left radius and the distal radioulnar joint.

4. A 29-year-old epileptic man falls onto his outstretched hand following a fit and injures his left shoulder. On examination the left deltoid appears hollow and the arm is held in internal rotation.

5. A 28-year-old cricketer presents with a painful phalanx. He cannot extend the terminal phalanx of his ring finger.

## 256. ANSWERS

1. **I - Femoral neck fracture**
The femoral neck is the commonest site of fractures in the elderly. There is usually a history of fall followed by pain in the hip. A shortened and externally rotated extremity is the key to diagnosis.

2. **J - Calcaneum fractures**
Fall from a height is the most common mechanism. Over 20% of these patients suffer associated injuries of the spine, pelvis or hip. Signs of compartment syndrome of the foot should always be checked (intense pain, extensive bruising and diminished sensibility).

3. **G - Galeazzi fracture dislocation**
This is the name given to fracture of the lower third radius with subluxation or dislocation of distal radioulnar joint. Prominence or tenderness over the lower end of ulna is the striking feature. In children, closed reduction is often successful; in adults, reduction is best achieved by open reduction and compression plating of the radius.

4. **B - Posterior shoulder dislocation**
It is rare, accounting for 2% of all shoulder dislocations. They occur usually following a fit or convulsion or an electric shock. The diagnosis is easily missed partly because a single AP view of the shoulder may look normal and partly because those attending the patient fail to think of it. The arm is held in internal rotation and is locked in that position. In the AP film the head of humerus looks abnormal (the light bulb sign). A lateral film is essential. In difficult cases CT scan is essential.

5. **H - Mallet finger**
It is usually due to avulsion of extensor tendon from its insertion into terminal phalanx and may be associated with a fracture. After a sudden flexion injury the terminal phalanx droops and cannot be straightened actively. Treatment consists of immobilising the terminal joint in slight hyperextension by means of a mallet finger splint which fixes the distal joint but leaves the proximal joint free. Occasionally it may be necessary to transfix the distal joint through the pulp with a k wire.

## 257. THEME: CONDITIONS OF THE HAND

OPTIONS

A. Scleroderma
B. Psoriasis
C. Volkmann's ischaemic contracture
D. Rheumatoid arthritis
E. Claw hand
F. Raynaud's phenomenon
G. Paronychia
H. Glomus tumour
I. Carpal tunnel syndrome

*For each of the patients described below, select the most appropriate diagnosis from the above list. Each option may be used once, more than once, or not at all.*

1. A 30-year-old female presents with a painful fingernail. On examination there is a small purple red spot beneath the nail. There is no history of any trauma.

2. A 32-year-old pregnant female presents with pain in her left hand worse at night. She also complains of pins and needles in her thumb and index finger.

3. A 26-year-old diabetic presents with a painful fingertip that throbs and is painful at night. The skin at the base and side of nail is red, tender and bulging.

4. A 25-year-old man presents with flexion deformity of the fingers in his right hand. The deformity is abolished by flexion of his wrist. He gives a history of neglected elbow trauma in the recent past.

5. A 40-year-old female presents with pain and stiffness in both her hands worse in the morning. On examination there is flexion deformity of her DIP joints, with the presence of firm, non tender nodules over the forearms.

## 257. ANSWERS

1. **H - Glomus tumour**

This rare tumour usually occurs around fine peripheral neurovascular structures and especially the nail beds of fingers or toes. A young adult presents with recurrent episodes of intense pain in the fingertip. A small bluish nodule may be seen under the nail; the area is sensitive to cold and very tender. X-rays sometimes show erosion of the underlying phalanx. Treatment is excision; the tumour is never larger than a pea and is easily shelled out of its fibrous capsule.

2. **I - Carpal tunnel syndrome**

This is the commonest cause of hand pain at night. Compression of median nerve under the flexor retinaculum produces the characteristic symptoms and signs. Pregnancy, the pill, myxoedema, distal radial fractures are some of the common aetiologies. Wrist splints worn at night may relieve nocturnal pain.

3. **G - Paronychia**

Infection under the nail fold is the commonest hand infection. The edge of nail fold becomes red and swollen and increasingly tender. A tiny abscess may form in the nail fold; if this is left untreated pus can spread under the nail.

Initially treatment with antibiotics may be effective. However, if pus is present it must be released by an incision at the corner of the nail fold in line with the edge of the nail. If pus has spread under the nail, part or the entire nail may need to be removed.

4. **C - Volkmann's ischaemic contracture**

Contracture of the forearm muscles may follow circulatory insufficiency due to injuries at or below the elbow. Shortening of the long flexors causes the fingers to be held in flexion; they can be straightened only when the wrist is flexed so as to relax the long flexors. If the disability is marked, some improvement may be obtained by lengthening the shortened tendons, or else by excising the dead muscles and restoring finger movement with tendon transfers.

5. **D - Rheumatoid arthritis**

This condition is more common in females. This may present with monoarthritis, polyarthritis or as a systemic involvement. Early morning stiffness may last for several hours. Swan neck or boutonniere deformity may occur in the fingers.

Systemic manifestations of RA are caused by vasculitis or nodules. Nodules are usually found on pressure areas, e.g., forearm, but may occur on tendon sheaths or in lungs, myocardium, pericardium or sclera.

## 258. THEME: SHOULDER JOINT PATHOLOGIES

OPTIONS

A. Supraspinatus tendonitis
B. Rupture of rotator cuff
C. Acute calcific tendonitis
D. Bicipital tendonitis
E. Adhesive capsulitis
F. Acromioclavicular joint arthritis
G. Subdeltoid bursitis
H. Dislocated shoulder
I. Fracture of proximal humerus
J. Rupture of biceps tendon

*For each of the patients described below, select the most appropriate diagnosis from the above list. Each option may be used once, more than once, or not at all.*

1. A 52-year-old man complains of pain and bruising in his upper arm while lifting a heavy weight. On attempted forceful flexion of the elbow, a prominent lump is felt in the lower arm.
2. A 64-year-old female complains of gradually increasing pain in the left shoulder, preventing her from sleeping on that side. On examination there is a lack of active and passive movements in all directions.
3. A 35-year-old male complains of sudden onset of pain in his right shoulder. There is no history of trauma. On examination the arm is held immobile and the joint is very tender to palpation or movement.
4. A 36-year-old swimmer complains of right shoulder pain after taking part in a competition. On examination there is tenderness along the anterior edge of acromion. On active abduction pain is aggravated as the arm traverses an arc of 60–120°.
5. A 56-year-old presents with pain in the left shoulder following a fall on his left side. He has been troubled with chronic pain in the same shoulder in the past. On examination there is tenderness on the lateral joint line and an attempt at active abduction produces a characteristic shrug. Passive abduction however is found to be full.

## 258. ANSWERS

1. **J - Rupture of biceps tendon**

Bicipital tendon rupture usually accompanies rotator cuff disruption. Patient is usually more than 50 years of age. The key to diagnosis is the rounded distal belly of biceps (Popeye muscle) on attempted flexion of the elbow. Isolated tears in the elderly need no treatment. However, if the rupture is a part of rotator cuff lesion, especially in the young and active, surgery is indicated.

2. **E - Adhesive capsulitis**

Adhesive capsulitis or frozen shoulder is a disorder characterized by progressive pain and stiffness of the shoulder that resolves spontaneously after about 18 months. The cardinal feature is loss of both active and passive movements in all directions. Treatment is usually conservative aiming to relieve pain and preventing further stiffness.

3. **C - Acute calcific tendonitis**

Acute shoulder pain with no history of trauma may follow deposition of calcium hydroxyapatite crystals in the rotator cuff. The cause is unknown and symptoms are due to florid vascular reaction which produces tension and swelling in the tendon.

4. **A - Supraspinatus tendonitis**

Also known as painful arc syndrome, it usually occurs in patients under 40 years of age, after vigorous or unaccustomed activity. The shoulder looks normal but is tender anteriorly. On active abduction scapulohumeral rhythm is disturbed and pain is aggravated in the arc between 60–120° (painful arc). The condition is often reversible; settling down gradually once the initiating activity is avoided.

5. **B - Rupture of rotator cuff**

The patient is usually elderly and gives a history of refractory chronic shoulder pain with increasing stiffness and weakness. The clinical presentation is secondary to loss of supraspinatus tendon function with weakness in shrugging movement of shoulder during abduction and inability to lift the arm. The passive abduction is full and once the arm has been lifted above a right angle the patient can keep it by using the deltoid (the abduction paradox). When the patient lowers it sideways, it suddenly drops (the drop arm sign).

## 259. THEME: DISORDERS OF ELBOW JOINT

OPTIONS

A. Tennis elbow
B. Golfer's elbow
C. Pulled elbow
D. Gout
E. Rheumatoid arthritis
F. Osteochondritis dissecans
G. Post traumatic stiffness
H. Tuberculosis

*For each of the patients described below, select the most appropriate diagnosis from the above list. Each option may be used once, more than once, or not at all.*

1. A 26-year-old presents with sudden onset pain and swelling of his left elbow. On examination the swelling and redness extends down into the forearm and there is restriction in movements of the joint.

2. A 31-year-old man presents with gradual onset pain of his right elbow. On examination there is localised tenderness over the lateral epicondyle. Pain is reproduced on active extension of the wrist against resistance.

3. A 13-year-old boy presents with pain in his left elbow aggravated by activity and relieved by rest. On examination there is swelling, effusion, tenderness over the capitellum and terminal restriction of movements. X-ray shows fragmentation of the capitellum.

4. A 28-year-old Asian man presents with long standing history of pain and stiffness of his left elbow. On examination there is marked restriction of elbow movements with wasting of peri articular muscles. X-ray shows periarticular osteoporosis and joint erosion.

## 259. ANSWERS

1. **D - Gout**

The elbow or precisely the olecranon bursa is a favourite site for gout. In an acute attack the area rapidly becomes painful, swollen and inflamed. The serum uric acid level may be raised and the bursal aspirate may contain urate crystals. The condition may be easily mistaken for cellulitis or joint infection.

2. **A - Tennis elbow**

Pain and tenderness over the lateral epicondyle (common extensor origin) is a common complaint among tennis players, but even more common in non players who perform similar activities involving forceful repetitive wrist extension. It is aggravated by movements such as pouring out tea, turning a stiff door handle, shaking hands or among tennis players due to faulty technique.

Golfer's elbow is similar to tennis elbow except that the flexor origin (medial epicondyle) is affected

3. **F - Osteochondritis dissecans (OCD)**

The capiteelum is one of the common sites of OCD. This is probably due to repetitive stress following prolonged or unaccustomed activity. The lesion may require CT or MRI for a diagnosis. Treatment is usually symptomatic; however, there might be a separated fragment from the capiteelum, which should be removed surgically.

4. **H - Tuberculosis**

The elbow is affected in about 10% patients of tuberculosis. The onset is insidious and the most striking physical sign is marked wasting. Aspiration, synovial biopsy and microbiological investigation confirm the diagnosis. Rest and antituberculosis therapy are essential.

## 260. THEME: WRIST PROBLEMS

OPTIONS

A. Drop wrist
B. Keinbock's disease
C. Rheumatoid arthritis
D. Osteoarthritis
E. De Quervain's disease
F. Ganglion cyst
G. Carpal tunnel syndrome

*For each of the patients described below, select the most appropriate diagnosis from the above list. Each option may be used once, more than once, or not at all.*

1. A 46-yr-old housewife presents with pain on the radial aspect of her left wrist. On examination, the tip of radial styloid is tender and Finkelstein's test is positive.

2. A 23-yr-old man presents with a painless swelling on the dorsal aspect of his right wrist. On examination, the lump is well defined, cystic and non tender.

3. A 36-yr-old man presents with aching and stiffness of the left wrist. There is no history of trauma. On examination, tenderness is mainly localised over the lunate bone and grip strength is diminished.

4. A 68-yr-old man presents with a complaint of diffuse pain around the base of his thumb. On examination there is swelling and tenderness around trapezio-metacarpal joint and X-ray shows a decreased joint space.

5. A 42-yr-old woman presents with complaint of burning pain in her left hand worse at night. She also complains of tingling and numbness. The symptoms are relieved by hanging the arm over the side or shaking the arm.

## 260. ANSWERS

1. **E - De Quervain's disease.** The extensor retinaculum contains six compartments which transmit tendons lined with synovium. Tenosynovitis can be caused by unaccustomed movement, overuse or repetitive minor trauma. The first dorsal compartment (abductor pollicis longus & extensor pollicis brevis) and the second dorsal compartment (extensor carpi radialis brevis) are most commonly affected. Finkelstein's test involves placing the patient's thumb across the palm in full flexion and turning the wrist sharply into adduction. A positive test is painful. Arthritis at base of thumb or scaphoid non union are important differentials.

2. **F - Ganglion cyst.** Ganglion cysts are the most common swellings of the wrists. They arise from leakage of synovial fluid from a joint or tendon sheath and contain a viscous fluid. The back of the wrist is the most common site; less frequently seen on the volar side. Treatment can be conservative and the lump can be safely left alone. If it is painful or symptoms of nerve compression are present, removal is justified.

3. **B - Keinbock's disease.** It is an ischaemic necrosis of lunate bone that usually follows chronic stress or injury. The patient usually a young adult, complains of ache and stiffness. Only occasionally there is a history of acute trauma. In later stages wrist movements are limited and painful. MRI is the most reliable way of detecting early changes. Later, X-ray may show either mottled or diffuse density of the bone. Early stages may resolve with splintage of wrist; however, in advanced cases, with collapse of lunate, a prosthesis or arthrodesis may help.

4. **D - Osteoarthritis.** OA of the trapezio-metacarpal joint is common in post menopausal women. It may be bilateral and as a part of generalised OA. X-ray shows narrowing of trapezio-metacarpal joint. Most patients can be treated with NSAIDs, local steroid injections and splintage. If these measures fail, operative treatment with excision of trapezius, silicon prosthesis or arthrodesis may be required.

5. **G - Carpal tunnel syndrome.** This is one of the commonest nerve entrapment syndromes. Usually the cause is unknown but the syndrome is common at the menopause, in RA, in pregnancy and in myxoedema. The history is most helpful in diagnosis. Pain and paraesthesia in distribution of median nerve, worse at night, is the classical feature. Sensory symptoms can be reproduced by percussion over the median nerve (Tinel's sign) or by holding the wrist fully flexed for a minute or two (Phalen's test). Electrodiagnostic tests may be required for confirmation.

## 261. THEME: HAND INJURIES

OPTIONS

A. Bennett's fracture
B. Mallet finger
C. Boutonniere deformity
D. Flexor digitorum profundus injury
E. Flexor digitorum superficialis injury
F. Ulnar collateral ligament injury
G. Median nerve injury
H. Radial nerve injury
I. Ulnar nerve injury

*For each of the patients described below, select the most appropriate diagnosis from the above list. Each option may be used once, more than once, or not at all.*

1. A 36-yr-old man presents with flexion deformity of the proximal interphalangeal joint with DIP joint in extension in his right index finger. He gives a history of direct trauma to the dorsal aspect of the same finger.

2. A 26-yr-old basketball player presents with drooping of the terminal phalanx of his right middle finger after being hit by the ball. He is now unable to extend the tip of his finger.

3. A 42-yr-old man presents with lacerations to the hand from a cut glass. He is unable to flex the affected finger as the unaffected fingers are held in extension.

4. A 26-yr-old man sustains injury to his left hand while skiing. He complains of pain around the base of his thumb. On examination, he has difficulty in abducting the thumb.

5. A 31-yr-old boxer presents with injury to his right thumb. There is tenderness over the base of his first metacarpal. X-ray shows an oblique fracture of the base of the metacarpal, extending into carpometacarpal joint.

## 261. ANSWERS

1. **C - Boutonniere's deformity**

The lesion presents as a flexion deformity of the DIP joint. It is due to interruption or stretching of the central slip of the extensor tendon where it inserts into the base of the middle phalanx; the usual causes are direct trauma or RA. Initially deformity is slight and passively correctable; later the soft tissues contract, resulting in fixed flexion of the proximal and hyperextension of DIP joints (cf. swan neck deformity, where the proximal interphalangeal joint is hyper extended and DIP is flexed).

2. **B - Mallet finger**

This results from injury to the extensor tendon of the terminal phalanx. It may be due to direct trauma but more often follows tendon rupture when the finger tip is forcibly bent during active extension, perhaps while tucking the blanket under the mattress or trying to catch a ball. The terminal joint is held flexed and the patient cannot straighten it, but passive movement is normal. An acute mallet finger should be splinted with the joint in extension for about 8 weeks.

3. **E - Flexor digitorum superficialis injuries**

Tendon injuries are common following wounds with sharp objects such as cut glass. Both the FDS and FDP tendons should be checked for discontinuity.

FDP is tested by holding the PIP joint straight and instructing the patient to bend the distal joint. FDS is tested by holding all the fingers together straight, then releasing one and asking patient to bend the proximal joint. Holding the fingers straight immobilises all the deep flexors (including that of the finger being tested), which have a common muscle belly.

4. **F - Ulnar collateral ligament injury**

This injury is commonly seen in skiers who fall out on the extended thumb, forcing it into hyper abduction. A small flake of bone may be pulled off at the same time. On examination, there is tenderness and swelling over the ulnar side of the thumb MCP joint. An X-ray is essential to exclude a fracture. Treatment is conservative for partial tears and operative with repair of the ligament for complete tears.

5. **A - Bennett's fracture**

This fracture occurs at the base of 1st metacarpal bone and is commonly due to punching, but the fracture is oblique, extends into the carpometacarpal joint and is unstable. The thumb looks short and carpometacarpal region swollen. X-ray shows the characteristic fracture. Treatment involves reduction and stabilising either with POP or K-wires.

## 262. THEME: PAINFUL FOOT CONDITION

OPTIONS

A. Stress fracture
B. Morton's neuroma
C. Plantar fasciitis
D. Avulsion fracture
E. Jones fracture
F. Metatarsalgia
G. Bunion
H. Gout
I. Freiberg's disease

*For each of the patients described below, select the most appropriate diagnosis from the above list. Each option may be used once, more than once, or not at all.*

1. A 35-year-old man presents with pain under the ball of his feet. The pain is present on weight bearing throughout the day. On examination, there is tenderness along the distal edge of the heel contact area.

2. A 62-year-old man presents with continual pain in his forefoot when walking. A bony lump is palpable in the region of 2nd metatarsal. X-ray shows a widened and flattened head of 2nd metatarsal.

3. A 28-year-old soldier complains of pain in his foot while weight bearing. An X-ray taken shows no abnormality. Tenderness is present on the base of 3rd and 4th metatarsals.

4. A 52-year-old woman complains of pain in her forefoot and burning and tingling radiation to the toes. On examination, tenderness is present in the 3rd intermetatarsal space.

5. A 32-year-old man presents with sudden onset of pain in his right foot. There is no history of trauma. On examination, the skin over the 1st MTP joint is red and shiny. It is very hot and tender to touch.

## 262. ANSWERS

1. **C - Plantar fasciitis**

The term plantar fasciitis is used as the condition may be associated with inflammatory disorders such as gout, ankylosing spondylitis and Reiter's disease in which enthesopathy is one of the defining pathological lesions. Often, however, there is no obvious abnormality. A calcaneum spur is often seen on an X-ray and is regarded as a traction lesion in the plantar ligament. Treatment is conservative; anti inflammatory drugs or local injection of corticosteroids.

2. **I - Freiberg's disease**

It is a crushing type of osteochondritis of the 2nd metatarsal head (rarely 3rd). A bony lump is palpable and MTP joint is tender. X–rays show the head to be too wide and flat, the neck thick and the joint space is increased. Treatment may be conservative with walking plaster or moulded sandal. If pain persists, operative synovectomy, debridement and trimming of metatarsal head can be considered.

3. **A - Stress fracture**

Stress fracture, usually of the 2nd or 3rd metatarsal occurs in young adults after unaccustomed activity or in women with postmenopausal osteoporosis. The X-ray appearance is at first normal, but later shows fusiform callus around a fine transverse fracture. Long before X-ray signs appear, a radioisotope scan will show increased activity. Treatment is either unnecessary or consists simply of rest.

4. **B - Morton's neuroma**

It is essentially an entrapment or compression syndrome affecting one of the digital nerves, but secondary thickening of the nerve creates the impression of a neuroma. The symptoms of pain, tingling and numbness may be aggravated by wearing tight shoes and removed by removing the shoes. If diagnosis is in doubt, a diagnostic blocking test can be performed, an injection of local anaesthetic beneath the transverse intermetatarsal ligament will relieve the pain.

5. **H - Gout**

Patients are usually men over 30 years of age. The sudden onset of pain lasts for a week or two before resolving completely. The attack may come on its own or may be precipitated by minor trauma, alcohol, intercurrent illness, operation. Common sites are MTP joint of big toe, ankle, finger joint, and olecranon bursa. Hyperuricaemia is present at some stage, however, not necessarily during an acute attack. The true diagnosis is established by finding the characteristic negatively birefringent urate crystals in the synovial fluid. Cellulitis, septic bursitis, infected bunion or septic arthritis are important differential diagnosis.

## 263. THEME: BACK PAIN

OPTIONS

A. Metastasis
B. Discitis
C. Prolapsed intervertebral disc
D. Spondylolisthesis
E. Facet joint arthrosis
F. Spondylolysis
G. TB of spine
H. Muscle strain
I. Osteoporotic collapse

*For each of the patients described below, select the most appropriate diagnosis from the above list. Each option may be used once, more than once, or not at all.*

1. A 32-year-old man presents with complaints of low back pain following a day of strenuous activity. On examination, he has stiff back and there are no nerve root signs.

2. Following a microdiscectomy for a prolapsed intervertebral disc, a 41-year-old presents with worsening back pain, generalised malaise and fever. On examination, his back is stiff, SLR is limited but neurological examination is normal. Blood test shows increased WBC, ESR and CRP.

3. A 26-year-old Asian man present with long standing history of ill health and backache. He complains of weakness of his legs and paraesthesia. On examination, there is tenderness and kyphotic deformity of the thoracic spine. X-ray shows collapse of vertebral bodies and blood investigations show a raised ESR.

4. A 41-year-old man presents with sudden onset low backache while lifting a heavy box. The pain radiated down to the buttocks and back of both lower limbs. He also complains of tingling and numbness in legs and feet.

5. An 86-year-old woman complains of backache which she recalls following a fall 2 weeks ago. On examination, there is tenderness over the mid thoracic spine. The neurological examination is normal.

## 263. ANSWERS

1. **H - Muscle strain or myofascial backache.** It is one of the most common causes of backache. It may follow bad posture at work or some strenuous activity. There is paraspinal tenderness and spasm. The neurological examination is normal which differentiates it from other sinister causes of backache. It usually responds to short period of rest and restricted activity followed by gradually increased exercise.

2. **B - Discitis.** The common sources of infection are (A) direct inoculation during invasive procedures (spinal injections and disc operation), (B) indirect haematogenous spread from a pelvic infection or a remote site. Localised pain is the cardinal symptom. Systemic signs such as pyrexia and tachycardia are present. WBC and ESR are usually raised. MRI is the definitive diagnostic tool as X-rays may be normal initially. Treatment consists of bed rest, pain relief and intravenous antibiotics.

3. **G - TB of the spine.** The spine is the most common site of skeletal TB. Blood borne infection usually settles in a vertebral body adjacent to the vertebral disc. Infection spreads to the disc space and adjacent vertebrae which collapse causing a kyphotic deformity. Clinical features range from mild paraparesis to complete paraplegia. The earliest signs on X-ray are local osteoporosis of two adjacent vertebrae and narrowing of the disc space. Later there is obvious bony destruction. CT/MRI are useful in the investigation of cord compression. Treatment is with anti-tuberculous therapy and bed rest. Operative treatment may be required to drain an abscess and stabilise the spine.

Important differentials are pyogenic infection and metastasis. Disc space collapse is typical of infection and disc preservation is typical of metastatic disease.

4. **C - Prolapsed intervertebral disc.** Acute disc prolapse usually occurs while lifting or stooping. There is acute backache and the patient is unable to straighten up. Both backache and sciatica are made worse by coughing or straining.

Cauda equina compression is rare but may result in urinary retention. On examination, SLR is restricted. Neurological examination may show weakness, diminished reflexes and sensory loss corresponding to the affected level. CT/MRI are important imaging modalities.

5. **I - Osteoporotic collapse.** Postmenopausal osteoporosis may result in one or more compression fractures of the thoracic spine. Kyphosis is seldom marked. Senile osteoporosis affects both men and women. Patients are usually over 75 years of age, often incapacitated by some other illness and lack exercise. They complain of backache and spinal deformity is marked. It is important to exclude metastatic disease. Treatment is symptomatic.

## 264. THEME: DIAGNOSIS OF BACK PAIN

OPTIONS

A. Spinal stenosis
B. Osteoarthritis
C. Osteomyelitis
D. Multiple myeloma
E. Metastasis
F. Ankylosing spondylitis
G. Paget's disease
H. Lupus
I. Reiter's disease

*For each of the patients described below, select the most appropriate diagnosis from the above list. Each option may be used once, more than once, or not at all.*

1. A 52-year-old man complains of aching, numbness and paraesthesia in his thighs and legs. It comes on after standing upright or walking for 5–10 minutes and is relieved by sitting, squatting or leaning forward.

2. A 72-year-old female treated for breast carcinoma complains of sudden onset backache. Neurological examination is normal. X-ray of the thoracic spine shows collapse of T8/T9 vertebral body with preservation of disc space.

3. A 46-year-old female presents with gradual onset weakness and backache. She is noted to have normocytic, normochromic anaemia and a remarkably raised ESR.

4. A 22-year-old male complains of backache and stiffness worse in the morning and after inactivity. On examination, there is tenderness present in the lower back and sacroiliac joint. Blood tests show elevated ESR and positive HLA-B27.

5. A 62-year-old man presents with low back-ache and pain in his hips. He is found to have elevated alkaline phosphatase. He is also hard of hearing.

## 264. ANSWERS

1. **A - Spinal stenosis**

The patients, usually men over 50 years, may have a history of disc prolapse, chronic backache or spinal operation. Patients prefer walking uphill, which flexes the spine, to downhill which extends it. CT or MRI may be required for measurements of spinal canal.

2. **E - Metastasis**

The skeleton is one of the commonest sites for secondary cancer, in patients over 50 years of age. Bone metastasis is seen more frequently than all primary malignant bone tumours. The commonest source is carcinoma of breast; next in frequency are carcinoma of the prostate, kidney, lung, thyroid, bladder and GIT. Commonest sites for bone metastasis are vertebrae, pelvis, proximal femur and humerus. Metastases are usually osteolytic and pathological fractures are common. Osteoblastic lesions are uncommon. They usually occur in prostatic carcinoma.

3. **D - Multiple myeloma**

It is a B cell lymphoproliferative disorder of the marrow. The patient, typically 45–65 years, presents with weakness, backache, bone pain or pathological fracture. Myeloma is one of the commonest causes of osteoporosis and vertebral compression fractures in men over 45 years of age. High ESR is a constant feature. Over half of the patients have Bence Jones proteins in their urine.

4. **F - Ankylosing spondylitis**

It is a generalised chronic inflammatory disease but its effects are seen mainly in the spine and sacroiliac joints. It is characterised by pain and stiffness in the back. Males are more frequently affected and usual age of onset is between 15 and 25 years. There is a strong association with genetic marker HLA-B27.

5. **G - Paget's disease**

It is characterised by enlargement and thickening of the bone but with an abnormal internal architecture. Bone is unusually brittle. Most people with disease are asymptomatic. When patients do present it is because of pain or deformity or some complications of the disease. Cranial nerve compression may lead to deafness, impaired vision or facial palsy. The most useful test is measurement of serum alkaline phosphatase level, which correlates with the activity and extent of disease. Drugs that suppress bone turnover, notably calcitonin and bisphosphonates are most effective when the disease is active and bone turnover is high.

## 265. THEME: PERIPHERAL NERVE INJURIES

OPTIONS

A. Suprascapular
B. Thoracodorsal
C. Axillary
D. Upper subscapular
E. Long thoracic
F. Median
G. Ulnar
H. Musculocutaneous
I. Radial

*For each of the patients described below, select the most appropriate nerve injury from the above list. Each option may be used once, more than once, or not at all.*

1. A 26-year-old presents with aching and weakness on lifting the arm following a surgery to remove a cervical rib. On examination there is winging of the scapula on attempts to push the shoulder forwards against resistance.
2. A 32-year-old presents with weakness in abduction of shoulder while recovering from a fractured clavicle. On examination there is mild wasting of supraspinatus and diminished power of abduction and external rotation.
3. A 16-year-old boy is seen in A&E following a fall from a tree and injury to the right shoulder. On examination the shoulder is painful with loss of normal rounded contour. Motor examination is not possible due to pain. Sensory examination however reveals an area of numbness over the lateral aspect of his right deltoid.
4. A drunken man is brought to A&E after being found in the street laid on his right arm. Once awake he is found to have wrist drop, weakness of his triceps and sensory loss over the first dorsal interroseous space.
5. A 31-year-old man involved in a RTA is found to have an elbow dislocation. On examination, the hand is held with ulnar fingers flexed and index straight. There is also loss of sensation over radial three and a half digits.

## 265. ANSWERS

1. **E - Long thoracic**

Root value is C5, C6, and C7. It may be damaged in shoulder or neck injuries or during operations such as first rib resection, transaxillary sympathectomy or radical mastectomy. Paralysis of serratus anterior results, which causes winging of scapula. The classic test for winging is to have the patient pushing forwards against the wall or thrusting the shoulder forwards against resistance.

2. **A - Suprascapular**

This arises from the upper trunk of the brachial plexus (C5, 6) and runs through the suprascapular notch to supply the supra and infraspinatus muscles. It may be injured in the fractures of clavicle and scapula, by direct blow or sudden traction, or simply by carrying heavy loads over the shoulder. There might be wasting of supraspinatus and weakness of abduction and external rotation. Treatment might require decompression by division of suprascapular ligament.

3. **C - Axillary**

Root value is C5, 6. It arises from the posterior cord of the brachial plexus. It supplies teres minor and deltoid muscles and a patch of skin over the muscle (regimental batch area). The patient complains of shoulder weakness and deltoid is wasted in chronic cases. Although abduction can be initiated (by supraspinatus), it cannot be maintained (weak deltoid). Nerve injury with fractures or dislocation recovers spontaneously in about 80% cases.

4. **I - Radial**

It may be injured at the elbow, in the upper arm or in the axilla. Low lesions are usually due to fractures or dislocation at elbow or due to a local wound. High lesions occur with fractures of the humerus or after prolonged tourniquet pressure. There is an obvious wrist drop as well as an inability to extend the MCP joint in high lesions. Wrist extension is preserved in low lesions as the branch to ECRL arises proximal to the elbow.

5. **F - Median**

It is most commonly injured near the wrist or high up in the forearm. Typically the hand is held with the ulnar fingers flexed and index straight (the pointing sign). There is also a characteristic pinch defect. Instead of pinching with the thumb and index finger-tips flexed, the patient pinches with the distal joints in full extension.

## 266. THEME: LOWER LIMB NERVE INJURIES

OPTIONS

A. Sciatic nerve
B. Tibial nerve
C. Common peroneal nerve
D. Femoral nerve
E. Lateral cutaneous nerve of thigh
F. Lateral plantar nerve
G. Medial plantar nerve
H. Pudendal nerve
I. Saphenous nerve
J. Sural nerve
K. Posterior tibial nerve

*For each of the patients described below, select the most appropriate nerve injury from the above list. Each option may be used once, more than once, or not at all.*

1. A 68-year-old male patient is found to have a foot drop following a total hip replacement surgery. On examination, there is weakness of ankle dorsiflexion and loss of sensation over the front and outer half of leg and dorsum of foot.

2. A 32-year-old male presents with complaints of numbness, tingling and burning sensation over the anterolateral aspect of his thigh. There is no history of any trauma.

3. A 21-year-old male involved in a RTA is diagnosed with fractures of his proximal tibia and fibula. On examination, he can neither dosiflex nor evert his foot. Sensation is lost over the front and outer half of the leg and dorsum of the foot.

4. A 19-year-old haemophilic presents with spontaneous onset of pain and swelling in front of his left thigh. On examination, the patient is unable to extend his knee and there is numbness of the anterior thigh and medial aspect of the leg.

5. A 48-year-old male presents with pain and sensory disturbance over the plantar surface of his foot. The pain is precipitated by prolonged weight bearing.

## 266. ANSWERS

1. **A - Sciatic nerve**

The incidence of overt sciatic nerve dysfunction is 0.5–3% following primary THR and about twice as high during revision. The peroneal portion of the nerve lies closest to the acetabulum and is most easily damaged. Careful examination would show abnormalities in the distribution of tibial nerve also. If there is any doubt about the level of the lesion, EMG and nerve conduction tests will help.

2. **E - Lateral cutaneous nerve of thigh**

This nerve can be compressed as it runs through the inguinal ligament just medial to ASIS. The patient complains of tingling and numbness over the anterolateral aspect of his thigh (meralgia paraesthetica).

3. **C - Common peroneal nerve**

This nerve is often damaged at the level of fibular neck by severe traction when the knee is forced into varus or by pressure from a splint or plaster cast, from lying with the leg externally rotated, by skin traction or by wounds. The patient has foot drop and can neither dorsiflex nor evert his foot. Sensation is lost over the front and outer half of the leg and dorsum of foot.

4. **D - Femoral nerve**

It can be injured by a gunshot wound, by pressure or traction during an operation or by bleeding into the thigh. Quadriceps action is affected and the knee reflex may be diminished.

5. **K - Posterior tibial nerve**

Pain and sensory disturbance over the plantar surface of the foot may be due to compression of the posterior tibial nerve behind and below the medial malleolus (tarsal tunnel syndrome). The pain is worse at night and the patient may seek relief by walking around or stamping his or her foot. Nerve conduction studies help in establishing a diagnosis.

## 267. THEME: CALCIUM HOMEOSTASIS

OPTIONS

A. Parathyroid carcinoma
B. Primary hyperparathyroidism
C. Secondary hyperparathyroidism
D. Multiple myeloma
E. Paget's disease
F. Hypocalciuric hypercalcaemia
G. Osteomalacia

*For each of the patients described below, select the most appropriate diagnosis from the above list. Each option may be used once, more than once, or not at all.*

1. A 62-year-old female presents with abdominal pain, fatigue and muscle weakness. She is found to have ↑ S. calcium, ↓ S.phosphate, and ↑ S. parathyroid levels. The urinary calcium levels are decreased.

2. A 33-year-old man presents with insidious onset of bone pains, backaches and muscle weakness. He is found to have a low serum calcium and phosphate, increased alkaline phosphatase and decreased urinary excretion of calcium.

3. A 54-year-old male presenting with gradual onset of bone pain and deformity of his legs is found to be deaf. He has normal levels of serum calcium and phosphate. However, the serum alkaline phosphatase is raised.

4. A 32-year-old man presenting with history of renal stones is found to have ↑ S. calcium. His PTH levels are found to be normal. His urinary calcium levels are decreased.

## 267. ANSWERS

1. **B - Primary hyperparathyroidism**
Parathyroid hormone acts on bones producing osteoclastic resorption thus elevating the plasma calcium. It also acts on the kidney by increasing calcium reabsorption, decreasing phosphate reabsorption and elevates 25-OH cholecalciferol. Excessive secretion of PTH may be primary (due to adenoma or hyperplasia), secondary (due to persistent hypocalcaemia) or tertiary (when secondary hyperplasia leads to autonomous overactivity). Diagnosis of primary hyperparathyroidism is based on ↑S. calcium, ↓ S. phosphate and ↑ S. PTH. Other causes of hypercalcaemia in which PTH levels are depressed should be excluded (multiple myeloma, metastatic disease, sarcoidism).

2. **G - Osteomalacia**
In this condition, bone tissue throughout the skeleton is incompletely calcified and therefore softened. Patients may complain of bone pain, backache and muscle weakness for many years before the diagnosis is made. X-rays show Looser's zones, a thin transverse band of rarefaction in an otherwise normal looking bone. Biochemically there is ↓S. calcium and phosphate, ↑S. alkaline phosphatase and ↓ urinary calcium levels. The Ca × P product is diminished (C.f. osteoporosis – normal alkaline phosphatase, normal S. phosphate and a normal Ca×P product).

3. **E - Paget's disease**
Most patients with Paget's are asymptomatic. They present with any of the complications of the disease which can include fractures, osteoarthritis, nerve compression and spinal stenosis, bone sarcoma or high output cardiac failure.

4. **F - Hypocalciuric hypercalcaemia**

## 268. THEME: CHILDHOOD EXTREMITY DISORDERS

OPTIONS

A. Chondromalacia patella
B. Slipped femoral epiphyses
C. Osgood-Schlatter disease
D. Non accidental injury
E. Sickle cell disease
F. Juvenile rheumatoid disease
G. Influenza
H. Reactive arthritis
I. Transient synovitis of the hip
J. Growing pains
K. Perthes disease

*For each of the patients described below, select the most appropriate diagnosis from the above list. Each option may be used once, more than once, or not at all.*

1. A 13-year-old girl presents with pain in her left hip and limping. She is found to be overweight for her age. On examination, there is limitation of flexion, abduction and internal rotation.

2. An 11-year-old boy complains of pain in his right knee after activity. There is no history of trauma. On examination, there is a tender lump palpable anteriorly over the proximal tibia.

3. A 4-year-old child presents with a painful limp. On examination, there is no fever, the left hip is tender and range of movements in the left hip are terminally restricted. The WBC, ESR and CRP are within normal limits. X-ray is normal.

4. A 6-year-old boy presents with complaints of pain in the left knee and a painful limp. On examination, the left hip is tender with restriction of movements especially abduction and internal rotation. X-ray shows an increased joint space.

5. A 14-year-old athlete complains of pain in the anterior aspect of her left knee. Her symptoms are aggravated by activity or climbing stairs. On examination, there is mild quadriceps wasting, effusion, and tenderness and crepitus on movement of patella.

## 268. ANSWERS

1. **B - Slipped femoral epiphyses.** This condition is common in boys, around puberty who are typically overweight or very tall and thin. The child presents with a painful limp and on examination the leg is externally rotated and may be shortened. A classic sign is the tendency to increasing external rotation as the hip is flexed. The most reliable X-ray sign is the tilting of femoral epiphyses backwards in a lateral way. If not treated appropriately, it may result in avascular necrosis, chondrolysis or coxa vara deformity.

2. **C - Osgood-Schlatter disease.** In this common disorder of adolescence, the tibial tubercle becomes painful and swollen. It is a traction injury of the apophysis into which the patellar tendon is inserted. Active extension of the knee against resistance is painful and X-rays may reveal fragmentation of the apophysis. Initially rest and plaster cast immobilisation for 6–8 weeks may be needed.

3. **I - Transient synovitis of the hip.** It is the commonest cause of hip pain in children. Patient presents with a painful limp and the cardinal sign is restriction of the movement with pain at the extreme of the range in all directions. Blood investigations and X-rays are normal, but USG may reveal a small joint effusion. Characteristically, symptoms last for 1–2 weeks and then subside spontaneously. Other important differentials which have to be excluded are: Perthes disease is the main worry. Acute symptoms last for > 2 weeks and X-ray may show increased joint space. Later characteristic X-ray changes may appear. Slipped epiphysis may present as irritable hip initially. X-ray may be normal. If age/build are suggestive, X-ray should be repeated. Septic arthritis/tuberculous synovitis—symptoms will last longer and child will be generally unwell. ESR and CRP may be elevated.

4. **K - Perthes disease.** It is a painful disorder of childhood characterised by avascular necrosis of the femoral head. The patient, typically a boy of 4–8 years, complains of pain and starts limping. All hip movements are painful but especially abduction and internal rotation. Initially, X-rays may be normal but later there is obvious increase in joint space as well as flattening and lateral displacement of the epiphysis, with rarefaction and widening of metaphysis.

5. **A - Chondromalacia patella.** This is a syndrome of anterior knee pain and patello-femoral tenderness and is common among adolescents and young adults. The patient complains of pain over the front of the knee or underneath the knee cap. Patello-femoral pain is elicited by pressing the patella against the femur and asking the patient to contract the quadriceps. Arthroscopy may be used to diagnose cartilage softening and is helpful in excluding other causes of anterior knee pain.

## 269. THEME: TREATMENT OF UPPER LIMB INJURIES

OPTIONS

A. Collar and cuff
B. Open reduction and K wire fixation
C. Buddy strapping
D. Sling
E. Open reduction and internal fixation
F. Closed reduction and cast immobilisation
G. Plaster cast immobilisation alone
H. Kocher's method
I. External fixation

*For each of the patients described below, select the most appropriate treatment from the above list. Each option may be used once, more than once, or not at all.*

1. An 8-year-old boy presents with a painful and swollen elbow after a fall on the outstretched hand. The X-ray shows an undisplaced supracondylar fracture of humerus.

2. A 32-year-man involved in a RTA presents with pain and swelling of his right forearm. X-ray shows displaced fracture of mid shaft of radius and ulna.

3. A 25-year-old man presents with a swollen tender finger. X-ray shows a transverse, undisplaced fracture of proximal phalanx.

4. A 44-year-old man involved in a RTA presents with compound fracture of his right tibia and fibula. The fracture is comminuted and the wound is found to be severely contaminated.

5. An 83-year-old lady presents with pain and swelling of right wrist after a fall on her outstretched hand. X-ray shows a moderately displaced fracture of distal radius.

## 269. ANSWERS

1. **G - Plaster cast immobilisation alone.** Supracondylar fractures are among the commonest fractures in children. They may be displaced or undisplaced. It is essential to check for neurovascular damage with these injuries. The fracture is seen most clearly in the lateral view. In an undisplaced fracture the 'fat pad sign' should raise suspicion. An undisplaced fracture is treated by immobilising the elbow in 90 degree flexion in a plaster cast supported by a sling. It is essential to obtain an X-ray 5–7 days later to check for any displacement. A displaced fracture is usually treated with reduction and K wire fixation.

2. **E - Open reduction and internal fixation.** Fracture of forearm bones can be treated by closed reduction in children because the tough periosteum tends to guide and then control the reduction. In adults closed reduction is difficult and re-displacement of cast almost invariable. Hence most surgeons opt for open reduction and internal fixation from the outset. The fragments are held by inter-fragmentary compression with plate and screws. Bone grafting is advisable if there is comminution of more than one third of the circumference.

3. **C - Buddy strapping.** The phalanx usually fractures transversely, often with forwards angulation, which may damage the flexor tendon sheath. Fractures at either end of phalanx may enter the joint. Stiffness is the main threat and if fracture is displaced, the finger may be deformed. Undisplaced fracture may be treated by functional splintage. The finger is strapped to its neighbour (buddy strapping) and movements are encouraged from the outset. Splintage is retained for 2–3 weeks. Displaced fractures must be reduced either with buddy strapping or malleable splint.

4. **I - External fixation.** All compound fractures no matter how trivial must be considered contaminated. It is important to try to prevent them from becoming infected. The four essentials are wound debridement, antibiotic prophylaxis, stabilisation of the fracture and wound cover. Stability of fracture is important in reducing the likelihood of infection and assisting in the recovery of soft tissues. The method of fixation depends on the degree of contamination, length of time from injury to operation and the amount of soft tissue damage. If there is no obvious contamination and the time lapse is less than 8 hrs, open fractures of all grades up to type III A can be treated as for closed injuries. More severe injuries will require an external fixation and debridement of the wound as the initial management.

5. **F - Closed reduction and cast immobilisation.** Colles fracture is recognised by the classical dinner fork deformity with prominence on the back of the wrist and a depression in the front. Unless the fracture is comminuted, the fracture can be treated by reduction and immobilisation in a below elbow POP cast. Extreme positions of flexion and ulnar deviation must be avoided; 20 degree in each direction is acceptable. For comminuted fractures, plaster immobilisation alone may be insufficient; this can be supplemented by percutaneous K wire fixation.

## 270. THEME: COMPLICATIONS OF FRACTURES

OPTIONS

A. Compartment syndrome
B. Infection
C. Gas gangrene
D. Haemarthrosis
E. Nerve injury
F. Pressure sores
G. Delayed union
H. Avascular necrosis
I. Osteoarthritis
J. Myositis ossificans
K. Algodystrophy

*For each of the patients described below, select the most appropriate complication from the above list. Each option may be used once, more than once, or not at all.*

1. A 32-year-old man sustained a comminuted fracture of the proximal tibia. He was treated in an above knee POP cast. He attends A&E with complaints of pain and altered sensation over his foot. Passive stretching of the toes was excruciatingly painful.
2. A 23-year-old man presents to A&E with OG II fracture of his left tibia with a contaminated wound. The wound is debrided and closed primarily. While in the ward the patient complains of intense pain and swelling around the wound. A brownish foul smelling discharge is seen from the wound.
3. A 36-year-old man complains of pain and swelling of his left elbow. He had sustained a posterior dislocation of his elbow 3 months ago. On examination, there is local swelling and soft tissue tenderness on the anterior aspect of the elbow. X-ray shows fluffy calcification in the soft tissues anteriorly.
4. An 82-year-old lady complains of burning pain in her right wrist and hand after having recovered from a distal radius fracture. On examination, the skin around her wrist is pale and atrophic and X-ray shows patchy rarefaction of the bone.
5. A 32-year-old man is being treated for a displaced fracture of his left scaphoid. Six months after the trauma the fracture has failed to unite and the patient complains of persistent pain. X-ray taken shows an increase in bone density of the scaphoid.

## 270. ANSWERS

1. **A - Compartment syndrome.** High risk injuries are fractures of the elbow, the forearm bones and proximal third of tibia; also multiple fractures of the foot or hand, crush injuries and circumferential burns. If the limb is unduly painful, swollen or tense, the muscles should be tested by stretching them. When the fingers or toes are passively hyperextended there is increased pain in the calf or forearm. The presence of a pulse does not exclude a diagnosis.

The threatened compartment must be promptly decompressed. Casts, bandages and dressing must be completely removed. Fasciotomy might be needed to relieve the compartment pressure.

2. **C - Gas gangrene.** This condition is produced by Clostridium infection. These are anaerobes that can survive and multiply in tissues with low oxygen tension; the prime site for infection therefore is dirty wounds with dead muscle that has been closed without adequate debridement. Clinical features appear within 24 hrs of the injury. It is essential to distinguish gas gangrene from anaerobic cellulitis in which superficial gas formation is abundant but toxaemia usually slight.

The mainstay of treatment is prompt decompression of the wound and removal of dead and necrotic tissue. In advanced cases, amputation may be required.

3. **J - Myositis ossificans.** Heterotrophic ossification in the muscles sometimes occurs after an injury, particularly dislocation of elbow or a blow to the brachialis, the deltoid or the quadriceps. By 8 weeks after injury the bony mass may be palpable and identified on X-ray. The worst treatment is to attack an injured and stiffish elbow with vigorous muscle stretching exercises; this is liable to precipitate the condition. The joint should be rested in a position of function until pain subsides. Gentle active movements can then begin.

4. **K - Algodystrophy.** Also known as complex regional pain syndrome, this condition may occur following fractures in the extremity. The patient complains of continuous burning pain with tenderness and stiffness of nearby joints. X-ray shows patchy rarefaction of the bone. The treatment should begin early with analgesics and active exercises. Amitriptyline may help to relieve the pain in some cases.

5. **H - Avascular necrosis.** Certain regions are notorious for their propensity to develop ischaemia and bone necrosis after injury. They are (1) head of femur, (2) proximal part of scaphoid, (3) lunate, and (4) body of talus. There are no symptoms associated with AVN but if fracture fails to unite or if the bone collapses the patient may complain of pain. Treatment becomes necessary when joint function is threatened.

## 271. THEME: CAUSES OF PATHOLOGICAL FRACTURES

OPTIONS

A. Osteogenesis imperfecta
B. Postmenopausal osteoporosis
C. Solitary bone cyst
D. Chronic infection
E. Paget's disease
F. Chondrosarcoma
G. Osteosarcoma
H. Metastasis
I. Metastatic bone disease

*For each of the patients described below, select the most appropriate cause of pathological fracture from the above list. Each option may be used once, more than once, or not at all.*

1. A 13-year-old boy presents with pain around his right shoulder after a simple fall. X-ray shows a well demarcated radiolucent area in the proximal humeral metaphysis with a fracture line running through it.

2. A 69-year-old lady being treated for breast carcinoma presents with sudden onset pain in her back. X-ray shows collapse of her T10 and T11 vertebrae.

3. A 3-year-old child presents with pain and swelling of his leg following a trivial fall. He is diagnosed with a fracture of his left tibia. He is also found to have thin and lax skin with a blue sclera.

4. A 23-year-old man presents with pain and swelling around his right knee. X-ray shows an area of osteolysis with periosteal elevation and sunburst appearance with a fracture line running through the cortex.

## 271. ANSWERS

1. **C - Solitary bone cyst**

This lesion appears during childhood, typically in the metaphyses of one of the long bones and most commonly in the proximal humerus or femur. X-ray shows a well demarcated radiolucent area in the metaphysis often extending up to the physeal plate; the cortex may be thin. Asymptomatic lesions can be left alone. Actively enlarging cysts however should be treated by aspiration of fluid from the cyst and injection of 80–160 mg of methyl prednisolone. If this does not help, the cavity should be cleaned by curettage and then packed with bone chips.

2. **H - Metastasis**

With any destructive bone lesion in a patient between 50–70 years of age, the differential diagnosis must include metastasis. The sudden appearance of backache or thigh pain in an elderly person is always suspicious. If X-ray does not show anything, a radionuclide scan might show an area of increased density.

3. **A - Osteogenesis imperfecta**

It is one of the commonest genetic disorders of bone. Abnormal synthesis and structural defects of type 1 collagen result in abnormalities of the bones, teeth, ligaments, sclera and skin. The defining clinical features are (1) osteopenia, (2) liability to fractures, (3) laxity of ligaments, (4) blue colouration of the sclera, (5) dentinogenesis imperfecta. X-rays show generalised osteopenia, thinning of the long bones, fractures in various stages of healing, vertebral compression and spinal deformity.

4. **G - Osteosarcoma**

It is highly malignant tumour arising within the bone and spreading rapidly outwards towards the periosteum and surrounding tissues. It is common in children and adolescents. It may affect any bone but most commonly involves the long bone metaphyses, especially around the knee and proximal end of the humerus.

X-ray shows osteolytic areas alternatively with osteoblastic areas. Once the cortex is breached and the tumour extends into the adjacent soft tissues, streaks of new bone appear, radially outwards from the cortex – the so-called sun burst effect. Where the tumour emerges from the cortex, reactive new bone forms at the angles of periosteal elevation (Codman's triangle). A biopsy should always be carried out before commencing the treatment; it must be carefully planned to allow for compete removal of the track when the tumour is excised.

## 272. THEME: TREATMENT OF BACK PAIN

OPTIONS

A. Rest, weight loss and analgesia
B. Physiotherapy
C. Lateral mass fusion
D. Surgical removal of prolapsed disc
E. Spinal decompression with laminectomy
F. Calcitonin
G. Nerve root decompression
H. Chemotherapy
I. Radiotherapy
J. Excision of the nidus

*For each of the patients described below, select the most appropriate treatment from the above list. Each option may be used once, more than once, or not at all.*

1. A 70-year-old man presents with low back pain, aching and numbness in his thighs and legs. He prefers to walk uphill than downhill. His activities are restricted. X-ray reveals a trefoil shaped lumbar spinal canal and osteoarthritic changes.

2. A 72-year-old man presents with chronic back pain. On examination, he is tender along his shoulders, ribs and back. Blood tests reveal a high calcium and urea. X-ray shows generalised osteoporosis and crushed vertebra.

3. A 30-year-old man presents with bone pain around the knee. X-ray shows bony destruction and periosteal elevation with subperiosteal new bone formation. Chest X-ray reveals nodules.

4. A 60-year-old man presents with chronic back pain. On examination, he has a large head and bowed shin. He is hard of hearing. X-ray shows sclerosis and osteoporosis. His blood tests show an elevated alkaline phosphatase.

5. A 20-year-old man presents with a painful shin. Aspirin seems to relieve the pain. X-ray shows a localised osteolytic lesion surrounded by a rim of sclerosis.

## 272. ANSWERS

1. **E - Spinal decompression with laminectomy**

Spinal stenosis is the term used to describe abnormal narrowing of the central canal, the lateral recess or the intervertebral foramina to the point where the intervertebral foramina are compressed. When this occurs the patient develops neurological symptoms and signs in the lower limbs. Treatment may require a wide laminectomy, if required, over sacral levels and outwards to clear the nerve root canals. This relieves the leg pain, but not the back pain and occasionally it actually increases instability.

2. **H - Chemotherapy**

Backache is one of the presenting features of multiple myeloma. It is one of the commonest causes of osteoporosis and vertebral compression fractures in men over 45 years of age. Over half the patients have Bence Jones proteins in their urine and serum protein electrophoresis shows an abnormal band.

Treatment involves pain control and treatment of pathological fractures if necessary. Specific therapy is with alkylating cytotoxic agents, e.g., melphalan. Corticosteroids are also used if bone pain is marked.

3. **H - Chemotherapy**

The clinical picture is suggestive of osteosarcoma with metastasis to the lungs. Treatment involves multi-agent chemotherapy for 8–12 weeks and then, provided the lesion is resectable and there are no skip lesions, a wide resection is carried out.

Pulmonary metastases, especially if they are small and peripherally situated may be completely resected with a wedge of lung tissue.

4. **F - Calcitonin**

The clinical features are classically suggestive of Paget's disease. Deafness may be due to cranial nerve compression or otosclerosis. Calcitonin is the most widely used drug. It reduces bone resorption by decreasing both the activity and the number of osteoclasts.

5. **J - Excision of the nidus**

Relief of pain with aspirin and X-ray feature of an osteolytic lesion surrounded by dense sclerosis, are diagnostic. The only effective treatment is complete removal of the nidus. If the excision is likely to weaken the bone, prophylactic internal fixation may be carried out.

## 273. THEME: BONE DISEASE

OPTIONS

A. Osteomalacia
B. Osteopetrosis
C. Paget's disease
D. Pathological fracture
E. Psoriatic arthropathy
F. Rickets
G. Acropachy
H. Hypertrophic pulmonary osteoarthropathy
I. Osteoarthritis
J. Osteoporosis

*For each of the patients described below, select the most appropriate diagnosis from the above list. Each option may be used once, more than once, or not at all.*

1. A 50-yr-old man, a chronic smoker complains of pain in both his wrists and forearms. On examination, there is finger clubbing and the forearms are very tender on palpation.

2. An 82-yr-old woman falls after attempting to stand from a chair. She is very tender in her right groin and her limb is shortened and externally rotated.

3. A 30-year-old woman is admitted to hospital with Bell's palsy. The skull X-ray shows marked thickening of the skull vault.

4. A 75-year-old man complains of difficulty in climbing stairs and of pain in his hips, knees and shoulder girdles. X-rays taken show Looser's zones in the pubic rami.

5. A 58-year-old man complains of sudden onset pain in his thoracic spine. On examination he looks thin and unwell with tenderness over the mid thoracic vertebrae. Chest X-ray reveals an area of consolidation.

## 273. ANSWERS

1. **H - Hypertrophic pulmonary osteoarthropathy**

Digital clubbing can be present in a wide range of pulmonary, hepatic and intestinal disorders. In some cases it is associated with HPOA where there is marked tenderness of lower end of radius and ulna. X-ray shows subperiosteal new bone formation. Bronchogenic carcinoma is the most common cause of HPOA with clubbing. Other causes are pleural tumours, lung abscesses and empyema.

2. **J - Osteoporosis**

The key here is an elderly lady with fracture of the lower extremity (proximal femur) associated with a very trivial trauma.

Osteoporosis can be classified as primary, in which no specific cause can be found but which is usually related to ageing processes and decreased gonadal activity, and secondary (due to a variety of endocrine, metabolic and neoplastic disorders).

3. **B - Osteopetrosis**

This is a disease characterised by thickened bones due to defective resorption by osteoclasts. In the skull the thickened bones may lead to compression neuropathies (optic, Bell's palsy).

In the severe autosomal recessive form, the marrow space is replaced with bone which results in anaemia, infection and early death. The less severe autosomal dominant variety (osteopetrosis tarda) is detected in family studies or is an incidental finding after the patient has had X-rays for a fracture.

4. **A - Osteomalacia**

Muscle aches and pain with proximal muscle weakness, causing difficulty in climbing stairs are characteristics of this condition.

Looser's zones, pseudo fractures or milkman's fractures are focal radiolucent bands that may be found on the concave side of femoral neck, pubic rami, ribs, clavicles and the scapulae.

5. **D - Pathological fracture**

The patient's clinical condition and the X-ray picture suggest the possibility of tuberculosis. Sudden onset pain in the back (without any trauma or fall) with tenderness could be due to involvement of the spine with the disease process leading to a pathological fracture.

## 274. THEME: BONY LESIONS

OPTIONS

A. Avascular necrosis
B. Osteochondroma
C. Paget's disease
D. Rickets
E. Osteosarcoma
F. Osteochondroma
G. Osteomalacia
H. Ewing's tumour
I. Fibrosarcoma

*For each of the patients described below, select the most appropriate diagnosis from the above list. Each option may be used once, more than once, or not at all.*

1. A 60-yr-old man undergoing treatment for Paget's disease complains of weight loss and pain around his right knee. On examination, there is marked wasting of the muscles around the knee with a raised ESR.

2. A patient treated with immunosuppressive drugs and steroids, for more than 10 years due to chronic renal problems, presents with severe hip pain. On examination, the rotational movements of the hip are markedly restricted.

3. A 65-yr-old man presents with gradually increasing bowing of his legs over the past few years. He is found to be partially deaf during history taking and examination.

4. A 31-yr-old man presents with mild discomfort and lump around his left knee. He accidentally discovered this lump after a fall playing football. The lump is found to be bony hard and nontender. The man is otherwise fit and well.

5. A 12-yr-old boy presented with pain around his right forearm, fever and weight loss. On examination, a soft but tender ill-defined mass is palpable over his right forearm.

## 274. ANSWERS

1. **E - Osteosarcoma**

Secondary osteosarcoma may occur in patients of Paget's disease or following irradiation of bone. Clue, as in this case, is the appearance of pain or swelling in a patient with long standing Paget's disease. In late cases, pathological fractures may occur. Extra-compartmental spread has usually already occurred by the time the disease is diagnosed.

2. **A - Avascular necrosis**

The femoral head is the commonest site of symptomatic osteonecrosis, mainly because of its peculiar blood supply, which renders it vulnerable to ischaemia from arterial cut off, venous stasis, intravascular thrombosis or a combination of these. Restriction of rotational movements of the hip is classical. Common non-traumatic causes of AVN include high dose steroids, alcohol abuse, Gaucher's disease, sickle cell disease, SLE, and coagulopathies.

3. **C - Paget's disease**

Bowing of legs and deafness are diagnostic features of this disease.

4. **B - Osteochondroma**

This is one of the commonest benign tumours of the bone. Usually found around the growing ends of long bones and the crest of ileum. Any further enlargement of the tumour after the end of growth period is suggestive of malignant transformation. On X-ray, the lesion looks smaller than it feels because the cartilage cap is not seen. Excision is only indicated for big lumps, pressure symptoms or malignant transformation.

5. **H - Ewing's tumour**

This tumour commonly occurs around the age of 10 and 20 years, in a tubular bone like tibia, fibula or clavicle. Generalised illness and pyrexia together with a warm, tender swelling and a raised ESR may suggest osteomyelitis, which is an important differential diagnosis and should always be ruled out. X-ray shows an area of destruction, which unlike that seen in osteosarcoma, is predominantly in the mid diaphysis. The prognosis is poor and radiotherapy may help.

## 275. THEME: HIP FRACTURES

OPTIONS

A. Hemiarthroplasty
B. Dynamic hip screw
C. Total hip replacement
D. Cannulated screws
E. Traction
F. Intramedullary hip screw
G. External fixator

*For each of the patients described below, select the most appropriate treatment from the above list. Each option may be used once, more than once, or not at all.*

1. A 65-yr-old woman with severe rheumatoid arthritis affecting both hips and knees falls in the bathroom and presents to A&E with a shortened and externally rotated left leg. X-ray shows intracapsular fracture of the neck of femur.

2. A 45-yr-old man riding a motorbike is hit by a car. X-ray shows an intracapsular fracture of the neck of the right femur extending as a spiral fracture of the proximal shaft of femur.

3. A 30-year-old pedestrian is hit by a car and injures his left hip. X-ray shows an intracapsular fracture of the neck of left femur.

4. A 75-year-old woman trips at home and presents with an extra capsular fracture of her right hip.

5. A 90-year-old man with severe COPD falls while walking. X-ray reveals an extra capsular fracture of the neck of femur.

## 275. ANSWERS

### 1. C - Total hip replacement

In elderly patients, the treatment of choice for intracapsular fractures is a hemi arthroplasty. However, patients with pre-existing arthritis in conditions like RA, AVN, and Paget's disease may benefit from having a total hip replacement, as the prosthetic head would not glide smoothly in a diseased acetabulum. Total hip replacement would also be beneficial in the rare case where the fracture extends into the acetabular floor.

### 2. F - Intramedullary hip screw

The fixation device to be used in this fracture should be able to fix both the neck and proximal shaft. An intramedullary hip screw is an ideal device since it combines an intramedullary nail for fixing the shaft of femur with a sliding screw extending into the head of femur to stabilise the neck.

### 3. D - Cannulated screws

In young or physiologically active patients internal fixation is the treatment of choice so as to preserve the natural head of femur. This should ideally be achieved as early as possible to minimise the chances of future AVN. Cannulated screws (at least 3) should be used to fix the fracture.

### 4. B - Dynamic hip screw

This is the treatment of choice for extra capsular fractures in all age groups.

### 5. A - Hemiarthroplasty

## 276. THEME: ABNORMALITIES OF SYNOVIAL FLUID

OPTIONS

A. Osteoarthritis
B. Psoriatic arthropathy
C. Rheumatic fever
D. Rheumatoid arthritis
E. Pyrophosphate arthropathy
F. Septic arthritis
G. Behcet's disease
H. Gonococcal arthritis
I. Gout

*For each of the patients described below, select the most appropriate diagnosis from the above list. Each option may be used once, more than once, or not at all.*

1. Synovial fluid is yellow and slightly cloudy with 3000 white cells/mL. Under the polarizing microscope there are positively birefringent crystals.

2. Synovial fluid is very turbid and contains > 5000 white cells/sq.mm. It has a low viscosity and light microscopy reveals Gram-positive cocci.

3. Synovial fluid is clear and colourless with a white cell count of 200/mL. It has a high viscosity.

4. Synovial fluid is yellow and slightly cloudy with 3000 white cells/mL. Under polarizing microscope there are negatively birefringent crystals.

5. Synovial fluid is turbid and contains > 50,000 white cells/sq.mm. It has low viscosity. On microscopy Gram-negative diplococci are present.

## 276. ANSWERS

1. **E - Pyrophosphate arthropathy**

Pseudo gout is due to deposition of calcium pyrophosphate dihydrate crystals in the synovial space. The crystals are positively birefringent under polarized light.

2. **F - Septic arthritis**

The fluid is very turbid and has many polymorphs and Gram-positive cocci. The organisms commonly found are Staphylococcus aureus and Streptococcus pyogenes.

3. **A - Osteoarthritis**

The white cell count is slightly elevated. The fluid is of high viscosity.

4. **I - Gout**

Crystals of monosodium urate in gout are negatively birefringent.

5. **H - Gonococcal arthritis**

The fluid characteristics suggest septic arthritis. Gram-negative diplococci suggest gonococcal disease.

## 277. THEME: DISORDERS OF THE FOOT

OPTIONS

A. Pes cavus
B. Pes planus
C. Plantar fasciitis
D. Charcot's joint
E. Morton's metatarsalgia
F. March fracture
G. Hammer toe
H. Kohler's disease
I. Sever's disease
J. Gout

*For each of the scenarios described below, select the most appropriate diagnosis from the list of options above. Each option may be used once, more than once, or not at all.*

1. A 5-year-old child presents with a three month history of pain in the right foot. The foot is swollen and painful. There is tenderness over the medial longitudinal arch.

2. A young lady presents with pain in the sole of her foot and on the dorsal aspect of her second toe for a few weeks duration. The proximal interphalangeal joint of the second toe appears flexed and there is a callosity overlying the joint. The metatarsophalangeal joint and the distal interphalangeal joint of the corresponding finger appear hyperextended.

3. An 8-year-old child presents with pain in his right heel. He is exquisitely tender over the calcaneum. Rest of the examination is normal.

4. A 24-year-old chap has recently joined the army. He presents to you with a painful right foot for 10 days duration. He has been walking with a limp. On examination, he is tender over the third metatarsal.

## 277. ANSWERS

1. **H - Kohler's disease**

This is osteochondritis of the navicular bone. It results in aseptic necrosis of bone.

2. **G - Hammer toe**

The description is classical. The pain is due to the callosity. If pain is severe, treatment is with excision arthrodesis.

3. **I - Sever's disease**

This is osteochondritis of the calcaneal epithesis. Pain and tenderness occur close to the insertion of the Achilles tendon. The condition is self limiting.

4. **F - March fracture**

This is a classical metatarsal stress fracture usually involving the 2nd or 3rd metatarsal, which occurs in young adults after a period of unaccustomed walking. The affected bone feels tender and thick. Initial X-ray may be false negative. Treatment is symptomatic.

## 278. THEME: DISORDERS OF THE FOOT

OPTIONS

A. Pes cavus
B. Pes planus
C. Plantar fasciitis
D. Charcot's joint
E. Morton's metatarsalgia
F. March fracture
G. Hammer toe
H. Hallux valgus
I. Sever's disease
J. Gout

*For each of the scenarios described below, select the most appropriate diagnosis from the list of options above. Each option may be used once, more than once, or not at all.*

1. A teenager sees his GP with a congenital deformity involving both feet with clawing of toes.

2. A 50-year-old male with a long history of diabetes presents with a grossly deformed left foot with some pain. The ankle appears boggy, swollen and unstable. He tells you that he has had diabetes for 25 years.

3. A 39-year-old lady presents with pain in both feet, but mainly the right side. Examination reveals tenderness over the metatarsophalangeal joint of the great toe on the right. There is lateral deviation of both great toes.

## 278. ANSWERS

1. **A - Pes cavus**

It is usually hereditary and can be associated with conditions like Charcot-Marie-Tooth disease.

2. **D - Charcot's joint**

This is a chronic, progressive and degenerative disease of one or more joints, characterized by swelling, instability of the joint, haemorrhage, heat, and atrophic and hypertrophic changes in the bone. It is due to a combination of avascular necrosis and neuropathy. It is also known as neurogenic arthropathy. The commonest cause is diabetes. Other causes include syringomyelia and syphilis.

3. **H - Hallux valgus**

A bunion is a common term for a medical condition known as hallux valgus. Hallux valgus is the tilting of the toe away from the mid-line of the body. It is usually characterized by a lump or bump that is red, swollen and/or painful on the inside of the foot in and around the big toe joint. There are many causes of bunions, but the primary one is tight, ill-fitting shoes, that constrict the forefoot over a long period of time. High heels and constricting forefoot shoe gear are the primary causes of hallux valgus.

## 279. THEME: DISORDERS OF THE HAND

OPTIONS

A. Ganglion
B. Heberden's nodes
C. Dupuytren's contracture
D. Osler's nodes
E. Carpal tunnel syndrome
F. Radian nerve dysfunction
G. De Quervain's tenosynovitis

*For each of the scenarios described below, select the most appropriate diagnosis from the list of options above. Each option may be used once, more than once, or not at all.*

1. A 50-year-old gentleman known to have epilepsy presents with pain in his right hand. Examination reveals semi flexed ring and little fingers in his right hand. He is unable to extend them completely. However, flexion is full. The skin over the back of the proximal interphalangeal joints is thickened.

2. A 50-year-old lady presents with pins and needles sensation in the right hand, which is worse at night. The patient describes episodes of getting out of bed at night and shaking her hand to relieve pain. She has only recently been diagnosed with hypothyroidism.

3. A 50-year-old lady presents with a month long history of pain and tenderness over the right wrist particularly around the base of the thumb. Finkelstein's test is positive.

## 279. ANSWERS

1. **C - Dupuytren's contracture**

This is a classical description again. The condition is inherited as an autosomal dominant trait and is more common in males. It is related to ageing, smoking, tuberculosis, epilepsy (favourite with the examiners), AIDS and cirrhosis (another favourite association). Myofibroblasts in the palmar fascia proliferate and contract. Initially, there is a nodular swelling in the palm. Cords running into the fingers contract causing a flexion deformity of the metacarpophalangeal and proximal interphalangeal joints. Thickening of the skin over the proximal interphalangeal joint (Garrod's knuckle pads) may be seen. Occasionally Peyronie's disease is associated.

2. **E - Carpal tunnel syndrome**

This is classically carpal tunnel syndrome, which is caused by entrapment of the median nerve within the carpal tunnel. It is associated with pregnancy, obesity, myxoedema, acromegaly and rheumatoid arthritis.

3. **G - De Quervain's tenosynovitis**

This is due to constriction of the extensor pollicis brevis and abductor pollicis longus tendons within the compartment beneath the extensor retinaculum. Finkelstein's test clinches the diagnosis. There is pain over the radial side of the wrist when the patient's thumb is grasped and the hand is quickly abducted ulnarward.